Lecture Notes in Computational Vision and Biomechanics

Editors

João Manuel R.S. Tavares
R.M. Natal Jorge

Address:
Faculdade de Engenharia
Universidade do Porto
Rua Dr. Roberto Frias, s/n
4200-465 Porto
Portugal
tavares@fe.up.pt, rnatal@fe.up.pt

Editorial Advisory Board

For further volumes:
http://www.springer.com/series/8910

Lecture Notes in Computational Vision and Biomechanics
Volume 5

The research related to the analysis of living structures (Biomechanics) has been a source of recent research in several distinct areas of science, for example, Mathematics, Mechanical Engineering, Physics, Informatics, Medicine and Sport. However, for its successful achievement, numerous research topics should be considered, such as image processing and analysis, geometric and numerical modeling, biomechanics, experimental analysis, mechanobiology and enhanced visualization, and their application to real cases must be developed and more investigation is needed. Additionally, enhanced hardware solutions and less invasive devices are demanded.

On the other hand, Image Analysis (Computational Vision) is used for the extraction of high level information from static images or dynamic image sequences. Examples of applications involving image analysis can be the study of motion of structures from image sequences, shape reconstruction from images and medical diagnosis. As a multidisciplinary area, Computational Vision considers techniques and methods from other disciplines, such as Artificial Intelligence, Signal Processing, Mathematics, Physics and Informatics. Despite the many research projects in this area, more robust and efficient methods of Computational Imaging are still demanded in many application domains in Medicine, and their validation in real scenarios is matter of urgency.

These two important and predominant branches of Science are increasingly considered to be strongly connected and related. Hence, the main goal of the LNCV&B book series consists of the provision of a comprehensive forum for discussion on the current state-of-the-art in these fields by emphasizing their connection. The book series covers (but is not limited to):

- Applications of Computational Vision and Biomechanics
- Biometrics and Biomedical Pattern Analysis
- Cellular Imaging and Cellular Mechanics
- Clinical Biomechanics
- Computational Bioimaging and Visualization
- Computational Biology in Biomedical Imaging
- Development of Biomechanical Devices
- Device and Technique Development for Biomedical Imaging
- Digital Geometry Algorithms for Computational Vision and Visualization
- Experimental Biomechanics
- Gait & Posture Mechanics
- Multiscale Analysis in Biomechanics
- Neuromuscular Biomechanics
- Numerical Methods for Living Tissues
- Numerical Simulation
- Software Development on Computational Vision and Biomechanics
- Grid and High Performance Computing for Computational Vision and Biomechanics
- Image-based Geometric Modeling and Mesh Generation
- Image Processing and Analysis
- Image Processing and Visualization in Biofluids
- Image Understanding
- Material Models
- Mechanobiology
- Medical Image Analysis
- Molecular Mechanics
- Multi-modal Image Systems
- Multiscale Biosensors in Biomedical Imaging
- Multiscale Devices and Biomems for Biomedical Imaging
- Musculoskeletal Biomechanics
- Sport Biomechanics
- Virtual Reality in Biomechanics
- Vision Systems

Begoña Calvo • Estefanía Peña
Editors

Patient-Specific Computational Modeling

Springer

Editors
Begoña Calvo
Department of Mechanical Engineering
University of Zaragoza
Zaragoza, Spain

Estefanía Peña
Department of Mechanical Engineering
University of Zaragoza
Zaragoza, Spain

ISSN 2212-9391 ISSN 2212-9413 (electronic)
Lecture Notes in Computational Vision and Biomechanics
ISBN 978-94-024-0552-1 ISBN 978-94-007-4552-0 (eBook)
DOI 10.1007/978-94-007-4552-0
Springer Dordrecht Heidelberg New York London

Printed on acid-free paper

Springer is part of Springer Science+Business Media (www.springer.com)

Preface

Patient-specific modeling of biological tissue is of vital importance for an accurate determination of the biomechanical effects of surgeries of select different clinical treatments. Consideration of realistic mechanical properties in combination with the most advanced constitutive laws, computational analysis techniques and available medical imaging techniques (CT, MRI,) provides a powerful tool for modeling biological structures. Simulation-based medicine and the development of complex computer models of biological structures are ubiquitous in modern biomedical engineering and clinical research. Despite the many investigations developed in this field, the exact mechanical behavior of the different biological structures and the causes of many of their pathologies are not completely understood. This is partially due to inherent limitations of experimental studies such as their high cost, difficulties associated with the capture of accurate measures of strain and stress and, especially, the difficult and sometimes impossible reproduction of certain natural, pathological or degenerative situations.

This book contains a small collection of invited chapters on patient-specific modeling and can be a significant contribution to the state-of-the-art in the field of Computational Biomechanics focused in the context of Patient Specific computational modeling with a total of seven chapters has been included. An operator insensitive method to reconstruct vascular bodies from Computer Tomography-Angiography (CT-A) data is given by Gasser in Chap. 1. The approach is based on beam- and shell-like deformable (active) contour models and facilitates a hex-dominated Finite Element mesh generation for an efficient numerical computation of mechanical field variables. Fernandez et al. present in Chap. 2 a suite of subject-specific musculoskeletal models that were developed using the framework of The International Union of Physiological Sciences (IUPS) Physiome Project that has been developed as a framework for creation, sharing and dissemination of multiscale mathematical models of human physiology. In Chap. 3, Creane et al. review the current state of the art in the clinical risk assessment for atherosclerotic plaque disruption and details the barriers yet to be overcome if patient specific computational modeling is to be used as a clinical tool. Heidenreich et al. describe a methodology for the modeling and simulation of human ischemic heart in Chap. 4. Recent advances in lower-cost, non-invasive imaging and computing power (surface scanning, Cone Beam Computerised Tomography (CBCT) and Magnetic Resonance (MRI)) to capture and process surface and internal structures to a high resolution are presented by Richmond et al. in Chap. 5. Borghi et al. describe in Chap. 6 a computational mechanics model of TAA based on patient-specific anatomical and flow conditions, acquired from Magnetic Resonance Imaging (MRI) and Computed Tomography (CT). The model has been applied to eight patients with TAAs at different locations of the aorta as well as a normal subject as a control case for comparison. Finally, Lanchares et al. present in Chap. 7 a patient-specific model of the eye for helping in different ophthalmologic surgical techniques. They present the usefulness of this model to help in surgical planning of incisional surgery for the correction of astigmatism, the numerical analysis of the process of accommodation and the numerical simulation of the scleral buckling technique for retinal detachment.

Finally, the editors greatly appreciate the effort, dedication and work of the authors. Their expertise and worldwide reputation in Biomechanics field have undoubtedly enriched the scientific discussion contained in the book chapters.

Zaragoza, Spain

Begoña Calvo
Estefanía Peña

Contents

Chapter 1
Bringing Vascular Biomechanics into Clinical Practice.
Simulation-Based Decisions for Elective Abdominal Aortic Aneurysms Repair

T. Christian Gasser

Abstract Vascular diseases are the leading cause of death in the industrialized countries and some of the associated risk factors are increasing. A multi-disciplinary approach including biomechanics is needed to better understand and more effectively treat these diseases. Despite the tremendous progress made in modeling the biomechanics of the vasculature, so far this research has accomplished only very limited clinical relevance or acceptance. Establishing vascular biomechanical simulations in the clinical work-flow requires integrating (i) a robust reconstruction of vascular bodies from medical images, (ii) a non-linear biomechanical analysis and (iii) a clinically relevant interpretation of the derived results. Such an approach is outlined for the biomechanical rupture risk assessment of Abdominal Aortic Aneurysms (AAAs), i.e. a local dilatation of the infrarenal aorta that may form through irreversible pathological remodeling of the aortic wall. Rupture of an AAA is a frequent cause of death in the elderly male population and assessing this risk plays a central role in the clinical management of aneurysms. Specifically, the present chapter details an operator-insensitive method to reconstruct vascular bodies from Computer Tomography-Angiography data. The approach is based on beam and shell-like deformable (active) contour models and allows a hexahedral-dominated mesh generation for an efficient Finite Element computation. Laboratory experiments and histo-mechanical constitutive modeling of AAA tissue are reviewed. Finally, the clinical application of the biomechanical rupture risk assessment is demonstrated through the especially developed software A4clinics. Most critically, individual biomechanical parameters are related to the 'average AAA patient', which in turn provides a biomechanics-based index for elective AAA repair indication.

T.C. Gasser (✉)
Department of Solid Mechanics, School of Engineering Sciences, The Royal Institute of Technology (KTH), Osquars Backe 1, 100 44 Stockholm, Sweden
e-mail: tg@hallf.kth.se
url: http://www-old.hallf.kth.se/~tg/vascumech/

B. Calvo, E. Peña (eds.), *Patient-Specific Computational Modeling*,
Lecture Notes in Computational Vision and Biomechanics 5,
DOI 10.1007/978-94-007-4552-0_1,

1.1 Introduction

Vascular diseases are the leading cause of death in the industrialized countries and associated risk factors like obesity, diabetes, and life expectancy are increasing. Current clinical options are somewhat limited, and clearly there is an urgent need for multi-disciplinary approaches to improve our current view of vascular diseases. It is generally accepted that biomechanical conditions play a key role in the genesis and development of vascular diseases (Humphrey, 2002) and the identification of the specific causative links between biomechanics and biochemistry may help advance our current view of physiology and pathology. Hence, biomechanics plays a fundamental role in better understanding the etiology, pathology, and natural history of several vascular diseases.

Computer simulations of biomechanical phenomena are potentially significant in order to explore, for instance, loads experienced by cells and extra-cellular components, the interaction between medical devices and biological material, drug delivery pathways, the interplay between structure and function of tissues, mechanotransduction and the like. Although, to some extent, traditional mechanics concepts are directly applicable to solve biomechanical problems, they remain a modeling challenge due to complex spatial domains, constitutive nonlinearities, and coupling among structural, fluid, chemical and electrical fields to mention a few. Specifically, the inherent property of biological tissue to adapt to mechanical and chemical environments remains a challenging modeling task. Likewise, sophisticated and robust numerical schemes are required to investigate entire biological organs adequately, i.e. to gain a comprehensive view of a biological process. On the other hand, the inter-patient variability of input parameters, such as loading conditions or constitutive properties, lowers the patient-specific predictability, and hence the clinical benefit, of numerical simulations. Finally, laboratory testing of biological material is somewhat limited, where challenges regarding material harvesting, specimen preparation and establishing adequate testing environments are particularly difficult.

Many biomechanical models have been developed for clinical applications with the objective of improving the diagnosis and treatment of diseases. Unfortunately these efforts have so far only resulted in very limited clinical relevance or acceptance of these models. This is especially true for vascular tissue biomechanics. Several groups around the globe have worked on modeling angioplasty without any clinical recognition at all so far. In a work published in 2002 (Holzapfel et al., 2002) about the potential benefits of the new approach, the following hope was expressed: "*The proposed approach provides a tool that has the potential* (i) *to improve procedural protocols and the design of interventional instruments on a lesion-specific basis, and* (ii) *to determine postangioplasty mechanical environments, which may be correlated with restenosis responses.*" Unfortunately, 10 years later none of these model implications became true, and, although this biomechanical model is thought to be state-of-the-art, it clearly failed clinical needs. Naturally, a simulation model represents the real object or process to a desired degree of complexity, which is largely defined by the model's intended purpose. Hence, model complexity must be driven by clinical needs and not solely by experimental observations. For instance, considering an anisotropic constitutive formulation is only justified if it improves the model from the patient's perspective.

The present chapter provides an interdisciplinary approach to the biomechanics of Abdominal Aortic Aneurysms (AAAs), i.e. a local dilation of the infrarenal aorta caused by proteolytic degradation of elastin and collagen in the aortic wall (Choke et al., 2005). An AAA ruptures if the mechanical stress exceeds the local wall strength, and is a frequent cause of death in elderly male population (The UK Small Aneurysm Trial Participants, 1998). Clinically, the risk of rupture is correlated with the aneurysm's maximum diameter, and surgical or endovascular AAA repair is indicated if the diameter exceeds 55 mm (The UK Small Aneurysm Trial Participants, 1998). However, the diameter criterion has clear limitations and mechanical parameters, such as Peak Wall Stress (PWS) (Fillinger et al., 2002; Heng et al., 2008; Venkatasubramaniam et al., 2004) and Peak Wall Rupture Risk (PWRR) (Gasser et al., 2010; Maier et al., 2010), have been found to be more reliable indices to assess AAA rupture risk. The computation of PWS and PWRR require a patient-specific reconstruction of AAAs from medical images, modeling the constitution of aneurysmatic tissues and solving a non-linear structural mechanical problem, where typically the non-linear Finite Element Method (FEM) (Zienkiewicz and Taylor, 2000a, 2000b, 2000c) is used.

Throughout this chapter we will follow such an approach and discuss the different steps in AAA model development. Specifically, Sect. 1.2 introduces an operator-insensitive method to segment AAAs from medical images, which is essential in order to develop meaningful biomechanical AAA models. Section 1.3 discusses different laboratory experiments of aneurysm tissue and provides mechanical properties and information regarding collagen formation in the AAA wall. In Sect. 1.4 different constitutive descriptions for AAA tissue are introduced, with the focus on histo-mechanical formulations, i.e. aiming at integrating the tissue's histology with its mechanics. Finally, Sect. 1.5 demonstrates how a biomechanical-based decision-making tool can be integrated in the clinical work-flow of AAA patients.

1.2 Image Reconstruction

1.2.1 Introduction

An artifact insensitive segmentation of all structural relevant components of the AAA is fundamental to provide appropriate geometrical information for reliable patient-specific FEM models. Computerized Tomography Angiography (CT-A) is the preferred imaging modality in AAA treatment and provides typically sufficient contrast for a threshold-based automatic segmentation of the lumen (Giachetti et al., 2003; Subasic et al., 2002). In contrast, an automatic identification of the aneurysm's exterior surface requires more sophisticated approaches and Deformable Models (DMs) (also known as active contour models) have been proposed in the literature

(Auer and Gasser, 2010; Delingette, 1999; de Bruijne et al., 2002, 2004; Olabarriaga et al., 2005). For the segmentation of the exterior surface many DMs use the luminal surface as their initial configuration. Typically, clinical relevant aneurysms (Hans et al., 2005) include an Intra-Luminal Thrombus (ILT), i.e. luminal and exterior surfaces may differ significantly, and this initialization may not be optimal.

Results from FEM simulations depend on the thickness of the AAA wall, which however can not be reliably recovered from CT-A data. Consequently, most approaches use a predefine wall thickness (Fillinger et al., 2003; Heng et al., 2008; Maier et al., 2010; Raghavan et al., 2005; Truijers et al., 2007; Venkatasubramaniam et al., 2004) that might include wall thinning effects of the underlying ITL (Gasser et al., 2010; Kazi et al., 2003).

The stability and efficiency of FEM simulations strongly depends on the quality and topology of the underlying FEM mesh. Although known to violate the inf–sup condition (or BB condition) condition (Wriggers, 2008), mixed tri-linear hexahedral elements (Simo and Taylor, 1991) have been widely applied in vascular biomechanics. In contrast to tetrahedral mesh generation, where Delaunay based approaches are widely used, hexahedral mesh generation is much more difficult and, to the author's best knowledge, no generally applicable and automatic method (algorithm) has been presented in the open literature, see, e.g., Sack and Urrutia (2000) for issues associated with hexahedral meshes.

In this section a hierarchical technique to generate FEM meshes from standard clinical CT-A data is discussed. The segmentation is based on a successive application of 2D and 3D DMs, and aneurysm wall and the ILT are discretized by hexahedral and hexahedral-dominated meshes, respectively. The proposed approach is characterized by minimal user interactions and implemented in A4clinics (VASCOPS GmbH, Patent No. PCT/EP2008/064157) and detailed elsewhere (Auer and Gasser, 2010).

1.2.2 Active Segmentation Model

A hierarchical application of 2D and 3D DMs is considered. Specifically, the 2D model provides a pre-segmentation of the lumen, which in turn is used for the final 3D segmentation of the lumen. Finally, the luminal surface serves as initial (starting) configuration for the segmentation of the exterior AAA surface. The proposed method cuts-off small bifurcating vessels like lumbar arteries, which otherwise would lead to a much too detailed FEM model. Using a DM for the luminal segmentation can process CT-A data with larger slice thicknesses and less contrast than it is required for threshold-based segmentation concepts. Finally, it is emphasized that 3D DMs provide an accurate segmentation without discriminating the out-of plane direction and facilitating the reconstruction of saccular formations; a typical result is shown in Fig. 1.1.

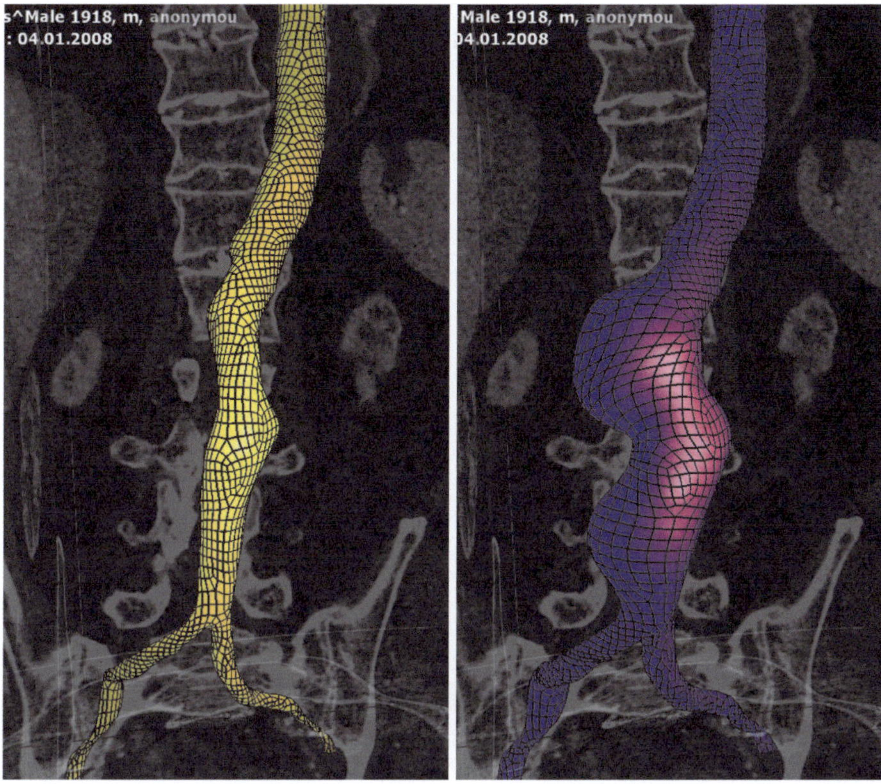

Fig. 1.1 3D reconstruction of the luminal (*left*) and exterior (*right*) surface of a particular AAA. Segmentation is based on DMs and the surfaces are represented by quadrilateral elements

1.2.2.1 Finite Element Formulation of the DMs

DMs are formulated based on elastic structural finite elements (Zienkiewicz and Taylor, 2000a). Specifically, theoretical concepts for frame and shell structures are used for 2D and 3D DMs, respectively. Here, each nodal point of the 2D DM has 3 degrees of freedom (2 translations $\mathbf{u} = \{u_1, u_2\}^\mathrm{T}$ and one rotation $\mathbf{w} = \{w\}$) whereas each nodal point of the 3D DM has 6 degrees of freedom (3 translations $\mathbf{u} = \{u_1, u_2, u_3\}^\mathrm{T}$ and 3 rotations $\mathbf{w} = \{w_1, w_2, w_3\}^\mathrm{T}$), see Fig. 1.2.

In order to derive the variational statement for a FEM implementation of the DMs, we consider stress resultants $\mathbf{q}$ (forces) and couples $\mathbf{m}$ (moments) distributed over a particular finite element Ω_e, i.e. $\mathbf{q} = \{q_1, q_2\}^\mathrm{T}$, $\mathbf{m} = \{m\}$ and $\mathbf{q} = \{q_1, q_2, q_3\}^\mathrm{T}$, $\mathbf{m} = \{m_1, m_2, m_3\}^\mathrm{T}$ for the 2D and 3D problems, respectively. Likewise, for each finite element the reference configuration $\mathbf{X}(\boldsymbol{\xi})$ is described with respect to the arc-length parameter $\boldsymbol{\xi}$ ($\boldsymbol{\xi} = \{\xi\}$ in 2D; $\boldsymbol{\xi} = \{\xi_1, \xi_2\}^\mathrm{T}$ in 3D), and the motion $\mathbf{x} = \mathbf{X}(\boldsymbol{\xi}) + \mathbf{u}(\mathbf{X}(\boldsymbol{\xi}), t)$ defines the element's spatial position over time t. Introducing admissible variations of the displacements and rotations, $\delta\mathbf{u}$ and $\delta\mathbf{w}$ say,

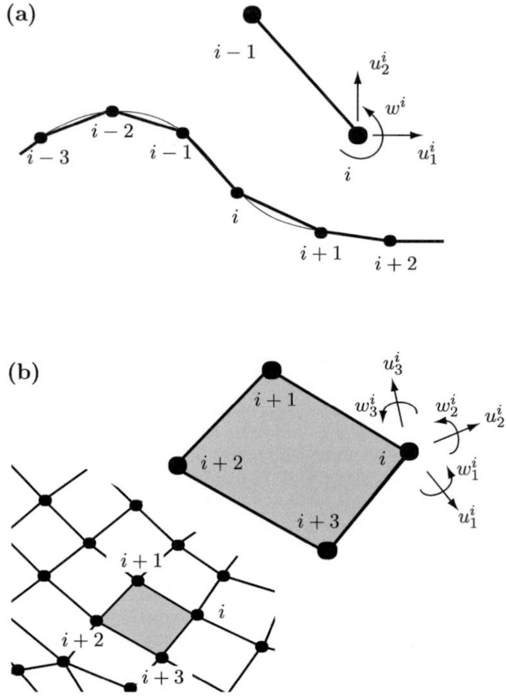

Fig. 1.2 Discrete representation of 2D and 3D Deformable Models (DMs) by frame and shell elements based on the Finite Element Method (FEM). (**a**) The 2D DM is assembled by frame elements, where each node has 2 translational and one rotational degree of freedom. (**b**) The 3D DM is assembled by shell elements, where each node has 3 translational and 3 rotational degrees of freedom. Figure taken from Auer and Gasser (2010)

the principle of virtual work (Oden and Reddy, 1976) reads

$$\underbrace{\int_{\Omega_e} (\delta\boldsymbol{\varepsilon} \cdot \mathbf{q} + \delta\boldsymbol{\kappa} \cdot \mathbf{m})\mathrm{d}\boldsymbol{\xi}}_{\delta\Pi_{\mathrm{int}}} - \underbrace{\int_{\Omega_e} \delta\mathbf{u} \cdot \overline{\mathbf{q}}\mathrm{d}\boldsymbol{\xi}}_{\delta\Pi_{\mathrm{ext}}} = 0, \tag{1.1}$$

where $\delta\boldsymbol{\varepsilon}$ and $\delta\boldsymbol{\kappa}$ are admissible variations of the strain measures $\boldsymbol{\varepsilon}$ and $\boldsymbol{\kappa}$, which are work-conjugate to the stress resultants $\mathbf{q}$ and $\mathbf{m}$. External loading acting on the finite element is denoted by $\overline{\mathbf{q}}$. In (1.1), $\delta\Pi_{\mathrm{int}}$ and $\delta\Pi_{\mathrm{ext}}$ are internal and external virtual works, which in turn define the associated internal $\mathbf{F}_{\mathrm{int}}$ and external $\mathbf{F}_{\mathrm{ext}}$ nodal forces (Zienkiewicz and Taylor, 2000a) acting on the finite element. The explicit relation between the stress resultants $\mathbf{q}$ and $\mathbf{m}$ and the strain measures $\boldsymbol{\varepsilon}$ and $\boldsymbol{\kappa}$ depends on the underlying FEM formulation and is well reported in the literature (Belytschko et al., 2000; Zienkiewicz and Taylor, 2000a, 2000b). It is emphasized that the proposed approach is founded on structural mechanics, which lead to predictable relations between the introduced algorithmic (structural) parameters and the response of the DM.

1.2.2.2 External Loadings Acting on DMs

External loadings $\overline{\mathbf{q}}$ (as introduced in (1.1)) are thought to arise from image data $\overline{\mathbf{q}}_\mathrm{i}$ and an internal pressure $\overline{\mathbf{q}}_\mathrm{p}$ acting on the DM. In addition external loading $\overline{\mathbf{q}}_\mathrm{v}$ due to viscosity is added to render a well-posed structural problem. Inertia effects are neglected.

Image forces $\overline{\mathbf{q}}_\mathrm{i}$ are defined as the inner product of the second spatial gradient of the image intensity $I = I(\mathbf{x})$ and the normal $\mathbf{n}$ onto the DM, i.e.

$$\overline{\mathbf{q}}_\mathrm{i} = \nabla^2 I \cdot \mathbf{n}. \tag{1.2}$$

The pressure $p(I)$ and the viscosity $\eta(I)$ are thought to dependent on the image intensity I, and the associated external loads were particularized according to

$$\overline{\mathbf{q}}_\mathrm{p} = p(I)\mathbf{n}, \qquad \overline{\mathbf{q}}_\mathrm{v} = \eta(I)\dot{\mathbf{x}} \tag{1.3}$$

with $\dot{\mathbf{x}}$ denoting the velocity of the DM and the explicit dependency on I reads

$$p(I) = \begin{cases} +\overline{p}, & I \in I_\mathrm{target} \\ -\overline{p}, & I \notin I_\mathrm{target} \end{cases} \quad \text{and} \quad \eta(I) = \overline{\eta}|\nabla I|^2, \tag{1.4}$$

where I_target denotes a intensity spectrum associated with the object to be segmented.

The pressure $\overline{p}$ can be changed by the user for instance if the model does not stop but overshoots the desired boundary. Relating the viscosity to the image gradient is thought to avoid oscillations of the DM if it approaches contours, i.e. where $\overline{\mathbf{q}}_\mathrm{i}$ increases.

1.2.2.3 Solving Strategy

The DM renders a non-linear system $\mathbf{F}_\mathrm{int} - \mathbf{F}_\mathrm{ext} = \mathbf{Ka}$ of algebraic equations (Zienkiewicz and Taylor, 2000a), where $\mathbf{K}$ denotes the diagonally populated global stiffness matrix and $\mathbf{a}$ defines the vector of unknowns (nodal degrees of freedom), i.e. $\mathbf{a} = \{u_1, u_2, w\}^\mathrm{T}$ and $\mathbf{a} = \{u_1, u_2, u_3, w_1, w_2, w_3\}^\mathrm{T}$ for a particular node of the 2D and 3D DM, respectively. This system is solved iteratively over time t until the DM successfully segments the object of interest from the remaining anatomical information of the image data.

1.2.3 Meshing

1.2.3.1 Surface Tessellation

The luminal pre-segmentation defines a structural (logical) point cloud of known correspondence between the different segmented contours. Hence, a simple and fast tessellation algorithm can be applied, where even vessel bifurcations can be addressed (Auer and Gasser, 2010). Finally, a sequence of local surface mesh improvements (Auer and Gasser, 2010) and Laplace smoothing (Field, 1988) is applied.

1.2.3.2 Volume Meshing

In a first step the aneurysm wall is meshed by a simple plastering step (Staten et al., 2005) from the exterior AAA surface towards the inside. Here, a predefined aneurysm wall thickness that depends on the thickness of the underlying ILT layer (Kazi et al., 2003; Raghavan et al., 2006) is used.

Since the luminal and the exterior surface meshes are logically identical, the ILT domain is split in a finite number of polyhedrals, which can be meshed by Whisker Weaving (Tautges et al., 1996) or any other method (Sack and Urrutia, 2000). The proposed meshing algorithm facilitates anisotropic meshing, where the radial mesh dimension can be defined independently. However, the algorithm does not support local mesh refinement and the mesh density in circumferential and axial directions can only be controlled by the mesh size of the 3D DMs. While this always gives a good control over the luminal surface of the mesh, the mesh size at the exterior surface is also affected by the object's topology, i.e. a thick thrombus causes a coarser mesh at the exterior surface. Note that the surface curvature is usually much lower behind a thick thrombus, and hence, a coarser mesh might be sufficient to capture the stress field in the aneurysm wall. The proposed meshing algorithm leads to large regions of structured mesh topology, which significantly reduces memory demands of the FEM problem. Finally, (volume constraint) *Laplace* smoothing and mesh optimization (Canann et al., 1998) is used to support finite deformation FEM analysis.

1.3 Laboratory Experiment

The laboratory experiment aims at collecting information about the mechanical properties and the histology of vascular tissue, and hence it provides basic input for constitutive modeling of AAA tissues.

1.3.1 Microscopy

Collagen is intrinsic birefringent and Polarized Light Microscopy (PLM) provides an ideal method for its detection and analysis (Lindeman et al., 2009; Vidal et al., 1982; Weber et al., 1990). Collagen fibers of decreasing thickness appear in red, orange, yellow, and green, and a correlation between collagen birefringence and its mechanical properties has been established (Long et al., 2004).

To analyze the collagen formation in AAA wall, anterior tissue samples were selected during elective open surgical repair. The collection and use of ILT material

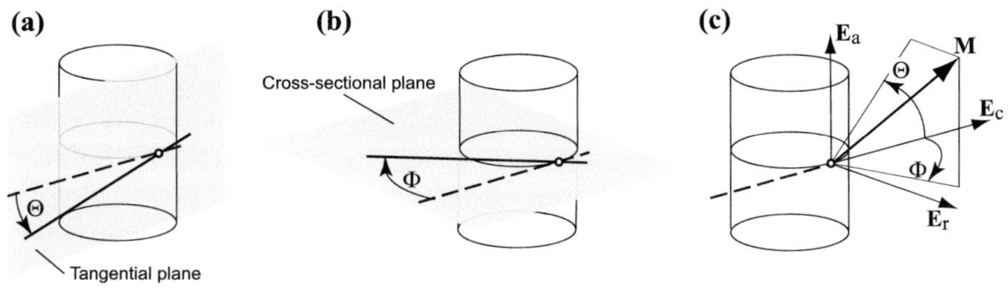

Fig. 1.3 Definition of the azimuthal angle θ (**a**) and the elevation angle ϕ (**b**) and their relation to the unit orientation vector **M** of a collagen fiber or a coherent bundle of fibers (**c**). The cylinder schematically represents the vessel with the dashed line denoting the circumferential direction. The azimuthal angle θ and the elevation angle ϕ are measured in planes in parallel (tangential plane) and perpendicular (cross-sectional plane) to the vessel axis, respectively. Both angles together define the three-dimensional orientation vector **M** of a collagen fiber within a Cartesian coordinate system $\mathbf{E}_c, \mathbf{E}_a, \mathbf{E}_r$, where the indices c, a and r denote the local circumferential, axial and radial directions, respectively

from human subjects was approved by the local ethics committee. Specimen were fixed, embedded in paraffin and sliced at a thickness of 7.0 micrometers. Finally, picrosirius red staining was used to enhance the birefringent properties of collagen, which improves the precision of measurement while preserving the optical axis of the unstained collagen fiber (Harold et al., 1981). Details of specimen preparation are given elsewhere (Gasser et al., 2012).

1.3.1.1 Method

The orientation of a collagen fiber, or a coherent bundle of fibers, in the three-dimensional space is uniquely defined by its azimuthal angle θ and its elevation angle ϕ that are measured by (in-plane) rotating and (out-of-plane) tilting the Universal Rotary Stage, respectively. See Fig. 1.3 for the definition of these angles. An artifact-free part of the slice was considered and the specimen edge was used as a reference for the collagen orientations; a typical microscopical image is shown in Fig. 1.4. Black regions correspond to collagen fibers perpendicular to the linear polarized light ray, and hence the appearance of the image changes during rotating and tilting the stage. The intensity of the non-extinguished (red) areas does not only depend on the angle of the collagen fibers with respect to the light ray but also on the amount of collagen in the tissue (Long et al., 2004).

To provide a statistically random selection, a 6 by 6 grid of measurement points was used, i.e. positions at which the collagen orientation was identified. Azimuthal θ and elevation ϕ angles were identified by sequentially rotating and tilting the specimen until the particular measurement point extinguished in the PLM (Harold et al., 1981).

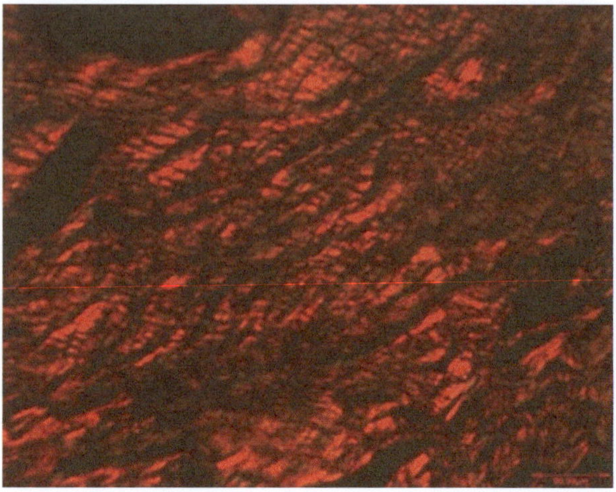

Fig. 1.4 Polarized Light Microscopy (PLM) image taken from the media of the Abdominal Aortic Aneurysm (AAA) wall

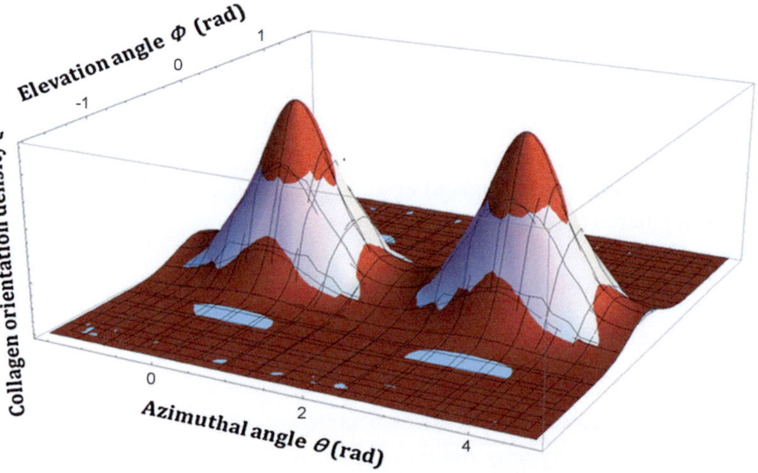

Fig. 1.5 Bingham distribution function (*red*) fitted to the experimentally measured fiber orientation distribution (*light-blue*) in the Abdominal Aortic Aneurysm (AAA) wall

1.3.1.2 Results

A comprehensive picture of collagen formation in the AAA wall is given by Fig. 1.5. Here, the measured data from all tissue samples were pooled, symmetrized and fitted to a Bingham distribution (Alastrué et al., 2010; Bingham, 1974)

$$\rho(\theta,\phi) = c^{-1}\exp\left[\kappa_1(\cos\theta\cos\phi)^2 + \kappa_2(\cos\phi\sin\theta)^2\right] \tag{1.5}$$

having the parameters $\kappa_1 = 11.6$ and $\kappa_2 = 9.7$. The normalization parameter c is used to normalize the collagen fiber density function, such that $\int_{\phi=-\pi/2}^{\pi/2}\int_{\theta=-\pi/2}^{\pi/2}\rho\,\cdot$

$\cos\phi \mathrm{d}\phi \mathrm{d}\theta = 1$ holds. This condition is satisfied for

$$c(\kappa_1, \kappa_2) = \sqrt{\pi} \sum_{i,j=0}^{\infty} \frac{\Gamma(i+\frac{1}{2})\Gamma(j+\frac{1}{2})\kappa_1^i \kappa_2^j}{\Gamma(i+j+\frac{3}{2}) i! j!} \tag{1.6}$$

where Γ and $i!$ denote the Euler gamma function and the factorial of i, respectively. Note that the Bingham distribution is symmetric, i.e. $\rho(\phi, \theta) = \rho(\phi + \pi, \theta + \pi)$ and able to capture a large spectrum of distributions. Details regarding the applied optimization method for parameter estimation are given elsewhere (Gasser et al., 2012).

Estimating the alignment of tissue samples that were taken during elective repair is naturally accompanied with significant uncertainty. The error in setting the longitudinal (or circumferential) direction by the surgeon was quantified by a random distribution within ± 15 degrees of specimen orientation. This uncertainty was considered when pooling the data. Further details are given in Gasser et al. (2012).

1.3.2 Planar Biaxial Testing

Planar biaxial testing of soft tissues is often required to fully characterize the inherent anisotropic properties of the tissue. To this end a tissue batch is biaxially loaded along its principal material axes. The motion of markers (ink dots) (see Fig. 1.6) is monitored with a high-resolution camera and used to compute the biaxial strain in the center of the specimen. Planar biaxial testing requires a sophisticated specimen fixation (hooks (Vande Geest et al., 2006a) and claps (Bursa and Zemanek, 2008) are used) and a careful setting of the orientation as well as the reference (unloaded) configuration of the test specimen. Either displacement or tension-based testing protocols are used (Bursa and Zemanek, 2008). Detailed results from biaxial testing of the AAA wall are given elsewhere (Vande Geest et al., 2006a), and simply put, individual specimens may show a remarkable anisotropy whereas mean population data demonstrates only a mild anisotropy of the AAA wall.

1.3.3 ILT Failure Testing

1.3.3.1 Method

ILT samples were harvested from AAAs during surgical elective repair and put in Dulbecco's Modified Eagle's Medium (DMEM). The collection and use of ILT material from human subjects was approved by the local ethics committee. Each ILT bulk tissue was first divided into the layers illustrated in Fig. 1.7 to gather tissue sheets from different structural layers. The thickness of the separated sheets ranged from 1.0 to 2.0 mm, and according to their location within the bulk ILT tissue,

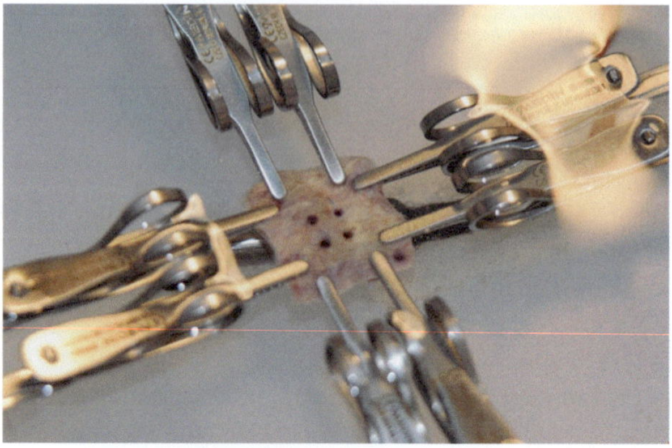

Fig. 1.6 Abdominal Aortic Aneurysm (AAA) wall specimen mounted in a planar biaxial testing device. Markers (ink dots) are used to compute the biaxial strain in the center of the specimen

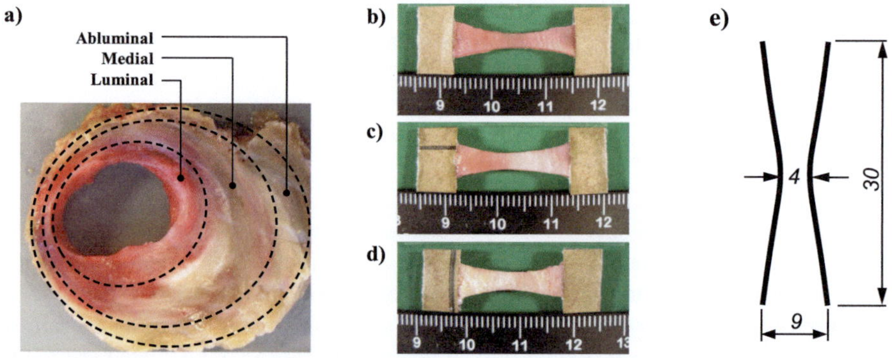

Fig. 1.7 Preparation of uniaxial test specimens. (**a**) Cross-section of the bulk ILT tissue harvested from elective AAA repair, where luminal, medial and abluminal layers are indicated. Sample uniaxial test specimens prepared from (**b**) luminal, (**c**) medial and (**d**) abluminal layers, respectively. (**e**) Dimensions of the pattern blade. Figure taken from Gasser et al. (2008)

they are labeled as luminal, medial and abluminal. From each sheet 4 uniaxial bone-shaped specimens, each oriented in circumferential direction, were punched out with an especially developed pattern blade (see Fig. 1.7e). To improve the fixation of the specimen in the testing machine, sand paper pieces were attached to their ends using super-adhesive glue.

Displacement controlled quasi-static and dynamic tensile testing were performed, where the load was measured by a 10N-load cell. During testing, ILT specimens were kept in DMEM (with supplements) at 37 °C and pH of 7.0 to ensure physiological conditions close to the in-vivo situation, see Fig. 1.8.

1.3.3.2 Results

The incompressible mechanical properties of ILT tissue were modeled by the one parameter Ogden-like strain energy function (1.7) (see Sect. 1.4.1), where the ma-

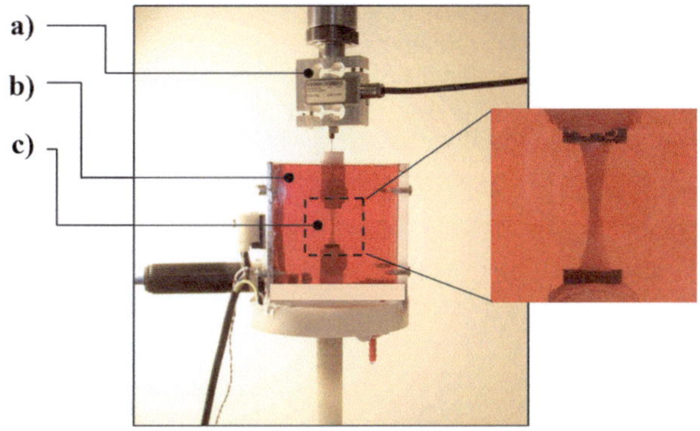

Fig. 1.8 Part of the testing equipment illustrating (**a**) the load-cell, (**b**) the tissue testing chamber filled with Dulbecco's Modified Eagle's Medium (DMEM) and (**c**) the test specimen fixed between the grips. Figure taken from Gasser et al. (2008)

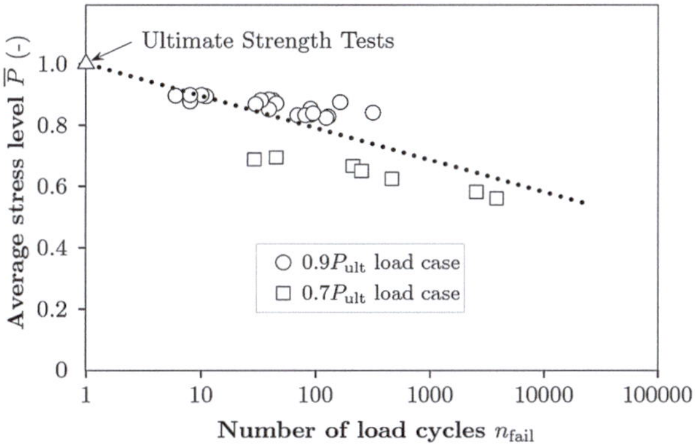

Fig. 1.9 S-N curve representing the vulnerability of ILT tissue against fatigue failure, i.e. decreasing strength with respect to the number of load cycles. Fatigue tests, where the ILT specimen failed during the experiment, are represented by (*circular* and *rectangular*) data points and the *dashed line* is defined by regression analysis. Figure taken from Gasser et al. (2008)

terial parameter c of the luminal, medial and abluminal ILT have been estimated to 2.62 kPa (SD 0.80), 1.98 kPa (SD 0.62) and 1.73 kPa (SD 0.64), respectively. Here, ILT's stiffness decreases about linearly by 44 % from the luminal to the abluminal tissue. For this parameter estimation plane stress FEM models were used to account for the non-homogeneous stress state of the bone-shaped specimens. Finally, the strength of the luminal, medial and abluminal ILT have been determined to 156.5 kPa (SD 57.9), 92.0 kPa (SD 37.5) and 47.7 kPa (SD 22.9), respectively. ILT fatigue effects are shown in Fig. 1.9. Specifically, the figure illustrates that at 60 % UTS stress-level the tissue fails at 10^4 cycles. Further results are given elsewhere (Gasser et al., 2008).

1.3.4 AAA-Wall Failure Testing

1.3.4.1 Method

Aneurysm tissue was harvested during elective open surgical repair. The collection and use of material from human subjects was approved by the local ethics

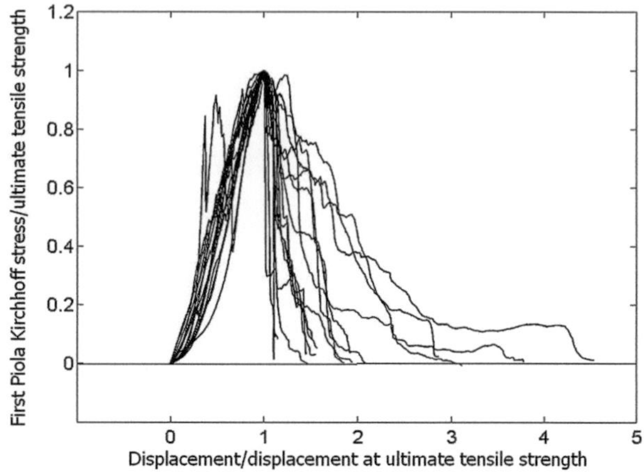

Fig. 1.10 Dimensionless stress versus stretch response of the wall from Abdominal Aortic Aneurysms (AAA). Data were recorded from uniaxial tension of bone-shaped specimens until failure

committee. The size of excised tissue patches allowed the preparation of a single longitudinally-aligned bone-shaped tensile specimen of dimensions similar as illustrated in Fig. 1.7e. Tensile testing without preconditioning at an elongation rate of 0.2 mm/s (average stretch rate of 0.008 s^{-1}) was performed until the specimen failed. Here, the specimen was entirely immersed in Ringer solution at $37 \pm 0.5°$ and further details regarding the testing protocol are given elsewhere (Forsell et al., 2012).

1.3.4.2 Results

The First Piola-Kirchhoff stress versus stretch response was calculated from the test results and a dimensionless plot is shown in Fig. 1.10. Results from 16 specimens (taken from 14 patients) showed an ultimate tensile strength of 437 (SD 319) kPa recorded at a stretch of 1.325 (SD 0.113).

1.4 Constitutive Modeling of AAA Tissue

Constitutive modeling of vascular tissue is an active field of research and numerous descriptions have been reported. However, the phenomenological approaches (Chuong and Fung, 1983; Fung et al., 1979; Humphrey, 1995; Takamizawa and Hayashi, 1987; Vaishnav et al., 1972) that have been successfully used to fit experimental data cannot allocate stress or strain to the different histological constituents in the vascular wall. Structural constitutive descriptions (Gasser, 2011; Gasser et al., 2006; Holzapfel et al., 2000; Lanir, 1983; Martufi and Gasser, 2011; Pena et al., 2011; Wuyts et al., 1995; Zulliger et al., 2004) overcome this limitation and integrate histological and mechanical information of the arterial wall. In addition to the mathematical description of mechanical properties an efficient and implicit numerical implementation (Gasser, 2011; Gasser and Forsell, 2011; Gasser and Holzapfel,

2002; Gasser et al., 2006) of constitutive formulations is beneficial for analyzing clinically relevant problems.

The extracellular matrix (ECM) provides an essential supporting scaffold for the structural and functional properties of vessel walls. The ECM mainly contains elastin, collagen, and proteoglycans (PGs) (Carey, 1991) and their three-dimensional organization is vital to accomplish proper physiological functions. The ECM, therefore, rather than being merely a system of scaffolding for the surrounding cells, is an active mechanical structure that controls the micro-mechanical and macro-mechanical environments to which vascular tissue is exposed. Specifically, a proper understanding of the mechanical properties of the ECM is critically important to estimate and quantify the amount of stress and/or strain transmitted from the macroscopic to the cellular levels of vascular tissue.

Collagen is one of the most dominant structural proteins in the ECM and critically involved in the gradual remodeling and weakening of the aneurysmal wall (Choke et al., 2005). Specifically, collagen fibrils (with diameter ranging from 50 to a few hundred of nanometers) are the basic building blocks of fibrous collagenous tissues (Fratzl, 2008), and their organization into suprafibrilar structures determines the tissue's macroscopic mechanical properties. Consequently, biomechanical (Gasser et al., 2006; He and Roach, 1996; MacSweeney et al., 1992) and clinical studies invariably show that the mechanics of the arterial wall essentially relies on fibrillar collagens in media and adventitia.

The late stage of AAA disease is characterized by irreversible pathological remodeling of the aortic wall connective tissue, which, amongst many others, involve degradation of the elastin and compensatory increased collagen synthesis, see Choke et al. (2005) and references therein. Consequently, the passive mechanical response of a larger AAA can be modeled as fibrous collagenous tissue with negligible contribution from the degraded and fragmented elastin. Information of collagen organization in the AAA wall permits a qualitative biomechanical understanding. However, the challenge is to relate it to engineering concepts and constitutive models, i.e. mathematical descriptions of biomechanical properties.

For soft biological tissues numerous constitutive models have been reported, where some of them, histo-mechanical constitutive models say, aim at integrating collagen fiber density and orientation. Specifically, the pioneering work by Lanir (1983) assumed macroscopic mechanical properties being governed by the arrangement of fibrous tissue components like collagen. According to his approach, the spatial orientation and undulation of collagen are the most influential micro-histological parameters that together with the fibers' constitution determine the macroscopic mechanical properties. Following such a structural approach the macroscopic mechanical tissue properties are derived through two numerical integrations, i.e. (i) over the undulation and (ii) over the fibers' spatial orientation. This requires extensive computations and makes the application of such an approach somewhat limited. However, either the use of phenomenological collagen fiber models or specific assumptions regarding the constitution and undulation of collagen can avoid the numerical integration over the undulation of collagen. Consequently, the biomechanics of an entire AAAs can be analyzed by such a two-scale approach within reasonable computational times.

1.4.1 *Elastic Model for the ILT*

An ILT is a complex structure, where aggregated platelets and other blood elements are trapped within a fibrin mesh traversed by a continuous network of interconnected canaliculi (Adolph et al., 1997). Mechanical testing has shown that ILT tissue can be regarded as an isotropic and linear material (Gasser et al., 2008; Vande Geest et al., 2006b; Wang et al., 2001), which withstands high deformations until failure (Di Martino et al., 1998; Gasser et al., 2008). Likewise, stiffness and strength decrease from inside to the outside (Gasser et al., 2008; Wang et al., 2001), whereas the time dependent (viscoelastic) properties remain constant across the thickness (van Dam et al., 2007). The incompressible mechanical properties of ILT tissue were modeled by the one-parameter Ogden-like strain energy function (Ogden, 1997)

$$\psi = c \sum_{i=1}^{3} (\lambda_i^4 - 1), \tag{1.7}$$

where λ_i denotes the i-th principal stretch and the material parameter c is determined through experimental data.

1.4.2 *Histo-mechanical Modeling of Collagenous Tissue*

Already 60 years ago Roach and Burton (1957) suggested that collagen had a main impact on the mechanical properties of arterial tissue at high strain levels. Since that time a direct correlation between the collagen content and the stiffness and strength has become generally accepted. Earlier observations indicated that the collagen-rich abdominal aorta was stiffer than the collagen-poor thoracic aorta (Bergel, 1961; Langewouters et al., 1984) and later regional variations of aortic properties were specifically documented, see Sokolis (2007) for example. Numerous further references are provided by the seminal works of Fung (1993) and Humphrey (2002). In addition to the volume fraction of collagen, its spatial arrangement, including the spread in orientations significantly affects the macroscopic mechanical properties (Gasser et al., 2006).

1.4.2.1 The CFPG-Complex

AAA wall tissue was regarded as a fibrous collagenous composite, where fibers of collagen reinforced an otherwise isotropic matrix material. Each collagen fiber is assembled by a bundle of collagen fibrils mutually interconnected by proteoglycan (PG) bridges (Scott, 2003, 2008) that provide interfibrillar load transition, see Fig. 1(b). Here, small proteoglycans like decorin bind noncovalently but specifically to the collagen fibril and cross-link adjacent collagen fibrils at about 60 nm intervals (Scott, 2003). Reversible deformability of the PG bridges is crucial to serve

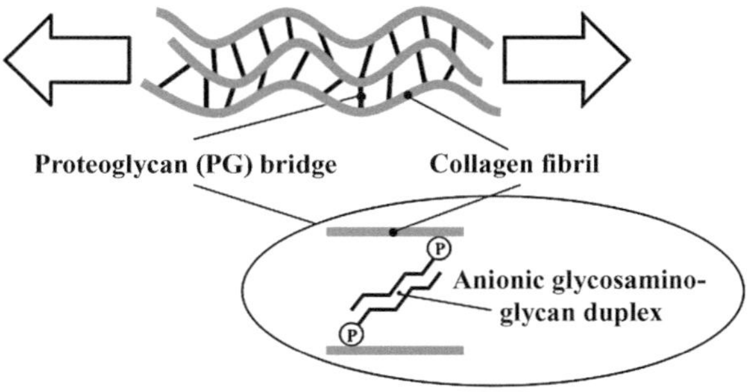

Fig. 1.11 Hierarchical structure of a collagen fiber, i.e. built up of undulated collagen fibrils that are interlinked by proteoglycan (PG) bridges

as shape-maintaining modules (Scott, 2003) and fast and slow deformation mechanisms have been identified. The fast (elastic) deformation is supported by the sudden extension of about 10 % of the L-iduronate (an elastic sugar) at a critical load of about 200 pN (Haverkamp et al., 2005). The slow (viscous) deformation is based on a sliding filament mechanisms of the twofold helix of the glycan (Scott, 2003). Alternatively, the close packing and cross-linking of collagen molecules in fibrils defines a virtually inextensible fiber, such that the strain within collagen fibrils is always much smaller than the macroscopic strain in collagenous tissues, which also points towards the existence of gliding processes occurring at the interfibrilar and/or the interfiber levels (Gupta et al., 2010).

The above described basic load carrying unit, Collagen Fibril PG-complex (CFPG-complex) say, is illustrated in Fig. 1.11. Stretching a collagen fiber involves continuous recruitment of collagen fibrils, which if straightened, start carrying load. Here, a straightening stretch λ_{st} defines the stretch beyond which the collagen fibril is stretched elastically, i.e. storing elastic energy in the CFPG-complex, i.e. in the collagen fibril itself and in the PG-rich matrix between the fibrils. Finally, the spatial orientation of collagen fibers is thought to be defined by the orientation density function $\rho(\mathbf{M})$.

1.4.2.2 Macroscopic Stress

Following Lanir (1983) we assume that the macroscopic Cauchy stress is defined by a superposition of individual collagen fiber contributions, i.e.

$$\boldsymbol{\sigma} = \frac{2}{\pi} \int_{\phi=0}^{\pi/2} \int_{\theta=0}^{\pi/2} \rho(\phi, \theta)\sigma(\lambda)\mathbf{m} \otimes \mathbf{m} \cos\phi \mathrm{d}\phi \mathrm{d}\theta + p\mathbf{I}, \qquad (1.8)$$

where $\mathbf{m} = \mathbf{FM}/|\mathbf{FM}|$ denotes the spatial orientation vector of the collagen fiber. In (1.8) the constitution of the collagen fiber is incorporated through its Cauchy stress $\sigma(\lambda)$. The relation $\sigma(\lambda) = \lambda P(\lambda)$ links the Cauchy stress to the First Piola-Kirchhoff stress P, where incompressibility of the collagen fiber was assumed. In (1.8) the term $p\mathbf{I}$ denotes the hydrostatic stress with the Lagrange parameter p that is defined by the problem's boundary conditions, i.e. cannot be computed from the tissue's constitutive law.

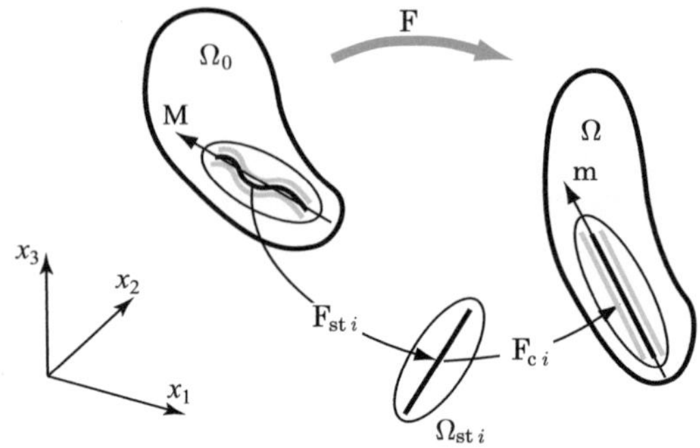

Fig. 1.12 Multiscale kinematics of the collagen-fiber-reinforced tissue. Configurational map, where the intermediate configuration $\Omega_{\mathrm{st}\,i}$ separates the straightening and stretching of the i-th collagen fibril. Figure taken from Martufi and Gasser (2011)

1.4.3 Elastic Multiscale Model for the AAA Wall

The model discussed in this section integrates the collagen's fibril and fiber levels with the tissue's continuum level. Specifically, cross-linked collagen fibrils are thought to form collagen fibers, which in turn are integrated over the unit sphere to define the tissue's macroscopic properties (Federico and Gasser, 2010; Lanir, 1983).

1.4.3.1 Kinematics

A fibrous tissue at finite deformations, where the unit direction vector **M** denotes the local collagen fiber direction in the reference configuration Ω_0 is considered, see Fig. 1.12. The deformation $\mathbf{F}_{\mathrm{st}\,i}$ straightens the i-th collagen fibril, i.e. it maps its crimped referential configuration into a straight but still unstressed intermediate configuration $\Omega_{\mathrm{st}\,i}$. In contrast the deformation $\mathbf{F}_{\mathrm{c}\,i}$ records deformation relative to $\Omega_{\mathrm{st}\,i}$ and maps the fibril to its spatial configuration Ω. Consequently, the intermediate configuration serves as a local reference configuration, with fibril stretch $\lambda_{\mathrm{c}\,i}$ and fibril tension $T_{\mathrm{c}\,i} = 0$, relative to which the fibril stretches elastically. According to multiplicative kinematics the continuum deformation is related to the introduced sub-deformations through $\mathbf{F} = \mathbf{F}_{\mathrm{c}\,i}\mathbf{F}_{\mathrm{st}\,i}$.

For simplicity and due to the lack of micro-structural data we assumed that the collagen fibrils straighten according to a symmetric triangular probability distribution (Kotz and vanDorp, 2004). Consequently, the first and last fibrils of a collagen fiber straighten at the fiber stretches of $\lambda_{\mathrm{min}} = 1$ and λ_{max} respectively. Elastin in the AAA wall is defragmented and collagen may determine the tissue's unloaded configuration, which in turn justifies setting $\lambda_{\mathrm{c}\,i} = 1$. Finally, affine deformation between the continuum and the collagen fiber, i.e. $\lambda = |\mathbf{FM}| = |\mathbf{m}|$, and incompressible macro-deformation ($\det \mathbf{F} = J = 1$), is considered.

1.4.3.2 Constitutive Description of the CFPG-Complex

Collagen fibrils have an approximately linear stress-stretch property (Miyazaki and Hayashi, 1999; Shen et al., 2008), which is nicely captured by the First Piola-

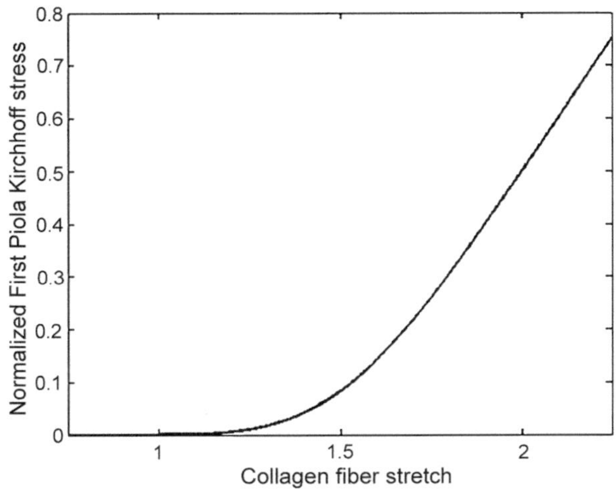

Fig. 1.13 Non-linear mechanical properties of a collagen fiber assembled from statistically-distributed collagen fibril proteoglycan-complexes (CFPG-complexes). Normalized First Piola-Kirchhoff stress as a function of the collagen fiber stretch is shown for $\lambda_{\max} = 2$. Figure taken from Martufi and Gasser (2011)

Kirchhoff stress $T_{ci} = k\lambda_{ci} \log \lambda_{ci}$ for the i-th CFPG-complex. Considering the continual recruitment of collagen fibrils gives (Martufi and Gasser, 2011)

$$T(\lambda) = k \int_0^{\lambda} \text{CDF}(\overline{\lambda}) \mathrm{d}\overline{\lambda}, \tag{1.9}$$

where $\text{CDF}(\overline{\lambda})$ denotes the Cumulative Density Function of the triangular probability distribution. Integrating $\text{CDF}(\overline{\lambda})$ and using the abbreviations $a = \lambda_{\max} - 1$ and $b = (\lambda_{\max} + 1)/2$ yields the piecewise analytical expressions for the First Piola-Kirchhoff stress

$$T(\lambda) = \begin{cases} 0, & 0 < \lambda \leq 1, \\ k\frac{2}{3a^2}(\lambda - 1)^3, & 1 < \lambda \leq b, \\ k[\lambda - \frac{2}{3a^2}(\lambda - \lambda_{\max})^3 - b], & b < \lambda \leq \lambda_{\max}, \\ k(\lambda - b), & \lambda_{\max} < \lambda \leq \infty. \end{cases} \tag{1.10}$$

This set of equations exhibits the typically non-linear property of soft biological tissues, as showed in Fig. 1.13. The numerical implementation of the models is detailed elsewhere (Martufi and Gasser, 2011).

1.4.3.3 Parameter Identification and Model Validation

Model parameters were identified from planar biaxial testing, where λ_c and λ_a denote the circumferential and axial stretches, respectively. Introducing the kinematics of the biaxial deformation of an incompressible solid, i.e. $\mathbf{F} = \text{diag}[\lambda_c, \lambda_a, (\lambda_c\lambda_a)^{-1}]$ and expressing the orientation of the collagen fiber through the Eulerian angles

Table 1.1 Model parameters used to predict the mean-population response of Abdominal Aortic Aneurysm (AAA) wall tissue (sr denotes steradian)

Bingham parameters	$\kappa_1 = 11.6$, $\kappa_1 = 9.7$
Collagen undulation parameters	$\lambda_{\max\text{c}} = 1.44$, $\lambda_{\max\text{a}} = 1.2$
CFPG-complex stiffness	$k = 2.0$ GPa/sr

$\mathbf{M} = [\cos\phi\cos\theta\ \sin\theta\ \sin\phi\cos\theta]^{\text{T}}$ (see Fig. 1.3), the circumferential σ_{c} and axial σ_{a} stresses read

$$\sigma_i = \frac{2}{\pi}\int_{\phi=0}^{\pi/2}\int_{\theta=0}^{\pi/2} \rho(\phi,\theta)\sigma(\lambda)(a_{ii} - a_{\text{rr}})\cos\phi \text{d}\phi\text{d}\theta; \quad i = \text{c, a}. \tag{1.11}$$

Here, $a_{\text{cc}}, a_{\text{aa}}, a_{\text{rr}}$ are the diagonal coefficients of the spatial tensor $\mathbf{a} = \mathbf{m} \otimes \mathbf{m} = (\mathbf{FM}) \otimes (\mathbf{FM})$ and $\sigma(\lambda) = \lambda T(\lambda)$, i.e. incompressibility of the collagen fiber was assumed. Equation (1.11) can be used to estimate constitutive parameters from biaxial experimental data.

Comprehensive experimental data of the AAA wall has been recorded from tension-based biaxial loading protocols (Vande Geest et al., 2006a). However, such data cannot directly be compared to predictions through (1.11), where the stretch rather than tension is prescribed. Hence, patient-specific model parameters that have been reported elsewhere (Ferruzzi et al., 2010) were used to generate synthetic experimental data. The synthetic data was then used to estimate constitutive parameters based on (1.11). In order to achieve a reasonable fit with the experimental data, it was essential that collagen fibers changed their constitution with respect to the their azimuthal alignment, and $\lambda_{\max} = \boldsymbol{\lambda}_{\max}\mathbf{M}$ with $\boldsymbol{\lambda}_{\max} = \text{diag}[\lambda_{\max\text{c}}, \lambda_{\max\text{a}}, (\lambda_{\max\text{c}}\lambda_{\max\text{a}})^{-1}]$ was considered. Finally, Fig. 1.14 shows model predictions and experimental data, where the parameters in Table 1.1 and a stretch ratio of $\lambda_{\text{c}}/\lambda_{\text{a}} = 2$ was used.

1.4.4 Inelastic Model for the AAA Wall

Understanding damage mechanisms of soft biological tissue is critical to the sensitive and specific characterization of tissue injury tolerance, including its implications on biological (physiological and pathological) responses. Such knowledge may help us to develop concepts, amongst others, that allow an accurate rupture risk assessment of Abdominal Aortic Aneurysms (AAAs) and vulnerable plaques, as it is crucial for clinical treatment planning, or to optimize the design of medical devices based on a proper understanding of short-term and long-term mutual interactions with biological tissues.

Exposing biological soft tissue to supraphysiological mechanical stresses rearranges the tissue's microstructure through irreversible deformations. Damage-related effects (such as, for tendon and ligament (Liao and Belkoff, 1999; Parry

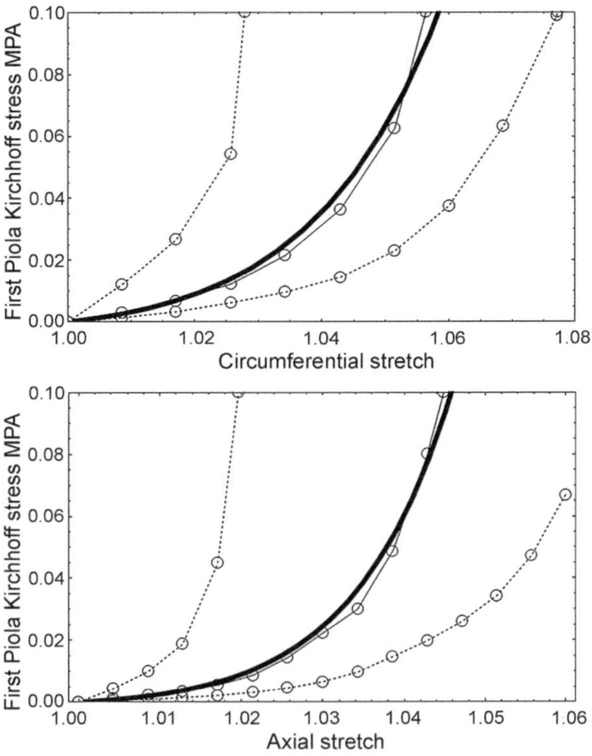

Fig. 1.14 Comparison between synthetic experimental and analytical stress-stretch response of the Abdominal Aortic Aneurysm (AAA) wall. Results are derived from a stretch-based biaxial loading protocol with a stretch ratio of $\lambda_c/\lambda_a = 2$. *Thick solid lines* show the analytical results, whereas the median and the 50 % quartile of the experimental data are illustrated by the *thin solid and dotted lines*, respectively

et al., 1978) and for vascular tissue (Emery et al., 1997a, 1997b; Oktay et al., 1991)) and plasticity-related effects (such as, for skin (Ridge and Wright, 1967), tendon and ligament (Abrahams, 1967; Parry et al., 1978; Sverdlik and Lanir, 2002) and vascular tissues (Oktay et al., 1991; Salunke and Topoleski, 1997)) have been documented, where experimental data were analyzed using macroscopic metrices like stress and strain. However, damage to soft biological tissue is defined by spatial localization of structural collagen damage, and microfailure well below ultimate failure at the tissue level, 51 ± 12 % of the ultimate strength for tendon tissue has been reported (Quinn and Winkelstein, 2008). Specifically, changes from small-angle X-ray scattering (SAXS) spectrum suggested that macroscopic tendon and ligament failure is preceded by damage from intrafibrillar sliding (Knörzer et al., 1986). Consequently, a macroscopic (single scale) view may be questionable in order to investigate and/or describe damage of soft biological tissue appropriately.

In conclusion, despite increasing experimental and analytical efforts to investigate failure-related irreversible effects of soft biological tissue, the underlying mechanisms are still poorly understood. There is still no clear definition of what damage is and conventional indicators of mechanical injury (such as visible failure and loss of stiffness) may not identify the tissue's tolerance to injury appropriately. Likewise, a macroscopic (single scale) view of tissues does not allow for an explicit description of individual collagen fibers, and hence, may fail to account for localized structural rearrangement of collagen fibrils at supraphysiological mechanical stress.

The present model uses a microfiber model approach and macroscopic tissue properties are derived by an integration over the unit sphere (Federico and Gasser, 2010; Lanir, 1983). Such an approach reflects salient features of the microstructure and supports the application of challenging constitutive models for collagen fibers. A simple straightening mechanism of collagen fibers is considered to account for their tension compression non-linearity, and a viscoplastic sliding mechanism is coupled with failure of collagen cross-links. The model is limited to strain stiffening, i.e. it cannot be applied to investigate macroscopic localization without additional regularization techniques.

1.4.4.1 Modeling Assumptions

The present model aims at capturing supraphysiological stress states and it is assumed that, at the straightening stretch λ_{st}, all collagen fibrils that constitute a collagen fiber straighten simultaneously. Specifically, the model does not consider a continuous recruitment of collagen fibrils, as it has been suggested in Sect. 1.4.3 and in the literature earlier (Martufi and Gasser, 2011; Wuyts et al., 1995; Zulliger et al., 2004). Stretching a collagen fiber beyond λ_{st} involves stretching of the collagen fibrils and shearing of interfibrillar material, as it is schematically illustrated in Fig. 1.15. Such a deformation mechanisms involves sliding of collagen fibrils relatively to each other, which is, to a great extent, defined by the elastic properties of the PG bridges.

The sliding of the PG bridge becomes irreversible if the overlap of the glycan chains decreases beyond a critical level, see Scott (2003) and references therein. Consequently, the physiological shape-maintaining deformation range of the PG bridge is exceeded and the collagen fibrils (within a collagen fiber) will be rearranged irreversibly. Note that this molecular mechanism, i.e. irreversible sliding of PG bridges, explains irreversible (plastic) effects known from macroscopic experimental testing of soft biological tissues (Abrahams, 1967; Oktay et al., 1991; Parry et al., 1978; Ridge and Wright, 1967; Salunke and Topoleski, 1997; Sverdlik and Lanir, 2002). At increasing stretch the PG bridges will slide apart (rupture), which weakens (damages) the collagen fiber due to loss of cross-links. Note that the sliding PG filament represents a slow (viscous) deformation mechanism (Scott, 2008), such that the loss of PG bridges is regarded as a continuous and time dependent process.

The above discussed deformation mechanisms of a collagen fiber, motivates the introduction of a 'stretch-based' constitutive concept, where irreversible (plastic) sliding of the collagen fibrils will not only define the fiber's irreversible elongation but also its state of damage. In other words, plastic deformation of the collagen fiber causes softening of the fiber. Note that at the molecular level it is very well understood that cross-links provide collagen fibrils with stiffness and strength (Buehler, 2008; Silver et al., 2003) and a similar reinforcement mechanism of collagen fibers is considered by the present model.

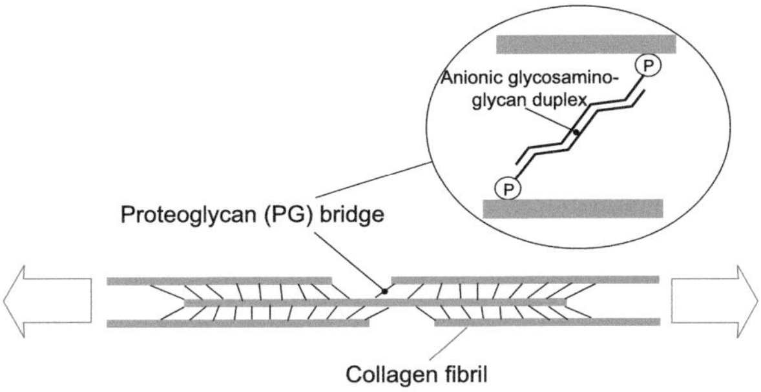

Fig. 1.15 Schematic load-carrying mechanisms of a collagen fiber assembled by a number of collagen fibrils. Load transition across collagen fibrils is provided by proteoglycan (PG) bridges. Figure taken from Gasser (2011)

1.4.4.2 Kinematics

Affine deformation between matrix and the collagen fiber is considered, which relates its total stretch $\lambda = \sqrt{\mathbf{M} \cdot \mathbf{C}\mathbf{M}} = |\mathbf{F}\mathbf{M}| = |\mathbf{m}|$ to the deformation of the matrix. Likewise, multiplicative kinematics are considered, i.e. $\mathbf{F} = \mathbf{F}_{\mathrm{el}}\mathbf{F}_{\mathrm{st}}$ with $\mathbf{F}_{\mathrm{el}}$ denoting the elastic deformation, i.e. deformation that reversibly stores strain energy.

1.4.4.3 Constitutive Model for the Collagen Fiber

Collagen fibers are thought to have no bending stiffness and at stretches below λ_{st} the stress in the fiber is zero. Exceeding λ_{st} a linear relation between the effective Second Piola-Kirchhoff stress $\widetilde{S}_{\mathrm{c\,st}}$ and the elastic stretch λ_{el} is assumed, i.e. $\widetilde{S}_{\mathrm{c\,st}} = c_{\mathrm{f}}\langle\lambda_{\mathrm{el}} - 1\rangle = c_{\mathrm{f}}\langle\lambda/\lambda_{\mathrm{st}} - 1\rangle$, where c_{f} and λ denotes the stiffness of the collagen fiber and its total stretch, respectively. The Macauley-brackets $\langle\bullet\rangle$ explicitly emphasize that a collagen fiber can only carry tensile load.

Considering incompressible elastic (micro-scale) deformation of the collagen fiber, the effective First Piola-Kirchhoff stress reads $\widetilde{P}_{\mathrm{c\,st}} = c_{\mathrm{f}}\langle\lambda_{\mathrm{el}}^2 - \lambda_{\mathrm{el}}\rangle$, which reveals the constitutive relation using work-conjugate variables.

The introduced stress $\widetilde{S}_{\mathrm{c\,st}}$ (and $\widetilde{P}_{\mathrm{c\,st}}$) is related to the intermediate configuration Ω_{st}, and for convenience a pull-back to the reference configuration Ω_0 is introduced. This mapping involves the particular micro-scale kinematics of the plastic deformation and, based on the above discussed sliding mechanism of the collagen fibrils, the plastic deformation gradient $\mathbf{F}_{\mathrm{st}}^{\mathrm{micro}} = \mathrm{diag}[\lambda_{\mathrm{st}}\ 1.0\ 1.0]$ with the micro-scale volume ratio $J_{\mathrm{st}}^{\mathrm{micro}} = \det \mathbf{F}_{\mathrm{st}}^{\mathrm{micro}} = \lambda_{\mathrm{st}}$, is considered. Note that during this plastic deformation the cross-section of the collagen fiber is kept constant, and hence, the pull-back of the stress to Ω_0 simply reads $\widetilde{S}_{\mathrm{c}} = \widetilde{S}_{\mathrm{c\,st}}$, with $\widetilde{S}_{\mathrm{c}}$ denoting the effective Second Piola-Kirchhoff stress with respect to Ω_0.

The state of damage of the collagen fiber is defined by an internal state (damage) variable d reflecting the loss of stiffness according to slid apart (broken) PG bridges. Thus the Second Piola-Kirchhoff stress of the collagen fiber reads

$$S_{\mathrm{c}} = (1-d)\widetilde{S}_{\mathrm{c}} = (1-d)c_{\mathrm{f}}\langle\lambda/\lambda_{\mathrm{st}} - 1\rangle. \tag{1.12}$$

For completeness, i.e. to model the development of λ_{st} and d, (1.12) needs to be enriched by plastic and damage constitutive relations, respectively.

Plastic Deformation Plastic deformation develops at large sliding of PG bridges, i.e. as soon as the overlap between the glycan chains of a PG bridge decrease beyond a critical level (Scott, 2003). The proposed model records plastic deformation by a monotonic increase of the straightening stretch $\lambda_{st0} \leq \lambda_{st} < \infty$, where λ_{st0} denotes the straightening stretch of the initial (not yet plastically deformed) collagen fiber. The initial straightening stretch λ_{st0} is thought to be a structural property defined by the continuous turn-over of collagen and determined by the biomechanical and biochemical environment that the tissue experiences in-vivo. Following the theory of plasticity (Lubliner, 1990; Simo and Hughes, 1998) we introduce an elastic threshold Y that classifies the following load cases,

$$\left.\begin{array}{ll} \widetilde{S}_c < Y & \text{elastic deformation,} \\ \widetilde{S}_c = Y & \text{plastic deformation,} \\ \widetilde{S}_c > Y & \text{to be ruled out.} \end{array}\right\} \tag{1.13}$$

At quasi-static loading conditions an ideal plastic response is considered with $Y = Y_0$ reflecting the elastic limit (in an effective Second Piola-Kirchhoff stress setting) of the collagen fiber. In contrast, time-dependent plastic loading is thought to induce a hardening effect, i.e. $Y = Y_0 + H$, where H reflects the increase of resistance against collagen fibril sliding due to the slow (viscous) sliding mechanism of the PG bridges. Likewise, any viscous inter-fibrilar material (fluid) would motivate a rate-dependent increase of resistance against collagen fibril sliding. Consequently, a viscoplastic behavior of the collagen fibers is considered, and (for simplicity) the first order rate equation

$$H = \eta \dot{\lambda}_{st} \tag{1.14}$$

defines the viscous hardening, with η denoting a material parameter.

Damage Accumulation As detailed above, larger irreversible (plastic) deformation of the collagen fiber causes failure of PG bridges, which in turn weakens the collagen fiber. The mechanical effect from ruptured PG bridges, i.e. the loss of stiffness of the collagen fiber is recorded by the damage parameter d, where an exponential relation

$$d = 1 - \exp\left[-a(\lambda_{st}/\lambda_{st0} - 1)^2\right] \tag{1.15}$$

with respect to the plastic deformation (reflected by $\lambda_{st}/\lambda_{st0}$) is considered. Equation (1.15) has the properties $d(\lambda_{st}/\lambda_{st0} = 1.0) = 0.0$ and $d(\lambda_{st}/\lambda_{st0} \to \infty) = 1.0$, and a denotes a material parameter. Specifically, small and large values of a define plastic-like and brittle-like failure of the collagen fiber, respectively.

Finally, it is noted that failure of PG bridges permits collagen fibrils to slide, which in turn activates the viscoplastic dissipative mechanisms of the collagen fiber. A similar experimental observation has been reported in the literature, where cross-linking of self-assembled type I collagen fibers reduces their viscoelastic dissipation (Silver et al., 2003). For an efficient numerical implementation of the models see elsewhere (Gasser, 2011).

Table 1.2 Material parameters estimated from a single macroscopic tensile test of tissue from the Abdominal Aortic Aneurysm (AAA) wall (sr denotes steradian)

Matrix material		
neoHookean parameter	c	0.02 MPa
Collagen fibers		
Straightening stretch	$\lambda_{\mathrm{st}\,0}$	1.08
Collagen fiber stiffness	c_{f}	0.23 MPa/sr
Elastic limit	Y_0	0.063 MPa/sr
Hardening viscosity	η	0.2 MPa s
Damage property	a	50.0

1.4.4.4 Parameter Identification and Model Validation

An implicit parameter estimation from macroscopic test data was used and a single test demonstrated basic model properties. To this end a collagen distribution model as suggested in Gasser et al. (2006) and with $b = 0.5$ was applied to the AAA wall. The introduced material parameters were set manually and led to a reasonable match between model and test results, see Fig. 1.16. Here, the set of material properties shown in Table 1.2 was considered.

By increasing the load beyond the toe region, a slightly non-linear relation between the First Piola-Kirchhoff stress and stretch is observed, before the collagen fibers gradually exceed their elastic limit and define a concave stress-stretch response, see Fig. 1.16. Gradually exceeding the collagen fibers' elastic limit defines a smooth transition from a convex to a concave curve, i.e. as it is typically observed in experimental data from vascular tissue.

Significant plastic deformation is required before the ultimate strength is reached. A further increase in stretch causes material instability, and the deformation becomes localized. In the strain softening region the results strongly depend on the test specimen's length, i.e. numerical and experimental responses can no longer be compared.

The impact of the stretch rate on the predictions is illustrated in Fig. 1.17, where continuous and cyclic increasing stretch was applied. According to the modeling assumptions, rate effects appear beyond the elastic limit, and as expected, a higher strain rate causes a higher ultimate strength at higher stretches, see particularly Fig. 1.17 (left). Cyclic stretching nicely illustrates the dissipation of the model and the accumulation of plastic deformations, i.e. the irreversible shift of the transition point from a matrix-material-dominated to a collagen-fiber-dominated behavior to higher values, see Fig. 1.17 (right). Note also that during the early phase of unloading (i.e. as long as the stress is above the quasi-static elastic limit) tissue damage increases. Finally, since preconditioning has been related to irreversible stretching of collagen fibers (Lokshin and Lanir, 2009), it is not surprising that the recorded curves in Fig. 1.17 (right) display typical features of tissue precondition.

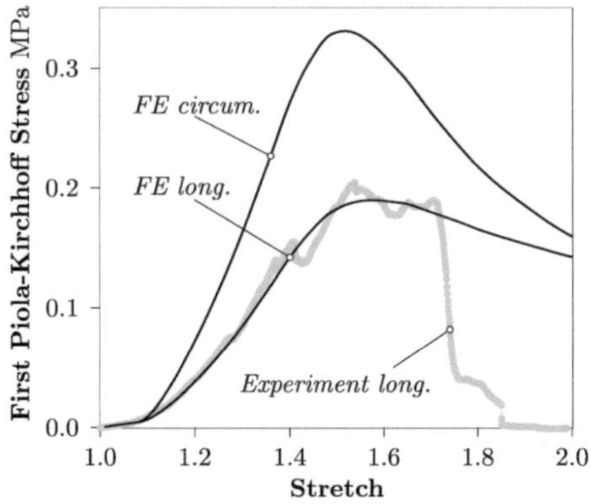

Fig. 1.16 Macroscopic constitutive response of Abdominal Aortic Aneurysm (AAA) wall tissue under uniaxial tension. Quasi-static model results (*solid black lines*) from tension along the circumferential and longitudinal directions using material properties given in Table 1.2. The *grey curve* illustrates the response from in-vitro experimental stretching of a single AAA wall specimen along the longitudinal direction. Figure taken from Gasser (2011)

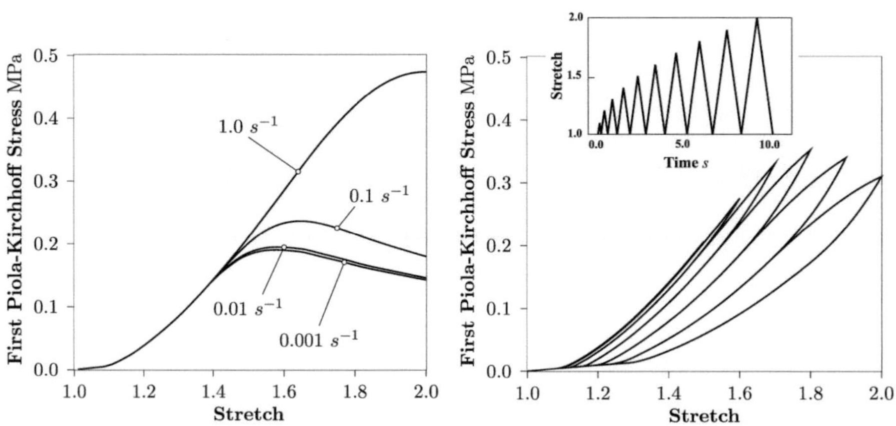

Fig. 1.17 Model predictions of tension along the longitudinal direction of Abdominal Aortic Aneurysm (AAA) wall tissue at different stretching conditions. *Left*: Continuous stretch at rates between 0.001 s^{-1} and 1.0 s^{-1}. *Right*: Cyclic stretches of $\lambda = 1.1, 1.2, \ldots, 2.0$ at a rate of ± 1.0 s^{-1}. Calculations are based on material properties given in Table 1.2. Figure taken from Gasser (2011)

1.5 Clinical Decision-Making Tool

1.5.1 Problem Definition

Rupture of AAAs account for a large number of deaths particularly in men above the age of 65 and elective repair (surgical or endovascular) is indicated if the risk of aneurysm rupture exceeds the interventional risks. Several studies investigated

AAA repair indication, where typically the maximum AAA diameter was aimed at quantifying AAA rupture risk. Based on results from these studies a maximum AAA diameter of 55 mm (or more) is accepted as AAA repair indication (The UK Small Aneurysm Trial Participants, 1998). However, the maximum diameter fails to describe AAA rupture risk patient-specifically (Brown, 1997), and hence, results from these studies do not directly apply to individual patients. Consequently, the maximum diameter of 55 millimeters describes the indication for a large number of patients, but not necessarily for an individual patient. Reported studies confirmed that fact and showed that 10 % (Nicholls et al., 1998) of small AAAs rupture, but 60 % (Darling et al., 1977) of large AAAs do not rupture during life time. In addition, due to the low prevalence of aneurysms in females, AAA repair indication in females is unclear. Consequently, the diameter criterion has clear limitations and other AAA rupture risk indicators have been suggested in the literature (Fillinger, 2007).

One of these alternative approaches, the biomechanical rupture risk assessment, progressed considerably through the last years. According to this concept the aneurysm wall will rupture as soon as the local mechanical stress overcomes the strength of the wall. Consequently, PWS (the maximum stress in the wall) and the PWRR (the maximum stress/strength ratio in the wall) are key biomechanical rupture risk indices. PWS and PWRR integrate a large number of well-known risk factors for AAA rupture as itemized in Table 1.3. Several independent studies demonstrated that PWS and PWRR are more reliable rupture risk indicators than the maximum diameter, i.e. they discriminate better between ruptured and non-ruptured AAAs (Fillinger et al., 2002; Gasser et al., 2010; Heng et al., 2008; Maier et al., 2010; Venkatasubramaniam et al., 2004). PWRR discriminates slightly better than PWS (Gasser et al., 2010; Maier et al., 2010). Despite the advantages of PWS and PWRR their meaning fits somehow difficult a clinical setting, and hence, the biomechanical rupture risk assessment is not applied in clinical practice. Finally, it is noted that weak (unreliable) diagnostic information puts patients at psychological stress that lowers their quality of life (Lindholt et al., 2000). This is considered one main reasons against the implementation of AAA screening programs.

This section summarizes the biomechanical rupture risk assessment and demonstrates its clinical application. Specifically, through a case study the patient-individual PWRR index is computed and translated to a (fictitious) aneurysm in the 'average AAA patient' at the same risk of rupture. This allows a clinically meaningful rupture risk assessment based on an individualized biomechanical analysis (Gasser, 2012).

1.5.2 Model Complexity

Beside the constitution of the aneurysm wall (Raghavan and Vorp, 2000) the Intra-Luminal Thrombus (ILT), which is found in most clinically relevant aneurysms (Hans et al., 2005), has characteristic solid mechanical properties (Gasser et al.,

Table 1.3 List of risk factors for AAA Rupture and their consideration (*marked as X*) through Peak Wall Stress (PWS) and Peak Wall Rupture Risk (PWRR) indices

	PWS	PWRR
Aneurysm size	X	X
Aneurysm shape, like asymmetry	X	X
Raised blood pressure	X	X
Wall weakening through the intra-luminal thrombus, diameter expansion, female gender and family history		X

2008; van Dam et al., 2007; Vande Geest et al., 2006b; Wang et al., 2001), and hence a profound structural impact (Li et al., 2008; Vorp et al., 1996) on the biomechanics of AAAs. ILT changes wall stress magnitude and distribution (Di Martino et al., 1998; Inzoli et al., 1993; Li et al., 2008; Mower et al., 1997; Wang et al., 2002), and hence, membrane-like or shell-like aneurysm models (Fillinger et al., 2003; Heng et al., 2008; Raghavan et al., 2005; Truijers et al., 2007; Venkatasubramaniam et al., 2004), which do not consider the ILT, will often fail to predict meaningful field variables. Despite the ILT is a porous structure that includes a considerable amount of (mobile) fluid, a single-phase simulation provides accurate quasi-static stress results (Polzer et al., 2012). Incompressible and large deformations are typical for vascular tissue and mixed FEM formulations based on hexahedral volume elements showed superior (Zienkiewicz and Taylor, 2000b) performance for these type of applications. The mixed (or reducible) FEM formulation uses a reducible set of nodal variables, e.g., to overcome volume locking phenomena, as they are known from incompressible materials (Zienkiewicz and Taylor, 2000a).

1.5.3 Clinical Work Flow

High-resolution medical imaging enables information for planning and performing surgical interventions. Besides a pure geometrical analysis of these image data, a detailed biomechanical analysis can be conducted. Such a method requires the following three work flow steps:

- Three-dimensional reconstruction of the AAA from image data.
- Defining and solving a Finite Element Method (FEM) problem.
- Analyzing and evaluating the computed data.

The FEM is a common numerical concept to solve engineering and other problems of the applied sciences and latest software (A4clinics, VASCOPS GmbH, Austria) allows it application to vascular medicine. The 3D reconstruction of the AAA from image data starts with a (rough) pre-segmentation of the lumen, which in turn is refined and used to segment the exterior surface of the AAA. Here, deformable contour models are used that present a precise capturing method with an expected reconstruction error in the range of one pixel of the in-plane image resolution (Auer and Gasser, 2010). A typical reconstructed AAA is shown in Fig. 1.18. Based on the derived reconstruction a meshing algorithm differentiates the aneurysmal tissue, i.e. the wall and the thrombus and splits it into a finite number of hexahedral-dominated finite elements. Most important, the derived three-dimensional reconstruction is insensitive to image artifacts, which is a basic requirement for a reliable biomechanical analysis.

The applied biomechanical model treats the aneurysm wall and the intra-luminal thrombus as separate soft tissue components (Gasser et al., 2010). Mean population data for the wall thickness is used and the reported thinning of the wall behind the thrombus (Kazi et al., 2003) is considered. The reconstructed AAA is enriched by mean-population constitutive tissue properties and loaded by the patient's mean arterial pressure (MAP), which in turn defines the FEM problem. Specifically, the model considers elasticity (Raghavan and Vorp, 2000) and strength (Vande Geest et al., 2006c) of the aneurysm wall, and elasticity (Gasser et al., 2008) of the intra-luminal thrombus. The tissues' constitutive models require parameters that have been identified from mechanical in-vitro experiments. Note that patient-specific information cannot be used at that modeling level and inter-patient variability of tissue parameters impacts the biomechanical analysis to some extent. A variation of tissue elasticity within the physiological rage leads to variability of about 5 % in PWS prediction (Di Martino and Vorp, 2003; Raghavan and Vorp, 2000). In contrast, a variation of wall thickness and tissue strength affects the predictions proportionally. Finally it is emphasized that the above outlined concept shows low variability among operators (Hyhlik-Dürr et al., 2011), which allows its integration in the clinical work flow.

1.5.3.1 Analyzing and Evaluating the Computed Data

The FEM model computes the mechanical stress in the aneurysm wall, i.e. the stress that is required to carry the MAP by the particular patient-specific geometry. The computed data is automatically analyzed and the maximum tensile stress in the wall is output through the PWS index. Similarly the largest stress/strength ratio is output through the PWRR index.

PWRR is related to the 'average AAA patient', which is defined by the mean PWRR observed in a larger cohort of patients. Specifically, the 'average AAA patient' can be expressed through the PWRR-diameter relation denoted by the thick solid line in Fig. 1.19. This curve reveals that the PWRR index of the 'average AAA patient' increases with respect to the maximum diameter, i.e. larger aneurysms are at higher risk. However, this functional relation between PWRR and diameter is significantly scattered (as indicated by the dotted lines in Fig. 1.19) and the individual patient may have higher or lower risk of rupture compared to an aneurysm of the same size in the 'average AAA patient'. Relating the PWRR index to the 'average AAA patient', i.e. the PWRR-diameter relation illustrated in Fig. 1.19, provides a rupture risk assessment within a clinical meaningful setting, as it is detailed by cases study below.

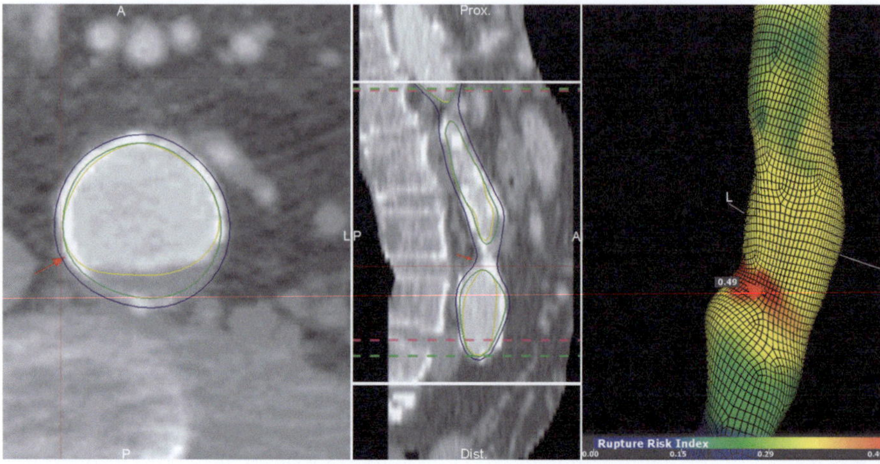

Fig. 1.18 Case study that uses a biomechanical model of an Abdominal Aortic Aneurysm (AAA) based on the Finite Element Method (FEM) to assess its risk of rupture. The FEM model considers geometry, blood pressure and the gender-specific strength of the wall. (*Left*) Three-dimensional reconstruction from Computer Tomography-Angiography (CT-A) images (transversal and sagittal views are displayed). The *red arrow* indicates the site of Peak Wall Rupture Risk (PWRR). (*Right*) Color-coded rupture risk index distribution plotted on top of the three-dimensional FEM model—*red areas* are under higher risk. The site of PWRR, i.e. the position of highest risk of rupture, is indicated by the *red arrow*

1.5.3.2 Case Study

The application of the biomechanical rupture risk analysis is best illustrated by a case study. For the present case we consider a female patient with an aneurysm of a maximum diameter of 42 mm and a blood pressure of 138/76 mmHg. The biomechanical analysis was carried-out with a standard laptop computer (Compaq 6910p) within 14 minutes. The distribution of wall rupture risk is shown in Fig. 1.18(b) and the biomechanical analysis computed a PWRR of 0.49. This information (diameter of 42 mm and a PWRR index of 0.49) is plotted in Fig. 1.18, which immediately illustrates that this individual AAA is at significantly higher risk than an aneurysm of the same size in the 'average AAA patient'. To better quantify the risk of rupture, the Rupture Risk Equivalent Diameter (RRED) is introduced. The RRED is a fictitious diameter that denotes the maximum diameter of an aneurysm in the 'average AAA patient' at the same risk of rupture, i.e. that has the same PWRR index. To this end the point representing the individual patient in diagram (Fig. 1.18) is shifted horizontally until the curve representing the 'average AAA patient' is intersected. For the present patient this gives a RRED of 56 mm, which means that the (biomechanically evaluated) risk of rupture for the individual patient compares to a 56 mm aneurysm in 'average AAA patient'. Consequently, AAA repair would be indicated.

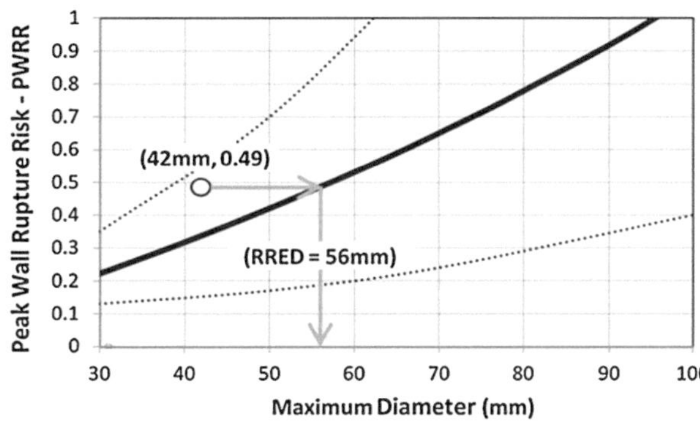

Fig. 1.19 Case study to demonstrate the biomechanical rupture risk assessment. The Peak Wall Rupture Risk (PWRR) index is translated into a Rupture Risk Equivalent Diameter (RRED) that relates the individual risk of rupture to the 'average AAA patient'. The *thick solid and dotted lines* denote mean value, and the 5 % and 95 % quartiles, respectively

1.6 Conclusions

Vascular biomechanics is critical in order to define new diagnostic and therapeutic methods that could have a significant influence on our medical understanding and even on the life style of human beings. Continued advances in computer technology and computational methods allow us nowadays to model patient-specific problems and to derive patient-individual information on a daily basis in clinical practice. In particular, the nonlinear FEM provides a powerful numerical tool with which to solve the 3D (coupled) mechanical problems that arise. It allows us to incorporate the nonlinear character of the related problems and combines synergetically with medical imaging. However, less attention has been paid to bringing this concept into clinical practice, and only a very few vascular simulation products are available for routine clinical applications.

Biomechanical models in the literature are typically overloaded with mechanical complexities but almost all of them fail to address clinical problems adequately, and hence, do not always enjoy clinician acceptance. A simulation model represents the real object or process to a desired degree of complexity and must be driven by clinical needs and not only by experimental observations. However, such models do not only require a careful selection and combination of modeling assumptions but also rigorous validation though longitudinal clinical trials.

A clinically meaningful biomechanical analysis of vascular bodies is characterized by an operator-insensitive reconstruction method, reliable constitutive description of vascular tissue and a straight-forward interpretation of the derived results. In this chapter the biomechanical rupture risk assessment of AAAs was used to demonstrate the integration of biomechanical simulations in the clinical work-flow of AAA patients. To this end a patient-specific FEM model translates numerous well-known risk factors for AAA rupture into the PWRR index. The meaning of the PWRR index is translated into the diameter of a biomechanically equivalent aneurysm in the 'average AAA patient', i.e. the RRED. The RRED links the individual rupture risk with conclusions drawn from earlier clinical studies, reporting indication for elective AAA repair.

The present chapter focused on structural aspects and it is known that aneurysm disease also alters the blow flow through the aorta (Taylor and Humphrey, 2009).

The enlarged lumen lowers the wall shear stress (Biasetti et al., 2009) and vortical structure dynamics differ remarkably between normal and aneurysmatic aortas (Biasetti et al., 2011). These hemodynamic alterations dictate the distribution of chemical species like thrombin (Biasetti et al., 2012), and the associated biological consequences are unknown. Finally, it is a fact that biomechanical models of the vasculature are characterized by numerous challenges, where the inherent property of biological tissue to adapt to mechanical and biochemical environments is mentioned specifically. Consequently, the key for improving biomechanical models is to understand these adaption mechanisms. This may also solve the current issues on how to consider residual strains and tissue inhomogeneities in a geometrically complex vascular body.

Acknowledgements The author is extremely thankful to Jacopo Biasetti for his valuable comments and proof reading the manuscript. This work has been financially supported by the Young Faculty Grant No. 2006-7568 provided by the Swedish Research Council, VINNOVA and the Swedish Foundation for Strategic Research, and the EC Seventh Framework Programme, Fighting Aneurysmal Disease (FAD-200647).

References

Abrahams M (1967) Mechanical behavior of tendon in vitro. A preliminary report. Med Biol Eng 5:433–443

Adolph R, Vorp DA, Steed DL, Webster MW, Kameneva MV, Watkins SC (1997) Cellular content and permeability of intraluminal thrombus in abdominal aortic aneurysm. J Vasc Surg 25:916–926

Alastrué V, Saez P, Martínez MA, Doblaré M (2010) On the use of the bingham statistical distribution in microsphere-based constitutive models for arterial tissue. Mech Res Commun 37:700–706

Auer M, Gasser TC (2010) Reconstruction and finite element mesh generation of abdominal aortic aneurysms from computerized tomography angiography data with minimal user interaction. IEEE Trans Med Imaging 29:1022–1028

Belytschko T, Liu WK, Moran B (2000) Nonlinear finite elements for continua and structures. Wiley, Chichester

Bergel DH (1961) The static elastic properties of the arterial wall. J Physiol 156:445–457

Biasetti J, Gasser TC, Auer M, Hedin U, Labruto F (2009) Hemodynamics conditions of the normal aorta compared to fusiform and saccular abdominal aortic aneurysms with emphasize on thrombus formation. Ann Biomed Eng 38:380–390

Biasetti J, Hussain F, Gasser TC (2011) Blood flow and coherent vortices in the normal and aneurysmatic aortas. A fluid dynamical approach to intra-luminal thrombus formation. J R Soc Interface 8:1449–1461

Biasetti J, Spazzini PG, Gasser TC (2012) An integrated fluido-chemical model towards modeling the formation of intra-luminal thrombus in abdominal aortic aneurysms. Submitted

Bingham C (1974) An antipodally symmetric distribution on the sphere. Ann Stat 2:1201–1225

Brown EJ (1997) Adhesive interactions in the immune system. Trends Cell Biol 7:289–295

Buehler MJ (2008) Hierarchical nanomechanics of collagen fibrils: atomistic and molecular modeling. In: Fratzl P (ed) Collagen—structure and mechanics. Chap. 8

Bursa J, Zemanek M (2008) Evaluation of biaxial tension tests of soft tissues. Stud Health Technol Inform 133:45–55

Canann SA, Tristano JR, Staten ML (1998) An approach to combined Laplacian and optimization-based smoothing for triangular, quadrilateral, and quad-dominant meshes. In: Proceedings of the 7th international meshing roundtable, pp 479–494
Carey D (1991) Control of growth and differentiation of vascular cells by extracellular matrix proteins. Annu Rev Physiol 53:161–177
Choke E, Cockerill G, Wilson WR, Sayed S, Dawson J, Loftus I, Thompson MM (2005) A review of biological factors implicated in abdominal aortic aneurysm rupture. Eur J Vasc Endovasc Surg 30:227–244
Chuong CJ, Fung YC (1983) Three-dimensional stress distribution in arteries. J Biomech Eng 105:268–274
Darling RC, Messina CR, Brewster DC, Ottinger LW (1977) Autopsy study of unoperated abdominal aortic aneurysms. Circulation 56:161–164
de Bruijne M, van Ginneken B, Niessen WJ, Antoine Maintz JB, Viergever MA (2002) Active shape model based segmentation of abdominal aortic aneurysms in CTA images. Proc SPIE Int Soc Opt Eng 4684:463–474
de Bruijne M, van Ginneken B, Viergever MA, Niessen WJ (2004) Interactive segmentation of abdominal aortic aneurysms in CTA images. Med Image Anal 8:127–138
Delingette H (1999) General object reconstruction based on simplex meshes. Int J Comput Vis 32:111–146
Di Martino ES, Vorp DA (2003) Effect of variation in intraluminal thrombus constitutive properties on abdominal aortic wall stress. Ann Biomed Eng 31:804–809
Di Martino ES, Mantero S, Inzoli F, Melissano G, Astore D, Chiesa R, Fumero R (1998) Biomechanics of abdominal aortic aneurysm in the presence of endoluminal thrombus: experimental characterization and structural static computational analysis. Eur J Vasc Endovasc Surg 15:290–299
Emery JL, Omens JH, McCulloch AD (1997a) Biaxial mechanics of the passively overstretched left ventricle. Am J Physiol 272:H2299–H2305
Emery JL, Omens JH, McCulloch AD (1997b) Strain softening in rat left ventricular myocardium. J Biomech Eng 119:6–12
Federico S, Gasser TC (2010) Non-linear elasticity of biological tissues with statistical fibre orientation. J R Soc Interface 7:955–966
Ferruzzi J, Vorp DA, Humphrey JD (2010) On constitutive descriptors of the biaxial mechanical behavior of human abdominal aorta and aneurysms. J R Soc Interface 8:435–540
Field D (1988) Laplacian smoothing and Delauney triangulation. Commun Appl Numer Methods 4:709–712
Fillinger MF (2007) Who should we operate on and how do we decide: predicting rupture and survival in patients with aortic aneurysm. Semin Vasc Surg 20:121–127
Fillinger MF, Raghavanand ML, Marra SP, Cronenwett J-L, Kennedy FE (2002) In vivo analysis of mechanical wall stress and abdominal aortic aneurysm rupture risk. J Vasc Surg 36:589–597
Fillinger MF, Marra SP, Raghavan ML, Kennedy FE (2003) Prediction of rupture risk in abdominal aortic aneurysm during observation: wall stress versus diameter. J Vasc Surg 37:724–732
Forsell C, Gasser TC, Swedenborg J, Roy J (2012) On the quasi-static damage of the abdominal aortic aneurysm wall at high stresses. Merging histological and mechanical data through a histo-mechanical constitutive model. Submitted
Fratzl P (ed) (2008) Collagen—structure and mechanics. Springer, New York
Fung YC (1993) Biomechanics. Mechanical properties of living tissues, 2nd edn. Springer, New York
Fung YC, Fronek K, Patitucci P (1979) Pseudoelasticity of arteries and the choice of its mathematical expression. Am J Physiol 237:H620–H631
Gasser TC (2011) An irreversible constitutive model for fibrous soft biological tissue: a 3d microfiber approach with demonstrative application to abdominal aortic aneurysms. Acta Biomater 7:2457–2466

Gasser TC (2012) Hard data about AAA. Can we predict the risk of rupture according to AAA morphology? In: CACVS 2012—controversies and updates in vascular surgery, Paris, France, January 19–21, 2012

Gasser TC, Auer M, Labruto F, Swedenborg J, Roy J (2010) Biomechanical rupture risk assessment of abdominal aortic aneurysms. Model complexity versus predictability of finite element simulations. Eur J Vasc Endovasc Surg 40:176–185

Gasser TC, Forsell C (2011) The numerical implementation of invariant-based viscoelastic formulations at finite strains. An anisotropic model for the passive myocardium. Computer methods in applied mechanics and engineering. Comput Methods Appl Mech Eng 200:3637–3645

Gasser TC, Gallinetti S, Xing X, Forsell C, Swedenborg J, Roy J (2012) Spatial orientation of collagen fibers in the abdominal aortic aneurysm wall and its relation to wall mechanics. Submitted

Gasser TC, Görgülü G, Folkesson M, Swedenborg J (2008) Failure properties of intra-luminal thrombus in abdominal aortic aneurysm under static and pulsating mechanical loads. J Vasc Surg 48:179–188

Gasser TC, Holzapfel GA (2002) A rate-independent elastoplastic constitutive model for (biological) fiber-reinforced composites at finite strains: continuum basis, algorithmic formulation and finite element implementation. Comput Mech 29:340–360

Gasser TC, Ogden RW, Holzapfel GA (2006) Hyperelastic modelling of arterial layers with distributed collagen fibre orientations. J R Soc Interface 3:15–35

Giachetti A, Tuveri M, Zanetti G (2003) Reconstruction and web distribution of measurable arterial models. Med Image Anal 7:79–93

Gupta HS, Seto J, Krauss S, Boesecke P, Screen HRC (2010) In situ multi-level analysis of viscoelastic deformation mechanisms in tendon collagen. J Struct Biol 169:1183–1191

Hans SS, Jareunpoon O, Balasubramaniam M, Zelenock GB (2005) Size and location of thrombus in intact and ruptured abdominal aortic aneurysms. J Vasc Surg 41:584–588

Harold SF, Canham PB, Strake J (1981) Orientation of collagen in the tunica adventitia of the human cerebral artery measured with polarized light and the universal stage. J Ultrastruct Res 77:133–145

Haverkamp R, Williams MW, Scott JE (2005) Stretching single molecules of connective tissue glycans to characterize their shape-maintaining elasticity. Biomacromols 6:1816–1818

He CM, Roach MR (1996) The composition and mechanical properties of abdominal aortic aneurysms. J Vasc Surg 20:6–13

Heng MS, Fagan MJ, Collier JW, Desai G, McCollum PT, Chetter IC (2008) Peak wall stress measurement in elective and acute abdominal aortic aneurysms. J Vasc Surg 47:17–22

Holzapfel GA, Gasser TC, Ogden RW (2000) A new constitutive framework for arterial wall mechanics and a comparative study of material models. J Elast 61:1–48

Holzapfel GA, Stadler M, Schulze-Bauer CAJ (2002) A layer-specific three-dimensional model for the simulation of balloon angioplasty using magnetic resonance imaging and mechanical testing. Ann Biomed Eng 30:753–767

Humphrey JD (1995) Mechanics of the arterial wall: review and directions. Crit Rev Biomed Eng 23:1–162

Humphrey JD (2002) Cardiovascular solid mechanics. Cells, tissues, and organs. Springer, New York

Hyhlik-Dürr A, Krieger T, Geisbüsch P, Kotelis D, Able T, Böckler D (2011) Reproducibility of deriving parameters of AAA rupture risk from patient-specific 3d finite element models. J Endovasc Ther 18:289–298

Inzoli F, Boschetti F, Zappa M, Longo T, Fumero R (1993) Biomechanical factors in abdominal aortic aneurysm rupture. Eur J Vasc Surg 7:667–674

Kazi M, Thyberg J, Religa P, Roy J, Eriksson P, Hedin U, Swedenborg J (2003) Influence of intraluminal thrombus on structural and cellular composition of abdominal aortic aneurysm wall. J Vasc Surg 38:1283–1292

Knörzer E, Folkhard W, Geercken W, Boschert C, Koch MH, Hilbert B, Krahl H, Mosler E, Nemetschek-Gansler H, Nemetschek T (1986) New aspects of the etiology of tendon rupture. An analysis of time-resolved dynamic-mechanical measurements using synchrotron radiation. Arch Orthop Trauma Surg 105:113–120

Kotz S, vanDorp JR (2004) Beyond beta: other continuous families of distributions with bounded support. World Scientific, Singapore

Langewouters GJ, Wesseling KH, Goedhard WJA (1984) The static elastic properties of 45 human thoracic and 20 abdominal aortas *in vitro* and the parameters of a new model. J Biomech 17:425–435

Lanir Y (1983) Constitutive equations for fibrous connective tissues. J Biomech 16:1–12

Li Z-Y, U-King-Im J, Tang TY, Soh E, See TC, Gillard JH (2008) Impact of calcification and intraluminal thrombus on the computed wall stresses of abdominal aortic aneurysm. J Vasc Surg 47:928–935

Liao H, Belkoff SM (1999) A failure model for ligaments. J Biomech 32:183–188

Lindeman JHN, Ashcroft BA, Beenakker J-WM, van Es M, Koekkoek NBR, Prins FA, Tielemans JF, Abdul-Hussien H, Bank RA, Oosterkamp TH (2009) Distinct defects in collagen microarchitecture underlie vessel-wall failure in advanced abdominal aneurysms and aneurysms in Marfan syndrome. Proc Natl Acad Sci USA 107:862–865

Lindholt JS, Vammen S, Fasting H, Henneberg EW (2000) Psychological consequences of screening for abdominal aortic aneurysm and conservative treatment of small abdominal aortic aneurysms. Eur J Vasc Endovasc Surg 20:79–83

Lokshin O, Lanir Y (2009) Viscoelasticity and preconditioning of rat skin under uniaxial stretch: microstructural constitutive characterization. J Biomed Eng 131:1031009

Long A, Rouet L, Bissery A, Rossignol P, Mouradian D, Sapoval M (2004) Compliance of abdominal aortic aneurysms: evaluation of tissue Doppler imaging. J Ultrasound Med Biol 30:1099–1108

Lubliner J (1990) Plasticity theory. Macmillan, New York

MacSweeney ST, Young G, Greenhalgh RM, Powell JT (1992) Mechanical properties of the aneurysmal aorta. Br J Surg 79:1281–1284

Maier A, Gee MW, Reeps C, Pongratz J, Eckstein HH, Wall WA (2010) Ia comparison of diameter, wall stress, and rupture potential index for abdominal aortic aneurysm rupture risk prediction. Ann Biomed Eng 38:3124–3134

Martufi G, Gasser TC (2011) A constitutive model for vascular tissue that integrates fibril, fiber and continuum levels. J Biomech 44:2544–2550

Miyazaki H, Hayashi K (1999) Tensile tests of collagen fibers obtained from the rabbit patellar tendon. Biomed Microdevices 2:151–157

Mower WR, Quiñones WJ, Gambhir SS (1997) Effect of intraluminal thrombus on abdominal aortic aneurysm wall stress. J Vasc Surg 33:602–608

Nicholls SC, Gardner JB, Meissner MH, Johansen HK (1998) Rupture in small abdominal aortic aneurysms. J Vasc Surg 28:884–888

Oden JT, Reddy JN (1976) Variational methods in theoretical mechanics. Springer, Heidelberg

Ogden RW (1997) Non-linear elastic deformations. Dover, New York

Oktay HS, Kang T, Humphrey JD, Bishop GG (1991) Changes in the mechanical behavior of arteries following balloon angioplasty. In: ASME 1991 biomechanics symposium, AMD, vol 120. Am Soc Mech Eng, New York

Olabarriaga SD, Rouet JM, Fradkin M, Breeuwer M, Niessen WJ (2005) Segmentation of thrombus in abdominal aortic aneurysms from CTA with nonparametric statistical grey level appearance modeling. IEEE Trans Med Imaging 24:477–485

Parry DAD, Barnes GRG, Craig AS (1978) A comparison of the size distribution of collagen fibrils in connective tissues as a function of age and a possible relation between fibril size distribution and mechanical properties. Proc R Soc Lond B 203:305–321

Pena J, Martínez MA, Pena E (2011) A formulation to model the nonlinear viscoelastic properties of the vascular tissue. Acta Mech 217:63–74

Polzer S, Gasser TC, Markert B, Bursa J, Skacel P (2012) Impact of poroelasticity of the intraluminal thrombus on the wall stress of abdominal aortic aneurysms. Submitted
Quinn KP, Winkelstein BA (2008) Altered collagen fiber kinematics define the onset of localized ligament damage during loading. J Appl Physiol 105:1881–1888
Raghavan ML, Vorp DA (2000) Toward a biomechanical tool to evaluate rupture potential of abdominal aortic aneurysm: identification of a finite strain constitutive model and evaluation of its applicability. J Biomech 33:475–482
Raghavan ML, Fillinger MF, Marra SP, Naegelein BP, Kennedy FE (2005) Automated methodology for determination of stress distribution in human abdominal aortic aneurysm. J Biomech Eng 127:868–871
Raghavan ML, Kratzberg J, Castro de Tolosa E, Hanaoka M, Walker P, da Silva E (2006) Regional distribution of wall thickness and failure properties of human abdominal aortic aneurysm. J Biomech 39:3010–3016
Ridge MD, Wright V (1967) Mechanical properties of skin: a bioengineering study of skin structure. J Appl Physiol 21:1602–1606
Roach MR, Burton AC (1957) The reason for the shape of the distensibility curve of arteries. Can J Biochem Physiol 35:681–690
Sack J-R, Urrutia J (eds) (2000) Handbook of computational geometry. Elsevier, Amsterdam
Salunke NV, Topoleski LDT (1997) Biomechanics of atherosclerotic plaque. Crit Rev Biomed Eng 25:243–285
Scott JE (2003) Elasticity in extracellular matrix 'shape modules' of tendon, cartilage, etc. A sliding proteoglycan-filament model. J Physiol 553:335–343
Scott JE (2008) Cartilage is held together by elastic glycan strings. Physiological and pathological implications. Biorheology 45:209–217
Shen ZL, Dodge MR, Kahn H, Ballarini R, Eppell SJ (2008) Stress-strain experiments on individual collagen fibrils. Biophys J 95:3956–3963
Silver FH, Freeman JW, Seehra GP (2003) Collagen self-assembly and the development of tendon mechanical properties. J Biomech 36:1529–1553
Simo JC, Hughes TJR (1998) Computational inelasticity. Springer, New York
Simo JC, Taylor RL (1991) Quasi-incompressible finite elasticity in principal stretches. Continuum basis and numerical algorithms. Comput Methods Appl Mech Eng 85:273–310
Sokolis DP (2007) Passive mechanical properties and structure of the aorta: segmental analysis. Acta Physiol 190:277–289
Staten ML, Owen SJ, Blacker TD (2005) Unconstrained paving & plastering: a new idea for all hexahedral mesh generation. In: Proc. 14th int meshing roundtable, pp 400–416
Subasic M, Loncaric S, Sorantin E (2002) 3-D image analysis of abdominal aortic aneurysm. Proc SPIE Int Soc Opt Eng 4684:1681–1689
Sverdlik A, Lanir Y (2002) Time-dependent mechanical behavior of sheep digital tendons, including the effects of preconditioning. J Biomech Eng (in press)
Takamizawa K, Hayashi K (1987) Strain energy density function and uniform strain hypothesis for arterial mechanics. J Biomech 20:7–17
Tautges TJ, Blacker T, Mitchell SA (1996) The whisker weaving algorithm: a connectivity-based method for constructing all–hexahedral finite element meshes. In: Proc. 4th int meshing roundtable, Sandia National Laboratories
Taylor CA, Humphrey JD (2009) Open problems in computational vascular biomechanics: hemodynamics and arterial wall mechanics. Comput Methods Appl Mech Eng 198:3514–3523
The UK Small Aneurysm Trial Participants (1998) Mortality results for randomised controlled trial of early elective surgery or ultrasonographic surveillance for small abdominal aortic aneurysms. Lancet 352:1649–1655
Truijers M, Pol JA, Schultzekool LJ, van Sterkenburg SM, Fillinger MF, Blankensteijn JD (2007) Wall stress analysis in small asymptomatic, symptomatic and ruptured abdominal aortic aneurysms. Eur J Vasc Endovasc Surg 33:401–407
Vaishnav RN, Young JT, Janicki JS, Patel DJ (1972) Nonlinear anisotropic elastic properties of the canine aorta. Biophys J 12:1008–1027

van Dam EA, Dams SD, Peters GWM, Rutten MCM, Schurink GWH, Buth J, van de Vosse FN (2007) Non-linear viscoelastic behavior of abdominal aortic aneurysm thrombus. Biomech Model Mechanobiol 7:127–137

Vande Geest JP, Sacks MS, Vorp DA (2006a) The effects of aneurysm on the biaxial mechanical behavior of human abdominal aorta. J Biomech 39(7):1324–1334

Vande Geest JP, Sacks MS, Vorp DA (2006b) A planar biaxial constitutive relation for the luminal layer of intra-luminal thrombus in abdominal aortic aneurysms. J Biomech 39:2347–2354

Vande Geest JP, Wang DHJ, Wisniewski SR, Makaroun MS, Vorp DA (2006c) Towards a noninvasive method for determination of patient-specific wall strength distribution in abdominal aortic aneurysms. Ann Biomed Eng 34:1098–1106

Venkatasubramaniam AK, Fagan MJ, Mehta T, Mylankal KJ, Ray B, Kuhan G, Chetter IC, McCollum PT (2004) A comparative study of aortic wall stress using finite element analysis for ruptured and non-ruptured abdominal aortic aneurysms. Eur J Vasc Surg 28:168–176

Vidal BC, Mello MLS, Pimentel ER (1982) Polarization microscopy and microspectrophotometry of sirius red, picrosirius and chlorantine fast red aggregates and of their complexes with collagen. Histochem J 14:857–878

Vorp DA, Mandarino WA, Webster MW, Gorcsan J (1996) Potential influence of intraluminal thrombus on abdominal aortic aneurysm as assessed by a new non-invasive method. Cardiovasc Surg 4:732–739

Wang DH, Makaroun MS, Webster MW, Vorp DA (2001) Mechanical properties and microstructure of intraluminal thrombus from abdominal aortic aneurysm. J Biomech Eng 123:536–539

Wang DH, Makaroun MS, Webster MW, Vorp DA (2002) Effect of intraluminal thrombus on wall stress in patient-specific models of abdominal aortic aneurysm. J Vasc Surg 36:598–604

Weber KT, Pick R, Silver MA, Moe GW, Janicki JS, Zucker IH, Armstrong PW (1990) Fibrillar collagen and remodeling of dilated canine left ventricle. Circulation 82:1387–1401

Wriggers P (2008) Nonlinear finite element methods. Springer, Berlin

Wuyts FL, Vanhuyse VJ, Langewouters GJ, Decraemer WF, Raman ER, Buyle S (1995) Elastic properties of human aortas in relation to age and atherosclerosis: a structural model. Phys Med Biol 40:1577–1597

Zienkiewicz OC, Taylor RL (2000a) The finite element method, vol 1: The basis, 5th edn. Butterworth Heinemann, Oxford

Zienkiewicz OC, Taylor RL (2000b) The finite element method, vol 2: Solid mechanics, 5th edn. Butterworth Heinemann, Oxford

Zienkiewicz OC, Taylor RL (2000c) The finite element method, vol 3: Fluid dynamics, 5th edn. Butterworth Heinemann, Oxford

Zulliger MA, Fridez P, Hayashi K, Stergiopulos N (2004) A strain energy function for arteries accounting for wall composition and structure. J Biomech 37:989–1000

Chapter 2
A Subject-Specific Framework to Inform Musculoskeletal Modeling: Outcomes from the IUPS Physiome Project

J. Fernandez, P. Hunter, V. Shim, and K. Mithraratne

Abstract The International Union of Physiological Sciences (IUPS) Physiome Project was established as a framework for creation, sharing and dissemination of multiscale mathematical models of human physiology. We present a suite of subject-specific musculoskeletal models that were developed using this framework. This process starts with subject-specific geometry development using high-order cubic Hermite elements suitable for describing the topology of complex musculoskeletal structures accurately. These geometries are able to be customized using free-form deformation techniques with data from Computed Tomography (CT), Magnetic Resonance Imaging (MRI) or anthropometric information derived from motion capture. We describe how the deformations of soft tissues are referred to a microstructural curvilinear coordinate system. The constitutive laws that describe the stress-strain behavior of soft tissue are also referred to this anatomically based material coordinate system. Finally, we highlight the finite deformation mechanics framework through a set of clinically relevant examples. These examples include the efficient creation of a subject's hip model from CT for implant testing with validation; customization of bone and muscle geometry; a hybrid free-form deformation and mechanics method for assessing gait; coupled blood flow and solid deformation of the lower limb to examine the influence of deep vein thrombosis and patellofemoral joint contact pressure following a vastus release and tibial medialization.

We also examine the recent focus on multiscale approaches and how this integrates with subject-specific musculoskeletal modeling. The Physiome Project is a computational framework for understanding human physiology by integrating computational models at all levels of biological organization. Recent developments in multiscale modeling have made use of the markup languages, ontologies, databases and software tools, developed as part of the Physiome Project. Using these markup languages, including AnatML, FieldML and CellML, we are able to take unique subject-specific information at the whole organ level, which informs micro level

J. Fernandez (✉) · P. Hunter · V. Shim · K. Mithraratne
Auckland Bioengineering Institute, The University of Auckland, 70 Symonds Street, Auckland 1010, New Zealand
e-mail: j.fernandez@auckland.ac.nz

B. Calvo, E. Peña (eds.), *Patient-Specific Computational Modeling*, Lecture Notes in Computational Vision and Biomechanics 5,
DOI 10.1007/978-94-007-4552-0_2, © Springer Science+Business Media Dordrecht 2012

models and in turn initiates cell level remodeling. The cell level information is then passed up the model hierarchy to inform change in micro level architecture and modification of material behavior at the macro level. We illustrate this multiscale approach by presenting a model of the knee joint to explore a possible pathway to osteoarthritis. This is initiated by abnormal loads at the whole knee coupled with a micro model of the cartilage-bone interface, which is linked to both cartilage and bone cell remodeling.

2.1 Challenges in Modeling

The challenges faced in subject-specific modeling are similar in all organ systems. In this chapter we focus on musculoskeletal modeling, which has strong links with orthopedics and physiotherapy where patient-based treatment is increasingly being sought in clinical practice. Some of these modeling challenges include: (i) how to model the anatomy and tissue structure efficiently and in a 'patient-specific' manner; (ii) how to define constitutive laws (stress-strain behavior) that capture experimentally observed mechanical behavior and are not over-parameterized; (iii) how to link the constitutive parameters to underlying tissue micro-structure such as the unique fiber distributions within different muscles and within individuals; (iv) how to couple the equations of large deformation mechanics to the equations representing other physical processes such as blood flow in the lower limb; (v) and how to link the spatial scales to inform tissue level behavior from cell processes such as active muscle contraction and tissue remodeling, which is specific to different disease states, age groups and can account for 'patient-specific' treatments. Figure 2.1 depicts the modeling approach adopted in this chapter whereby a subset of geometries is derived from a database; microstructural information such as fiber fields are described within soft tissues; geometries are customized to individual profiles; macro level solid mechanics analysis is performed; solid stress from various activities is coupled to fluid flows; and the macro level solutions are used as boundary conditions for micro level models.

2.2 Geometry Development

One goal of the IUPS Physiome project (Hunter, 2004) was to develop a database of anatomically-based geometries as the first step in computational mechanics. Figure 2.2 shows how this database was developed from a number of sources including an anatomical skeleton model (SOMSO, www.somso.de), scanned using a Polhemus laser scanner and the soft tissues digitized from the Visible Man (VM) (Ackerman, 1998). The Somso skeleton allowed for accurate depiction of the complex joint articular surfaces at the end of the bones and attachment points, while the VM high resolution images provided information about the detailed three-dimensional relationships between muscles, tendons, ligaments and other organs.

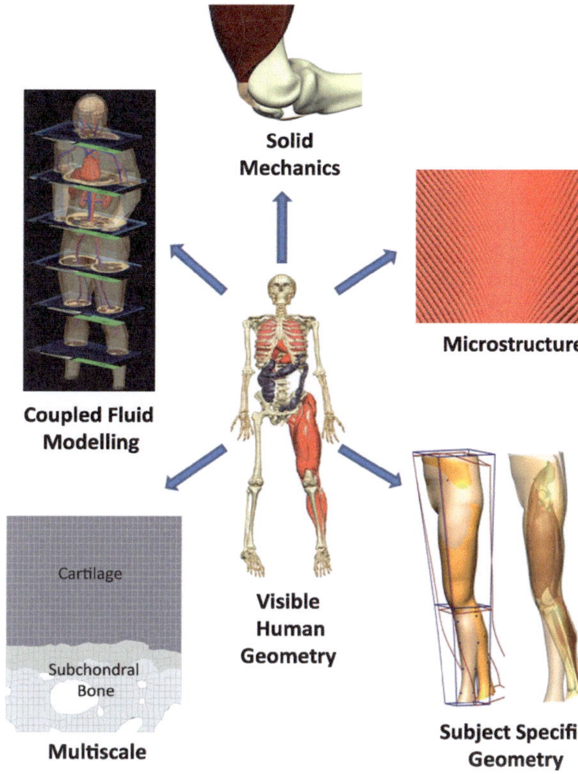

Fig. 2.1 Modeling framework used to simulate the musculoskeletal system. A database of generic geometries is developed from the Visible Human dataset; free-form deformation methods are used to customize the models using subject-specific data; microstructural material information is obtained from imaging and experiment; solid mechanics simulations predict spatial stress and strain in response to physiologically-based boundary conditions; whole organ models are mapped to micro mechanics using multiscale methods; and embedded vessel networks coupled to solid mechanics are used to predict fluid flows

These were collected in a supine reference pose as this was the position the data were imaged. Over the last 10 years additional images have been collected from the Visible Female (Spitzer et al., 1995) which is sliced at every 0.33 mm (as opposed to 1 mm for the VM) providing greater detail around the knee joint region where structures like the menisci and cartilage are typically a few millimeters thick. Additional imaging modalities have also been used including Magnetic Resonance Imaging (MRI) and Computed Tomography (CT) to add to the growing collection of data. The additional modalities offer further benefits by allowing customization of generic models and validation of model mechanics by comparison with Tagged MRI, dynamic X-ray (fluoroscopy) and dynamic ultrasound. The geometries are being collected into hierarchical modeling ontologies (Hunter and Borg, 2003) to facilitate data exchange among scientists contributing to the Physiome Project. The collected datasets utilize AnatML (www.physiome.org.nz/anatml_viewer), a markup language describing the linkages between the different structures using definitions from Grey's anatomy (Gray, 2008) and Anatomica (FCAT, 2011).

Once the raw segmented data is acquired, a set of 3D parameterized FE meshes suitable for mechanics are developed. The three-dimensional FE meshes have basis (or shape) functions determined from the tensor product of 1D interpolation func-

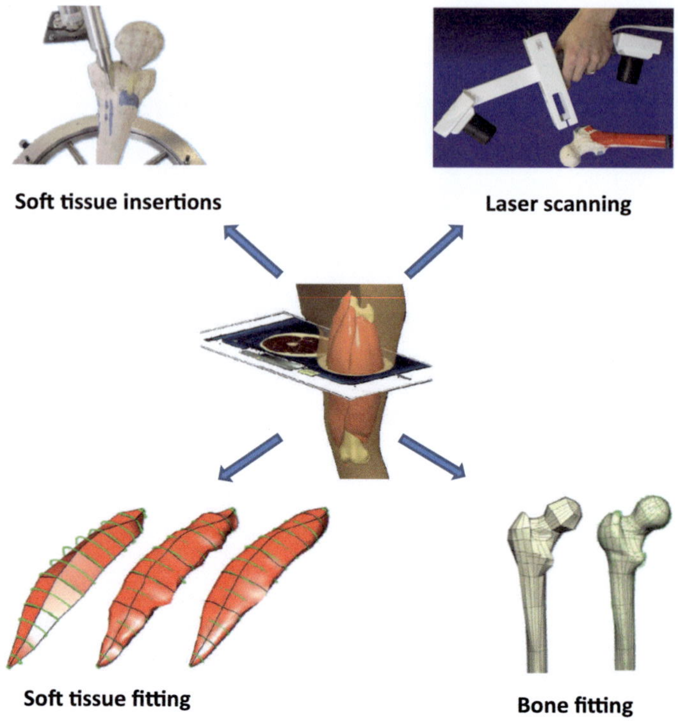

Fig. 2.2 A subset of the lower limb model derived from the Visible Man dataset with bone geometry and soft tissue insertions from a physical Somso model. The process of fitting the rectus femoris (quadriceps) muscle and femur (thigh) bone to data is illustrated

tions. These four 1D cubic Hermite basis functions are given by

$$\begin{aligned} \Psi_1^0(\xi) &= 1 - 3\xi^2 + 2\xi^3; \qquad \Psi_2^0(\xi) = \xi^2(3 - 2\xi); \\ \Psi_1^1(\xi) &= \xi(\xi - 1)^2; \qquad \Psi_2^1(\xi) = \xi^2(\xi - 1), \end{aligned} \tag{2.1}$$

where ξ is the normalized local or element coordinate which is defined from 0 to 1. These cubic Hermite elements differ from the usual Lagrange family finite elements in that they preserve both the continuity of the nodal values (C^0 continuity), and their first derivatives (C^1 continuity). This provides many advantages in constructing a finite element geometry, particularly of biological structures such as muscles and other organs that typically have smooth surfaces (Wriggers et al., 2001). Moreover, the realistic geometries are useful in such applications as virtual surgery and medical education. Another attractive feature of cubic Hermite elements is that fewer numbers of elements are required for complex geometries. C^1-continuous interpolation also provides a smooth change in the surface normal across element boundaries and this provides numerical benefits when solving contact mechanics problem. Interpolation of the spatial coordinates of line elements in space with cubic Hermite basis functions is given by

$$u(\xi) = \Psi_1^0(\xi)u_1 + \Psi_2^0(\xi)u_2 + \Psi_1^1(\xi).\frac{du}{ds}\bigg|_1 L + \Psi_2^1(\xi).\frac{du}{ds}\bigg|_2 L, \tag{2.2}$$

where u is x, y or z if the field is geometry and du/ds is the derivative of the spatial coordinate with respect to a measure of distance, chosen to be arc-length here. Subscripts 1 and 2 refer to node numbers and superscripts 0 and 1 are the zeroth and first derivatives, respectively. L is the physical arc length along the curve. To ensure we have continuity with respect to arc-length we enforce the condition that the magnitude of du/ds should be 1. The interpolation can be any field in general such as stress, temperature or fiber information and more details can be found in Fernandez et al. (2004).

Now that we have established the element primitive we fit the elements to segmented data using a least-squares fitting procedure. We employ a face fitting routine for surfaces of the volume mesh and define a face objective function, $F(u_n)$, consisting of two components, namely the data error and a smoothing constraint given by

$$F(u_n) = \sum_{d=1}^{N} w_d \left\| u(\xi_{1d}, \xi_{2d}) - z_d \right\|^2 + F_s(u_n), \tag{2.3}$$

where the data error is the summation of the square of the distances between each data point, z_d, and its orthogonal projection $u(\xi_{1d}, \xi_{2d})$ on the relevant face. Each point can be weighted based on importance using w_d. The smoothing constraint, $F_s(u_n)$, is appended to the objective function as a penalty function defined by

$$\begin{aligned} F_s(u_n) = \int_0^1 \int_0^1 \Bigg\{ & \alpha_1 \left\| \frac{\partial u}{\partial \xi_1} \right\|^2 + \alpha_2 \left\| \frac{\partial u}{\partial \xi_2} \right\|^2 + \alpha_3 \left\| \frac{\partial^2 u}{\partial \xi_1^2} \right\|^2 + \alpha_4 \left\| \frac{\partial^2 u}{\partial \xi_2^2} \right\|^2 \\ & + \alpha_5 \left\| \frac{\partial^2 u}{\partial \xi_1 \partial \xi_2} \right\|^2 \Bigg\} d\xi_1 d\xi_2, \end{aligned} \tag{2.4}$$

which is the second order Sobolev norm (Bradley et al., 1997) used as the smoothing constraint to account for sparse and scattered data. Constants α_i $(i = 1, \ldots, 5)$ are the Sobolev weights (penalty parameters) and each term has a distinct effect on the final shape of the fitted object. The first two terms (α_1, α_2) control the arc-length, while the third and fourth terms (α_3, α_4) control the arc-curvature in the ξ_1 and ξ_2 directions, respectively. The last term (α_5) represents the face area. For instance, if the weight associated with the cross-derivative term is set to a relatively higher value, one might end up with a smaller face area. All Sobolev weights must be at least an order lower than the weight associated with the data error component, w_d, which is usually taken as 1.0.

We highlight two examples of model fitting depicted in Fig. 2.2. If the data set is sparse, such as shown with the rectus femoris muscle (one of the quadriceps) and if the Sobolev weights are all set to have minimal effect then the fitting will produce an oscillatory shape in the muscle. This is an artifact arising from the data being dense in the radial direction but sparse in the longitudinal direction. If, however, we place more weight on the curvature in the longitudinal direction and increase smoothing on the face area we arrive at a more anatomically correct shape. This shows that the Sobolev weights can account for incomplete or non-uniform data sets. In the second example we have a bone to fit (the femur) with a uniform and dense cloud of data from a scanned source. There is usually less need to increase Sobolev smoothing parameters in such a case as the data is sufficient and homogeneously distributed for an accurate fit. However, if we want to place more emphasis on a particular region such as the greater and lesser trochanters then we can increase the data point weights for those features. The fitting algorithm will then ensure a better fit in those regions.

2.3 Combining Sparse Data Sets

Situations may arise when only a limited amount of geometric data is available, such as when the knee is imaged using MRI but we want a whole limb model. Another situation, which may limit data availability, is when excessive imaging is undesirable such as when ionizing radiation from CT is involved. Subject specific finite element models require a complete dataset and therefore a new method of supplementing patient CT images with images from the Visible Human CT was developed (Shim et al., 2007). This method uses the previously described cubic Hermite elements and least squares fitting procedures. Figure 2.3 outlines the method starting with dividing the patient CT and Visible Human CT into the same number of anatomically defined regions. Second, within each region we transformed slices from the Visible Human CT slice to the patient CT slice using landmarks at the beginning and end of each region. Third, we selected a minimal number of slices within each region of the Visible Human CT to transform and fill the gaps in the patient CT set. It was found that with only 12 CT slices we were able to generate smooth and accurate meshes of the proximal femur with a geometric root mean square (RMS) error of less than 1 mm and peak errors less than 8 mm. We tested this method on three patient data sets, generating FE meshes of the pelvis using only 10 CT slices with an overall RMS error less than 3 mm. Considering that linear meshes usually require about 70–100 pelvic CT slices (in axial mode) to generate FE models, our method has brought a significant data reduction to the automatic mesh generation step.

Using this technique we validated the resulting finite element model developed from hybrid CT data with mechanical experiments (Shim et al., 2008) as shown in Fig. 2.4. Three cadaveric embalmed pelvises were strain gauged and FE models were generated from the CT scans. Material properties for cancellous bone were obtained from the CT scans and assigned to the FE mesh using a spatially varying field embedded inside the mesh while the mechanical characteristics of other materials used in the model were obtained from the literature. For each pelvis, five different

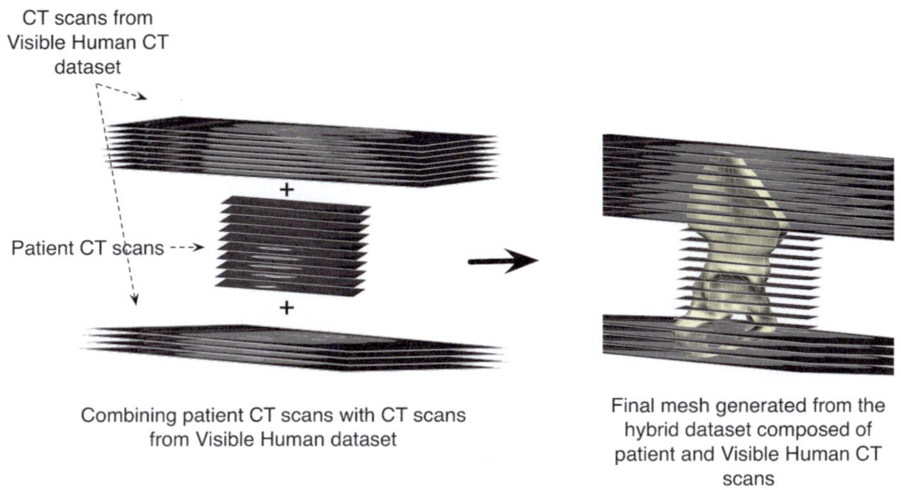

Fig. 2.3 A finite element mesh of the pelvis developed from a hybrid CT dataset comprising both patient and visible human data

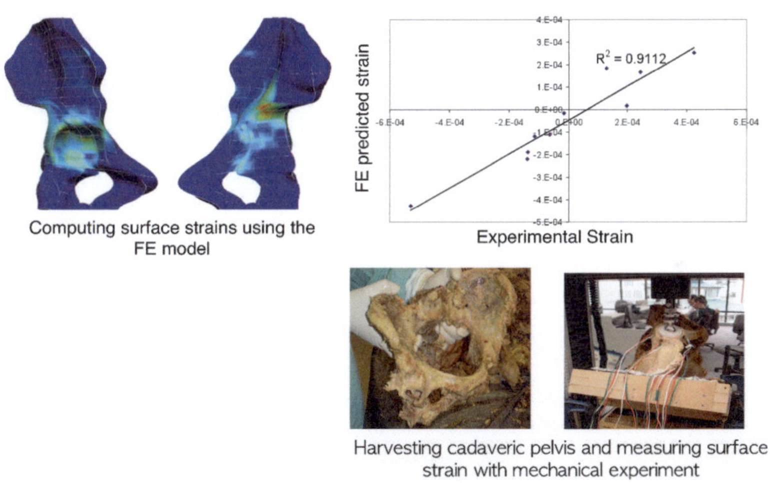

Fig. 2.4 Experimental setup of the pelvic validation trial for the hybrid finite element model. Shown are the FE surface strains, mechanical rig and comparison between experimental and predicted strain

FE meshes with a varying number of patient CT slices (8–12) were generated to determine how many patient CT slices were needed for good accuracy. All five mesh types showed good agreement between the model and experimental strains with an R^2 of 0.9. Meshes generated with incomplete data sets showed very similar stress distributions to those obtained from the FE mesh generated with complete data sets.

2.4 Subject-Specific Customization

A database of geometries is extremely useful for sharing and disseminating models amongst the scientific community, especially using the popular Visible Human dataset. They can be used to study population-based mechanics primarily in healthy individuals. However, when studying diseased joints, pathology leading to deformed geometry (such as cerebral palsy) or for focused studies aimed at predicting the outcomes of intervention a subject-specific geometry is required. The original database of geometries serves as a good basis to morph and fit to patient data obtained from MRI, CT or motion capture. We utilize a technique, based on free-form, to rapidly morph complex geometries using only a few control points (Fernandez et al., 2005).

The "host-mesh" fitting method described below is a free-form deformation technique used to perform geometric transformations consisting of both Euclidean (translation and rotation) and Affine (Euclidean plus scaling and shearing) operations on arbitrary parameterized meshes. The structure of the host mesh is a parallelepiped in these examples, but can in general be any shape. The size of the host mesh is determined from experience, however, as a general rule it should be close to the size of the object being deformed and the number of degrees freedom of the host mesh depends on the control the user wishes to have over the deformation and object anatomy. The object being morphed is embedded within the host and when the host is morphed the object within it also undergoes the same transformation. For most cases one to three-element host meshes will suffice to provide enough degrees of freedom to control its deformation. We demonstrate this method in a couple of scenarios shown in Fig. 2.5 including changing the articular features of femoral bone, changing the attachments of ligaments and morphing the rectus femoris muscle.

The host-mesh technique permits morphing of anatomical geometries given a limited number of data points. This is most useful where only a limited data set is available, such as a partial MRI or CT, or only discrete measures can be obtained (such as motion capture). The quality of fit can be controlled through weighting the data points (placing more weight on important regions) or through constraining the host that the body lies within. A useful illustration is the femur, which is known to vary between patients and is influenced by gender (with females having a wider quadriceps angle) and pathology (such as children with cerebral palsy with highly curved femurs). When performing finite element analyses the resulting stress distribution is influenced by the geometric profile and so obtaining a quick fit is desirable when performing large population studies. In this case 24 landmark points were identified from a CT-scanned femur but could also be obtained from other modalities. Each data point represents a distinct extremity such as a peak or groove in the bone. The host was divided into 3 segments (elements) for separate control of the shaft, proximal and distal ends. Greater freedom was allowed for the femur ends while the shaft, which had limited data available, was allowed only to radially expand, twist and lengthen. The blue markers indicate the landmark points and the red markers show their desired final positions. The undeformed host (blue) was distorted to the red host in order to minimize the distance between the blue and red markers in a weighted least squares sense. The fitting procedure used to distort

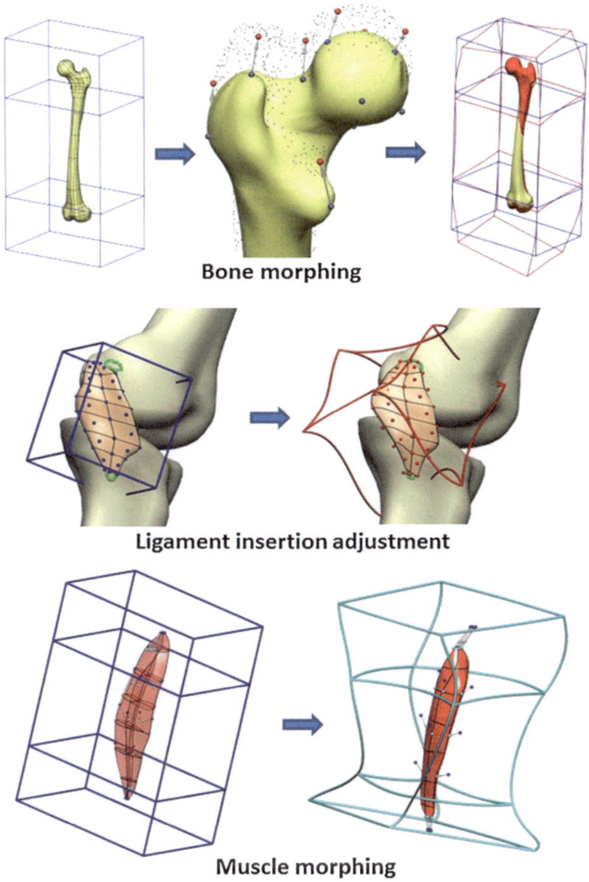

Fig. 2.5 Host-mesh customization of the femur (*top*), medial collateral ligament insertion (*middle*) and rectus femoris muscle (*bottom*)

the mesh in order to minimize the data error is identical to that described in (2.3) and (2.4) for fitting.

The host mesh can also be used to adjust small features while maintaining the remaining geometric shape. Ligament attachments vary between patients, as observed in MRI, and can be modified due to surgery to correct pathology. Illustrated in Fig. 2.5 is a new ligament attachment specified by green markers on the femur. The medial collateral ligament was morphed so as to match the insertion into the femur while maintaining the original ligament origin at the tibia. In this example only a sparse set of data existed (the insertion points), so we increased the Sobolev smoothing to assist the fit by placing weights on the host-mesh curvature. This ensured that the new ligament was not distorted.

Soft tissues can come in a variety of deformed poses and shape depending on the orientation the subject is imaged. While muscles typically have textbook profiles defined based on cadaveric studies it may be useful to rapidly customize a generic muscle to another subject. Here we have chosen an extreme example whereby the generic rectus femoris muscle (one of the quadriceps) derived from the Visible Male is customized to a subset of points taken from the Visible Female dataset. Muscle size is useful because it affects the force generation capacity in computation. We identified a set of landmarks at the ends of the muscle and radially along the length of the axis (a total of 20 points). The same sites were located on the female muscle set using Visible Female images and we performed the fit to minimize the distance between the marker sets. The resulting mesh closely resembled the female muscle and to check we performed a least squares fit against the fully segmented female muscle giving an RMS of less than 3 mm.

2.5 Mechanics

Once we have the desired geometry we aim to predict the finite deformation given a material property description and boundary conditions (Nash and Hunter, 2000). Modeling mechanics is presented in the context of the patellar joint, which is further elaborated in Sect. 2.8 with applications. Figure 2.6 shows the first step, which is to identify the muscle shapes and fiber orientations in the quadriceps. This may be done using Diffusion Tensor Imaging or Ultrasound. For this work we participated in a complete cadaver dissection to learn about muscle anatomy, ligament and tendon insertions and surface fiber orientations. The muscles were photographed and a mapping of surface fiber orientation was extruded through the muscle volume. This was fitted as finite element field information and is shown for the rectus femoris muscle (with bi-pennation angle).This was repeated for all the quadriceps and hamstring muscles. This process draws on the fitting procedures described in Sect. 2.2.

Second, we solved for soft tissue deformation due to muscle contraction in the complete patellar complex. The virtual work statement for the problem at hand in the absence of body forces can be written as

$$\int_{V_0} \frac{1}{J} T^{\alpha\beta} F_\beta^j \frac{\partial \delta u_j}{\partial \upsilon_\alpha} dV_0 = \int_{S_c} f_c \delta u_j^c dS_c, \tag{2.5}$$

since the muscles were undergoing large deformation (greater than 10 % strain). V_0 is the undeformed volume and S_c is the surface in contact used to account for the interaction between muscles and between the patella cartilage and femoral condyles. δu_j is the virtual displacement, δu_j^c is the variation of the contact gap and $F_\beta^j = \partial x_j / \partial \upsilon_\beta$ is the deformation gradient tensor which maps between the deformed spatial coordinates x_j, and material coordinates, υ_β. The Jacobian, J, is the determinant of the deformation gradient tensor, F and f_c is the frictionless contact force, which is implemented using a penalty based method with the complete details described in Fernandez and Hunter (2005). $T^{\alpha\beta}$ is the 2nd Piola-Kirchoff stress tensor,

$$T^{\alpha\beta} = \frac{\partial W}{\partial E_{\alpha\beta}} + pa_\upsilon^{\alpha\beta} + T_0 \delta_1^\alpha \delta_1^\beta, \tag{2.6}$$

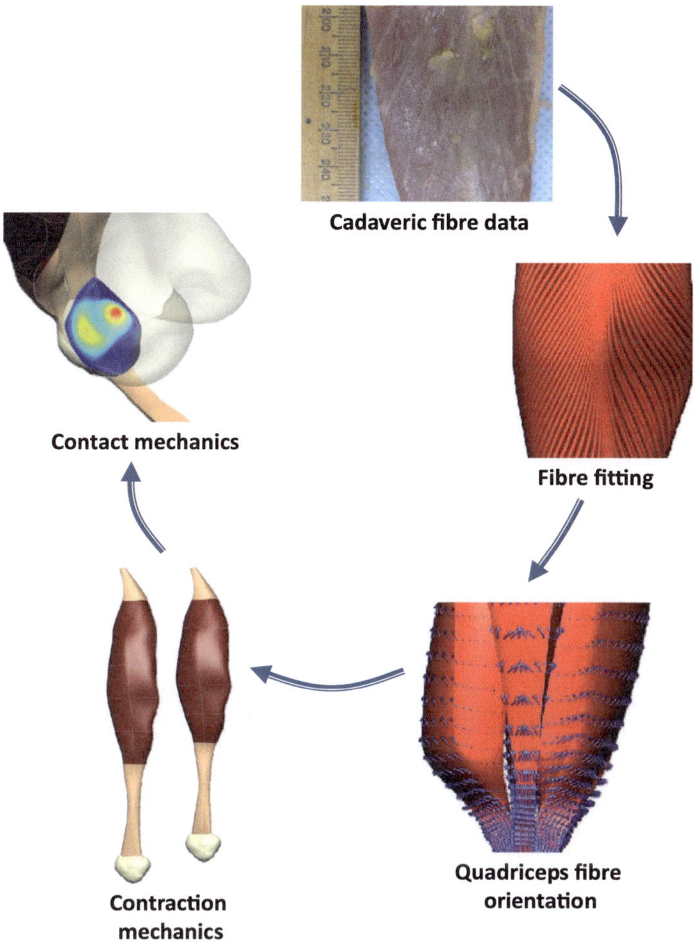

Fig. 2.6 Mechanics framework for the patellofemoral joint starting with a representation of fiber information from a cadaver, which is described as a field within a finite element mesh and repeated for the full set of quadriceps muscles. A muscle contraction is simulated, which shortens the muscle and pulls on the patella and the resulting patellar cartilage contact stress is predicted

and defined with respect to the undeformed curvilinear material coordinate system, ν_α. W is a strain energy density function and $E_{\alpha\beta}$ are the Green-Lagrange strain components. The hydrostatic pressure, p, arises in order to satisfy volume conservation and T_0 is the second Piola Kirchoff equivalent of the Cauchy active stress (muscle contraction). The contravariant metric tensor $a_\upsilon^{\alpha\beta} = \partial\upsilon_\alpha/\partial x_k.\ \partial\upsilon_\beta/\partial x_k$ is the inverse of the right Cauchy deformation tensor (covariant metric tensor).

We have used a number of constitutive laws depending on the availability of experimental data and modeling assumptions. A 'St-Venant Kirchoff' strain energy density function, a particular case of hyperelastic materials for a homogeneous isotropic material, was used for bone and cartilage, and for tendon we adopted a transversely isotropic version of the well-known Mooney Rivlen material (Rivlin, 1948) with information derived from the literature. With muscle, however, we have available a number of instruments to perform muscle experiments and so have adopted a micro-structurally based constitutive law, the 'pole-zero' law (Hunter, 1995) for passive muscle,

$$W = k_{\alpha\beta} \frac{E_{\alpha\beta}^2}{|a_{\alpha\beta} - E_{\alpha\beta}|^{b_{\alpha\beta}}}, \tag{2.7}$$

where W is a strain energy density function, $E_{\alpha\beta}$ are Green's strain components referred to a microstructural fiber axis, $a_{\alpha\beta}$ are the strain limits (poles) and $k_{\alpha\beta}$, $b_{\alpha\beta}$ are the scaling and curvature control parameters, respectively.

Those models that include some form of active muscle behavior have been based on one of three approaches: (i) rheological models based upon Hill-type relationships (Hill, 1938) and have been shown to be more reliable in predicting forces and comparing with experiments; (ii) models employing physiological reasoning and 'cross-bridge' kinetics via Huxley-based models (Huxley, 1957); (iii) the final group is a recent addition and links the macro and micro scales by having low-order variable models of the whole muscle via approximations of the 'cross-bridge' theory maintaining biophysically meaningful variables. Examples include the 'distribution moment' model by Zahalak (2000) and the HMT model of Hunter et al. (1998). Here we used the model of Hunter and add a contractile force in the fiber direction to simulate muscle action given by

$$\sigma_0(\lambda, \mathrm{Ca}_{actn}) = \frac{(\mathrm{Ca}_{actn}.[\mathrm{Ca}^{2+}]_{\max})^h}{(\mathrm{Ca}_{actn}.[\mathrm{Ca}^{2+}]_{\max})^h + (c_{50})^h} \sigma_{ref}\big[1 + \beta(\lambda - 1)\big], \tag{2.8}$$

where σ_0 is the active tension added to the fiber direction and given by the calcium-tension derived from the 'fading-memory' model, which is based on the hill type model (Hunter, 1995). Ca_{actn} is the level of activation (non-dimensional calcium value), λ is the sarcomere stretch length, $[\mathrm{Ca}^{2+}]_{\max}$ is the intracellular calcium concentration for maximum activation, c_{50} is the concentration at which isometric tension is 50 % of its maximum, h is the hill coefficient, T_{ref} is the active isometric tension when $\lambda = 1$ and β is the slope parameter.

The model was driven by a combination of patellofemoral kinematics (derived from motion capture) and simulated muscle contraction, which shortens the muscle and pulls on the patella via the tendon resulting in patellar cartilage contact stress. The model was solved as a series of quasi-static steps.

2.6 Coupling Mechanics and Free-Form Deformation

The free-form deformation (FFD) technique (host-mesh fitting) is a useful tool for customization and rapidly transforming body shapes into different poses. This has the benefit of being able to compute muscle length change given only kinematics

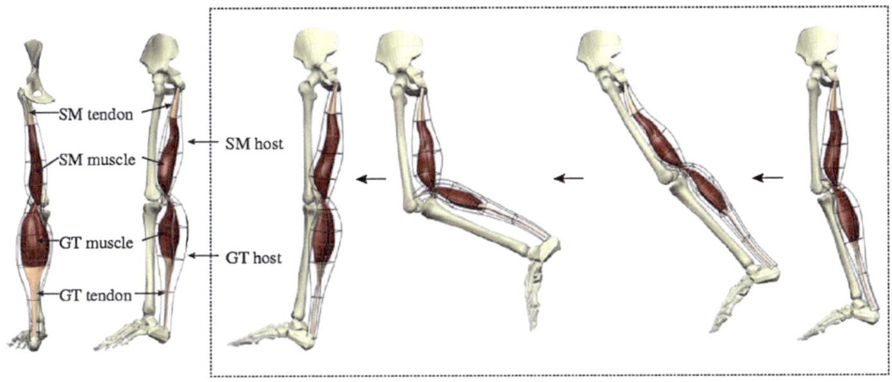

Fig. 2.7 Hybrid host-mesh mechanics of the semimembranosus and semitendinosus muscles during gait

from sources such as motion capture and X-ray fluoroscopy. However, while efficient it does not take into account the wrapping of muscle around bones and other muscles, or the different lengthening of tendon and muscle due to material stiffness. We have coupled the original FFD method with the mechanics framework previously established to solve mechanics on a coarse representation of a muscle (a host-mesh), which in turn passes on this deformation to the detailed muscle inside (Fernandez et al., 2005). In this way different regions of the muscle will undergo varying degrees of deformation providing physiologically accurate shapes. If the host mesh is close to the actual embedded muscle then the volume of the muscle is also preserved. More importantly, the muscles inside will interact with other surrounding tissues and so account for sliding between muscles and with bone.

The deformed lower limb bones and stance of cerebral palsy (CP) children fully utilize the subject-specific customization tools as the new bone shapes are substantially different in profile to a healthy generic model. First, we customize the geometry to the patient including the complete muscle bundle. Figure 2.7 highlights the technique for the hamstrings (semimembranosus, semitendinosus) and the gastrocnemius as these muscles are typically lengthened by surgeons and cross the knee joint. We then collect motion capture data from both a healthy control and CP patient. A host mesh similar in shape and size is placed around each muscle and material properties are assigned based on the location of tendon and the muscle belly. Computed kinematics are used to drive the model and change the location of the muscle attachment points. A mechanics deformation problem consisting of relatively fewer degrees of freedom is solved using displacement based boundary conditions while ensuring that the embedded muscles do not penetrate one another. In a subsequent step the shape of the embedded muscle is updated and the new muscle lengths are computed.

The host-mesh can also make reasonable predictions of muscle lengths and shape changes using purely geometric constraints (Oberhofer et al., 2009). This offers attractive benefits to those in the animation industry where efficient methods of morphing characters to anatomically-correct poses may assist artists. Figure 2.8 shows

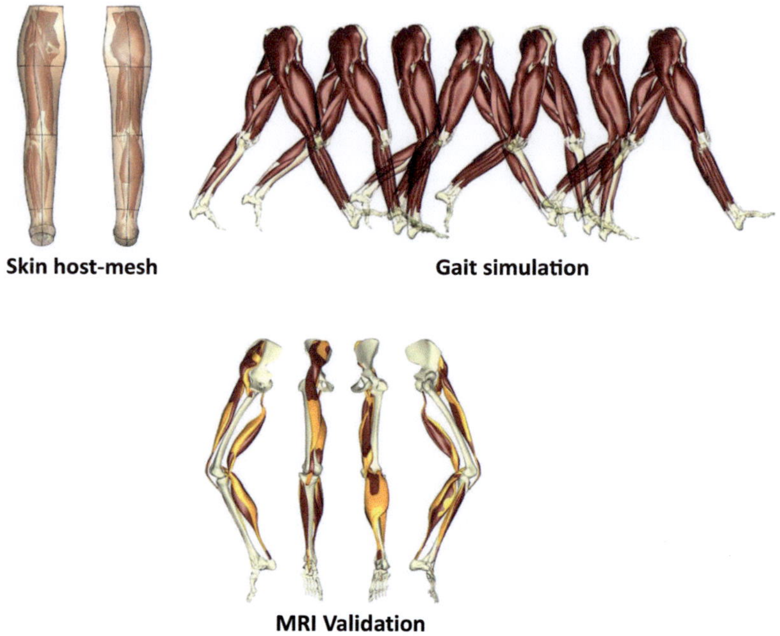

Fig. 2.8 Skin host-mesh fitting used to deform the complete lower limb muscle set (*red muscles*) during gait and validation against MRI derived muscles (*yellow muscles*)

a skin-shaped host mesh used to accurately deform 20 muscles of the lower limb by using information from the surrounding skin. In this case the host mesh was taken to be the volume defined by the actual skin, as opposed to the simpler shapes previously used, and the muscles were embedded within. Deformation driven by motion capture data produced a realistic walking simulation and we evaluated the shape changes of 5 muscles by comparing the predicted deformations with magnetic resonance image data in two lower limb positions (15° and 45° flexion). The predicted muscle positions shown in red were compared with MRI derived muscle shapes (shown in yellow) producing an average RMS error of 3.7 mm, which shows an excellent fit for muscle shapes predicted without mechanics.

2.7 Evaluating Compression in Deep Vein Thrombosis

Deep vein thrombosis (DVT), which is characterized by the formation of thrombi in deep veins, is a well-known problem following long haul flights (economy class syndrome) or extended hospital stays. The common factor is prolonged immobility and it is associated with other complications including chronic venous insufficiency and pulmonary embolism. The three main thrombogenic factors are stasis, hypercoagulability and injury to the vessel wall with the main treatments being either medicinal (anticoagulents) or mechanical (static or intermittent compression). We shall examine static compression due to its low cost and popularity among air travelers using this technique through compressive stockings. Despite its use the effect of compression is not fully understood. It is believed to cause reduction in deep vessel cross-section area, which in turn results in increased flow velocities. Another hypothesis is that shear stress and cyclic strain can influence cellular mechanisms to dissolve fibrin and prevent thrombus formation. A number of studies (Downie et al., 2007, 2008) have looked at modeling external compression and resulting blood flow in deep veins. All these models, however, have either employed images (e.g. MRI) directly (Dai et al., 1999; Downie et al., 2007, 2008; Narracott et al., 2007) or used the deformation of 2D continuum models (plane strain analysis) of surrounding soft tissue structures to reconstruct the deformed (collapsed) geometry of vessels. The computational model presented here is a 3D soft tissue continuum model undergoing large deformations (finite elasticity) due to applied external compression with a 1D flow network of major deep vessels embedded within the 3D continuum. Coupling between fluid and soft tissue is achieved via the vessel wall constitutive equation that describes the relationship between vessel radius and the transmural pressure. The latter is the difference between the fluid pressure and soft tissue hydrostatic pressure which arises due to the incompressibility of the soft tissue material.

The solid mechanics framework previously described is now extended to include a coupled one-dimensional blood flow network. The patient-specific geometry of both the soft tissue continuum and vein network is anatomically based and was developed using data derived from magnetic resonance images (MRI) using the fitting techniques previously described. The soft tissue includes all the muscles, subcutaneous fat layers and skin. The combined tissue mass was treated as an incompressible hyperelastic material with homogeneous isotropic properties. The mechanical characteristics of the tissue was described using a quadratic Mooney-Rivlin constitutive model with the coefficients $C_{10} = C_{20} = 10$ kPa (Meier and Blickhan, 2000). The computational flow model was the 1D Navier-Stokes equation comprising continuity and momentum relations given by

$$\frac{\partial R}{\partial t} + V\frac{\partial R}{\partial x} + \frac{R}{2}.\frac{\partial V}{\partial x} = 0 \quad \text{and} \tag{2.9}$$

$$\frac{\partial V}{\partial t} + (2\alpha - 1)V\frac{\partial V}{\partial x} + 2(\alpha - 1)\frac{V^2}{R}.\frac{\partial R}{\partial x} + \frac{1}{\rho_f}\frac{\partial P}{\partial x} + \left(\frac{2\nu\alpha}{\alpha - 1}\right)\frac{V}{R^2} = 0, \tag{2.10}$$

where R is the radius of the vessel, V is the mean velocity and P is the fluid pressure. ρ_f and ν are fluid density and kinematic viscosity respectively. α is the velocity profile parameter and the velocity profile is given by

$$u = \left(\frac{\gamma + 2}{\gamma}\right).V.\left[1 - \left(\frac{r}{R}\right)^{\gamma}\right] \quad \text{and} \quad \gamma = \frac{2 - \alpha}{\alpha - 1}. \tag{2.11}$$

The constitutive equation of the vein wall which describes the mechanical characteristics (vessel radius–transmural pressure relationship) was defined as a cubic polynomial of radius ratio R/R_0 by fitting the experimental data (Dobrin et al., 1988) obtained from a canine femoral vein,

$$P_{tr} = (P - p) = a\left(\frac{R}{R_0}\right)^3 + b\left(\frac{R}{R_0}\right)^2 + c\left(\frac{R}{R_0}\right), \tag{2.12}$$

where P_{tr} is the transmural pressure (difference between fluid and hydrostatic pressures), R_0 is the uncollapsed (reference) radius and a, b and c are the polynomial fitting coefficients.

Once compression is applied, the transmural pressure is computed as the difference between the fluid and soft tissue hydrostatic pressure. The latter arises due to the incompressibility of the soft tissue material. Transient flow governing equations are solved using the McCormack finite difference method (Anderson, 1995). The vascular network geometry was reconstructed with respect to the deformed soft tissue continuum to examine the degree of reduction in vessel cross-section area caused by gross deformation of the tissue continuum (without taking the hydrostatic pressure effects into account).

Simulation results from the computational model show a reasonably good agreement with the results reported in the literature on the degree of deformation in vein cross-section area estimated using MRI (Downie et al., 2008). The mean radius change of the venous network due to the gross deformation was found be insignificant (less than 2 %). The hydrostatic pressure distribution in response to the application of external compression is depicted in Fig. 2.9. The distribution of hydrostatic pressure was obtained by fitting it as a tri-linear FE field. The fitted hydrostatic pressure field was then interpolated to determine the external pressure acting on the vessel wall at each finite difference grid point of the venous flow network. The reduction in cross-section area at 1.0 ml/s based on a MRI study (Narracott et al., 2007) has been reported to be about 62 ± 10 %. The predicted value from this study compares reasonably well with the experimental data. Simulations also showed that increase in mean flow velocity due to compression resulted in increased wall shear stress (WSS), which stimulates endothelial cell activation and influences the release of tissue plasminogen activator (t-PA), which then converts plasminogen to active plasmin which dissolves fibrin and prevents thrombus formation.

2.8 Mechanics of the Patella

The patellar is a component of the knee that focuses the quadriceps muscles onto the tibia to enable the extensor action of the knee. Despite its role as a pivot to increase the moment arm (increasing the efficiency of the quadriceps) relatively less attention has been focused on its mechanics compared to the tibiofemoral joint. We have used the above framework to create the first fully 3D patellar integrated into a 3D continuum of muscles, tendons and ligaments to investigate the influence on joint loading from the action of muscle contraction (Fernandez and Hunter, 2005). Such a model has the potential to inform non-invasive treatment strategies on a patient basis

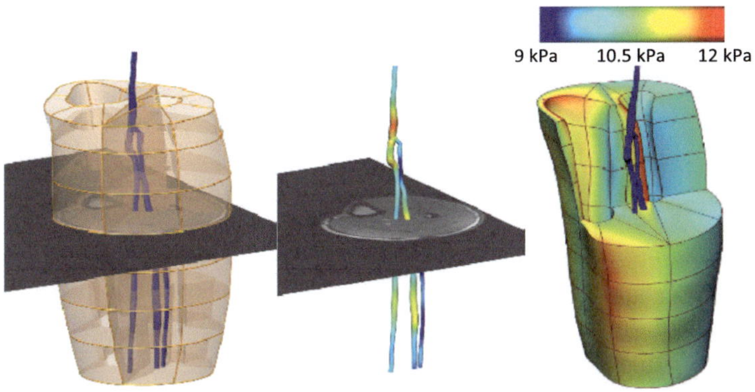

Fig. 2.9 Fitted 1D cubic FE mesh of the flow network embedded within 3D soft tissue (*left*); Radius field (cubic Hermite) in the flow network (*middle*); and hydrostatic pressure distribution of the calf at deformed state (*right*) [scale: 9 kPa (*blue*)–12 kPa (*red*)]

or predict the possible outcomes of surgery intervention such as a vastus lateralis release.

Figure 2.10 shows a knee joint from a healthy subject's MR data including muscles, ligaments, cartilage and bones. A generic model of the soft tissue was customized to the MR data and the bone was further divided into cortical and cancellous bone. Material properties were assigned to the bone regions using a grid point method independent of the mesh resolution using the 'St Venant Kirchoff' constitutive law. The fiber distribution was derived from a cadaveric study whereby the surfaces of fibers were taken from images and projected on the muscles. This has recently been extended by including fiber direction estimates using Diffusion Tensor Imaging sequences in an MRI. The motion of the tibia was derived from motion capture experiments and the patellar movement was controlled by the tension in the patellar ligament, contraction of the muscle tissues and contact with the femoral condyles. The model predicted the contact force, surface cartilage pressure and patellar kinematics in response to a healthy loading. Specifically, for normal gait we got two distinct regions of contact at contralateral toe-off (the highest loading point during gait) with a large contact area on the lateral facet and a small contact region on the medial facet. The peak in red represents 10 MPa.

We simulated two orthopedic procedures recommended for the alleviation of patellofemoral pain, the vastus lateralis (VL) release and the medialization of the tibial tubercle (as part of a Maquet procedure). The VL release works by excising a small region of muscle that inserts into the lateral portion of the patellar. Given the lateral facet is the most loaded (with the largest face) it is most often associated with osteoarthritis. The load on the lateral side is now reduced, which is exhibited by a medial shift in the cartilage contact pressure map. The original pressure distribution showed two distinct contact regions (with a peak on the lateral side). This has now migrated towards the middle and the two sites of contact have merged to form a single central contact patch. Patellar kinematics was relatively unchanged except for a slight increase in medial tilt.

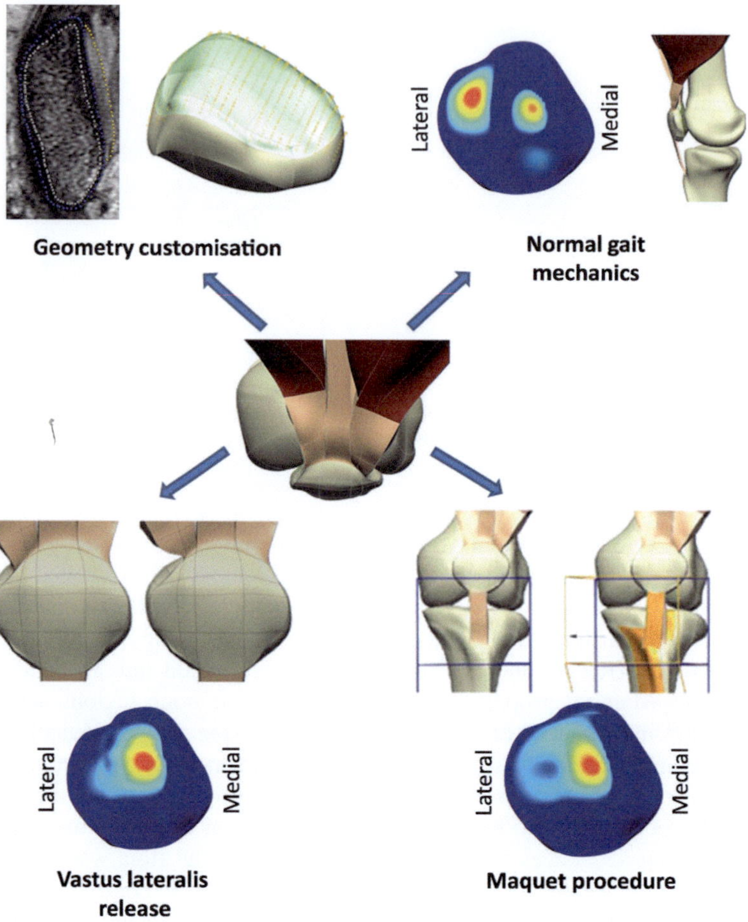

Fig. 2.10 Patient-specific customization of patella containing accurate topological descriptions of cancellous bone, cortical bone and articular cartilage; simulation of healthy gait showing contact pressure at contralateral toe-off; simulating a vastus lateralis release producing significant medial migration in patellar contact; and Maquet procedure predicting minor medial shift in patellar contact

Next we investigated medialization of the patellar tendon attachment point (part of the Maquet procedure) and used the host-mesh technique to morph the patella tendon insertion site (the tibial tuberosity) medially. In this case the contact pattern also migrated medially but some contact still remained on the lateral side. Patellar kinematics showed an increase in medial translation and medial tilt. The two simulations show that the Maquet procedure, which is generally more invasive, is more subtle in the contact redistribution but leads to more altered kinematics. In contrast, the VL release can be performed via key hole surgery (less invasive) has a subtle effect on kinematics but is better at completely alleviating loading from the lateral facet by directly affecting the muscle force.

2.9 Coupled Bone Cartilage Mechanics

The initiation of osteoarthritis has been linked to the onset and progression of pathologic mechanisms at the cartilage-bone interface. In order to evaluate this process we have developed a multiscale model using the open-source ontologies developed for the Physiome Project with cartilage and bone descriptions at the cellular, micro and macro levels. In this way we can effectively model the influence of whole body loadings at the macro level, the influence of bone organization and architecture at the micro level and have cell level processes determine bone and cartilage remodeling. Cell information is then passed up the spatial scales to modify micro architecture and provide a macro spatial characterization of cartilage inflammation. Figure 2.11 shows this framework being used to explore a common link with a widely reported knee injury (Anterior Cruciate Ligament Deficiency—ACDL) to proinflammatory mediators as a possible pathway to initiate osteoarthritis.

To simulate remodeling we designated the healthy strain state (normal gait) as homeostatic equilibrium, where bone and cartilage are maintained and no remodeling occurs. We then simulated the altered cartilage strains due to loading from ACLD. The difference between the homeostatic and ACLD strains was the excitation for bone remodeling to initiate. Micro models of cartilage (seen as red cubes in Fig. 2.11) are spatially placed across the bone cartilage interface to capture an average strain in that 1 mm^3 region. For each micro model, the average strain was then applied to the surface of the detailed micro bone-cartilage model and we modeled the propagation through the cartilage, zone of calcified cartilage (ZCC) and subchondral bone regions. The micro model was repeatedly run with each simulation representing a week's worth of loading. After each simulation the geometry was remodeled (through calling a cell level model) and the simulations were conducted again with the new bone architecture producing new strain patterns in both the bone, ZCC and cartilage. For both the macro and micro models, the bones and cartilage were treated as deformable linear elastic materials with the Young's modulus and Poisson's ratios for cartilage ($E = 10$ MPa, $\nu = 0.46$), ZCC ($E = 100$ MPa, $\nu = 0.3$) and bone ($E = 1$ GPa, $\nu = 0.3$). The micro FE model had a depth of 450 μm for cartilage, 200 μm for the zone of calcified cartilage (ZCC) and 350 μm for subchondral bone.

The micro model was informed by the parameters obtained from two cell models. A bone remodeling algorithm (Pivonka et al., 2008) based on the RANK-RANKL-OPG pathway, which predicts the number of active osteoblasts (to deposit bone) and osteoclasts (to absorb bone) implemented in CellML (Garny et al., 2008). The cell model used micro strains as excitation to predict temporal concentrations of osteoblasts and osteoclasts over their life cycle, from precursor cells to active working cells and finally apoptosis (cell death). The osteocyte sensors are strategically placed at numerical integration points within each element and inform the FE nodes excitation signal used to drive remodeling. Each node then calls the CellML bone model to determine the osteoblast/osteoclast numbers to provide the rate of remodeling, which is directioned normal to each surface. Similarly, a cartilage damage prediction model was developed based on the work of Nam et al. (2009), which quantitatively describes the action of nuclear factor-kappa B (NF-κB) signaling cascade

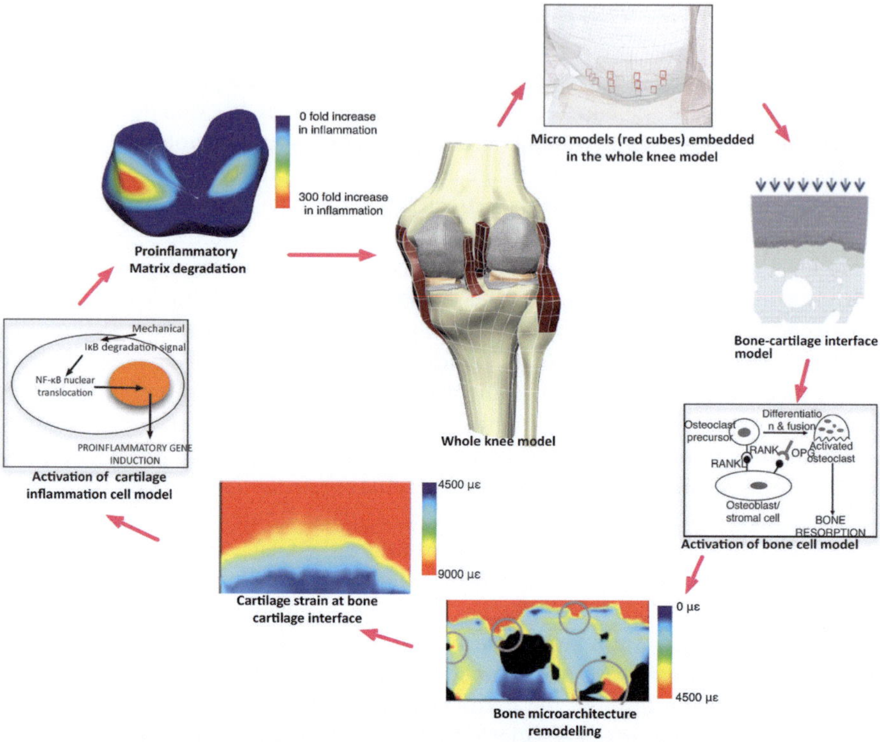

Fig. 2.11 The multiscale framework used in this study depicting the coupled links from the whole continuum knee model to the macro and cell level descriptions

under mechanical stimulation. Peak cartilage strains were used to activate NF-κB pathway, leading to induction of proinflammatory genes

This remodeling approach accounted for both bone growth and bone shape evolution enhancing the ZCC undulating profile and tidemark irregularity. This pattern resembles the finger-like structures that are reported to form during the progression of osteoarthritis (Zizak et al., 2003). The peak strain is also 15–20 % higher in the ACLD knee at the ZCC interface with higher strain closer to the ZCC interface compared to the normal knee. The increase in cartilage strains increased the production of inflammatory cytokines. The findings in this study may explain why altered or traumatic subchondral bone loadings can initiate a degenerative cycle in the cartilage matrix.

2.10 Conclusions

The modeling framework presented in this chapter demonstrates a collection of techniques that can be used to aid patient-specific analysis using computational methods.

This chapter primarily demonstrates efforts towards efficient methods of building subject-specific geometries. However, accurate boundary conditions and material properties are necessary before results can be used with confidence. Patient derived geometries are paramount for both bone and soft tissue when informing clinical decisions. Accurate descriptions of bone provide correct anatomical surface topology and articular features. This is especially important for diseased states like cerebral palsy, which differ significantly from the healthy condition, or when informing implant design for patient surgery. Furthermore, predicting joint contact areas requires accurate models of joint articulations. The anatomical axis is also influenced by the curvature of bone shaft, which in turn allows for accurate moment arm predictions and more meaningful muscle force estimates. Improved soft tissue profiles are important for volume prediction of muscle, which is used to estimate cross-sectional area and hence predict the power generation capacity. Finally, advances in multiscale modeling are being driven by increasing availability of information at all spatial scales. The methods presented here ensure that organ level models are more subject orientated when informing meso and micro descriptions.

Acknowledgements The authors would like to thank all members, past and present, of the Auckland Bioengineering Institute (ABI) musculoskeletal group who have contributed to the presented works, especially, Dr. Katja Oberhofer for her work with host mesh fitting of muscles and Dr. Iain Anderson for his work with patient-specific modeling of hips. This chapter was written with the financial assistance of an Aotearoa bioengineering fellowship awarded to J. Fernandez, a Wishbone Trust grant awarded to V. Shim and a FRST grant awarded to K. Mithraratne and P. Hunter (UOAX0712 and UOAX1006).

References

Ackerman MJ (1998) The visible human project. Proc IEEE 86(3):504–511

Anderson J (1995) Computational fluid dynamics—the basics with applications. McGraw-Hill, New York

Bradley CP, Pullan AJ, Hunter PJ (1997) Geometric modeling of the human torso using cubic Hermite elements. Ann Biomed Eng 25(1):96–111

Dai GH, Gertler JP, Kamm RD (1999) The effects of external compression on venous blood flow and tissue deformation in the lower leg. J Biomech Eng 121(6):557–564

Dobrin PB, Littooy FN et al (1988) Mechanical and histological changes in canine vein grafts. J Surg Res 44:259–265

Downie SP et al (2007) Role of MRI in investigating the effects of elastic compression stockings on the deformation of the superficial and deep veins in the lower leg. J Magn Reson Imaging 26(1):80–85

Downie SP et al (2008) Effects of elastic compression stockings on wall shear stress in deep and superficial veins of the calf. Am J Physiol, Heart Circ Physiol 294(5):H2112–H2120

FCAT (Federative Committee on Anatomical Terminology) (2011) Terminologia anatomica. International anatomical terminology, 2nd edn. Thieme, Stuttgart

Fernandez JW et al (2005) A cerebral palsy assessment tool using anatomically based geometries and free-form deformation. Biomech Model Mechanobiol 4(1):39–56

Fernandez JW, Hunter PJ (2005) An anatomically based patient-specific finite element model of patella articulation: towards a diagnostic tool. Biomech Model Mechanobiol 4(1):20–38

Fernandez JW et al (2004) Anatomically based geometric modeling of the musculo-skeletal system and other organs. Biomech Model Mechanobiol 2(3):139–155

Garny A et al (2008) CellML and associated tools and techniques. Philos Trans R Soc, Math Phys Eng Sci 366(1878):3017–3043
Gray H (2008) Gray's anatomy: the anatomical basis of clinical practice, 40th edn. Churchill Livingstone/Elsevier, Edinburgh/Amsterdam
Hill AV (1938) The heat of shortening and the dynamic constants of muscle. Proc R Soc Lond B, Biol Sci 126(843):136–195
Hunter PJ (1995) Myocardial constitutive laws for continuum mechanics models of the heart. Adv Exp Med Biol 382:303–318
Hunter PJ (1995) Myocardial constitutive laws for continuum models of the heart. In: Sideman S, Beyar R (eds) Molecular and subcellular cardiology. Springer, New York, pp 303–318
Hunter PJ (2004) The IUPS physiome project: a framework for computational physiology. Prog Biophys Mol Biol 85(2–3):551–569
Hunter PJ, Borg TK (2003) Integration from proteins to organs: the physiome project. Nat Rev Mol Cell Biol 4(3):237–243
Hunter PJ, McCulloch AD, ter Keurs HE (1998) Modeling the mechanical properties of cardiac muscle. Prog Biophys Mol Biol 69(2–3):289–331
Huxley AF (1957) Muscle structure and theories of contraction. Progress in biophysics & molecular biology, vol 7. 255 pp
Meier P, Blickhan R (2000) In: Herzog W (ed) Skeletal muscle mechanics: from mechanism to function. Wiley, Bognor Regis, pp 207–224
Nam J et al (2009) Biomechanical thresholds regulate inflammation through the NF-kappa B pathway: experiments and modeling. PLoS ONE 4(4):e5262
Narracott AJ et al (2007) Influence of intermittent compression cuff design on calf deformation: computational results. In: 2007 annual international conference of the IEEE Engineering in Medicine and Biology Society, pp 6335–6338
Nash MP, Hunter PJ (2000) Computational mechanics of the heart—from tissue structure to ventricular function. J Elast 61(1–3):113–141
Oberhofer K et al (2009) Anatomically-based musculoskeletal modeling: prediction and validation of muscle deformation during walking. Vis Comput 25(9):843–851
Pivonka P et al (2008) Model structure and control of bone remodeling: a theoretical study. Bone 43(2):249–263
Rivlin RS (1948) Large elastic deformations of isotropic materials. 1. Fundamental concepts. Philos Trans R Soc Lond Ser A, Math Phys Sci 240(822):459–508
Shim VB et al (2007) The use of sparse CT datasets for auto-generating accurate FE models of the femur and pelvis. J Biomech 40(1):26–35
Shim VB et al (2008) Development and validation of patient-specific finite element models of the hemipelvis generated from a sparse CT data set. J Biomech Eng 130(5):051010
Spitzer VM et al (1995) The visible-human (male and female). Radiology, vol 197. 533 pp
Wriggers P, Krstulovic-Opara L, Korelc J (2001) Smooth C-1-interpolations for two-dimensional frictional contact problems. Int J Numer Methods Eng 51(12):1469–1495
Zahalak GI (2000) The two-state cross-bridge model of muscle is an asymptotic limit of multi-state models. J Theor Biol 204(1):67–82
Zizak I et al (2003) Characteristics of mineral particles in the human bone/cartilage interface. J Struct Biol 141(3):208–217

Chapter 3
Patient Specific Computational Modeling in Cardiovascular Mechanics

Arthur Creane, Daniel J. Kelly, and Caitríona Lally

Abstract Diseases of the cardiovascular system are leading causes of morbidity and mortality worldwide. Computational modeling of cardiovascular mechanics has contributed to the understanding of cardiovascular disease etiology and risk evaluation. Patient specific finite element models of disease sites such as atherosclerotic plaques and aneurysms have provided important insights into their biomechanics, including identification of the characteristics of vulnerable locations.

Current clinical risk assessment for atherosclerotic plaque disruption is based on the stenosis produced by the lesion; however it has been found that the magnitude of stenosis does not correlate with the plaque's vulnerability. Likewise evaluation of the likelihood of aneurysm rupture is based mainly on diameter measurements; however this criterion has also been called into question. Plaque and aneurysm rupture are often fatal events and thus improved clinical indicators for them are required. Patient specific finite element models of these disease sites may provide improved indicators of vulnerability based on biomechanical principles. Proposed indicators in the literature include measures of maximal stress and stress/strength ratios, additionally geometric measures such as plaque curvature or vessel asymmetry have also been developed as potential indicators.

In recent years, model complexity has increased from 2D studies to 3D models with multiple components. Current technical challenges which are being addressed in the literature include the estimation of the stress free reference configuration of arteries from the deformed *in vivo* configuration present in medical images and the inclusion of residual stresses in the arterial wall. Furthermore anisotropic constitutive models with artery specific preferred material directions are being implemented in these complex geometries using stress or strain based fiber remodeling algorithms and geometric systems. This chapter reviews the current state of the art in the area and details the barriers yet to be overcome if patient specific computational mod-

---

A. Creane · C. Lally (✉)
School of Mechanical and Manufacturing Engineering, Dublin City University, Dublin 9, Ireland
e-mail: triona.lally@dcu.ie

D.J. Kelly · C. Lally
Trinity Centre for Bioengineering, School of Engineering, Trinity College, Dublin 2, Ireland

B. Calvo, E. Peña (eds.), *Patient-Specific Computational Modeling*,
Lecture Notes in Computational Vision and Biomechanics 5,
DOI 10.1007/978-94-007-4552-0_3,

eling is to be used as a clinical tool. These include trade-offs between automation, model complexity, computation time and reproducibility.

3.1 Introduction

Diseases of the cardiovascular system are leading causes of morbidity and mortality worldwide. Computational modeling of cardiovascular mechanics has contributed to the understanding of cardiovascular disease etiology and risk evaluation. In particular, patient specific finite element models of atherosclerotic plaques and aneurysms have provided important insights into their biomechanics, including identification of vulnerable characteristics.

Atherosclerotic plaques develop in several areas of the arterial tree. Common locations include the coronary arteries, the carotid arteries and other peripheral arteries such as the iliac arteries. Growth of plaques can restrict blood flow and cause ischemia, however they often develop silently and have no clinical symptoms (Naghavi, 2003; Schaar et al., 2004). Rupture of these so-called 'vulnerable' plaques can therefore be a sudden and destructive event. Embolic particles may be released into the lumen which then travel downstream and block blood vessels with smaller cross-sections. Depending on the location, this can lead to stroke or myocardial infarction. Like plaque, aneurysms develop in a number of locations in the arterial system and can remain clinically silent throughout the life of an individual. Aneurysm rupture compromises the integrity of the vessel wall and in a cerebral aneurysm this may cause a stroke, while rupture of an abdominal aortic aneurysm (AAA) leads to massive hemorrhage due to the large blood flow rate in the aorta. Both plaque and aneurysm rupture are therefore often fatal events.

Current clinical risk assessment for atherosclerotic plaque disruption is based on the stenosis produced by the lesion; however it has been found that the magnitude of stenosis does not correlate with the likelihood of plaque rupture (Golledge et al., 2000). Similarly, evaluation of the likelihood of aneurysm rupture (both saccular and fusiform) is based mainly on diameter measurements; however this criterion has also been called into question (Ma et al., 2004; Vorp, 2007). Improved indicators of plaque and aneurysm rupture are therefore necessary. While aneurysm and plaque rupture involve considerably different processes, they are both mechanical events. Engineering principles can therefore be used to predict the likelihood of rupture and considerable investigation in this area has taken place. The basic premise is that if the stress at a location in a material (plaque or aneurysm) exceeds its strength then failure (rupture) will occur. Developing patient specific finite element (FE) models provides a means of predicting this stress (see Fig. 3.1) where the geometry of the diseased artery is determined from *in vivo* imaging modalities such as CT or MRI, while the strength of the material can be estimated from *ex vivo* characterization and statistical methods (Vande Geest et al., 2006).

An artery is composed of many different structures (endothelial cells, smooth muscle cells, elastin and collagen). These components are not distributed evenly throughout the arterial wall nor are their orientations constant throughout the wall.

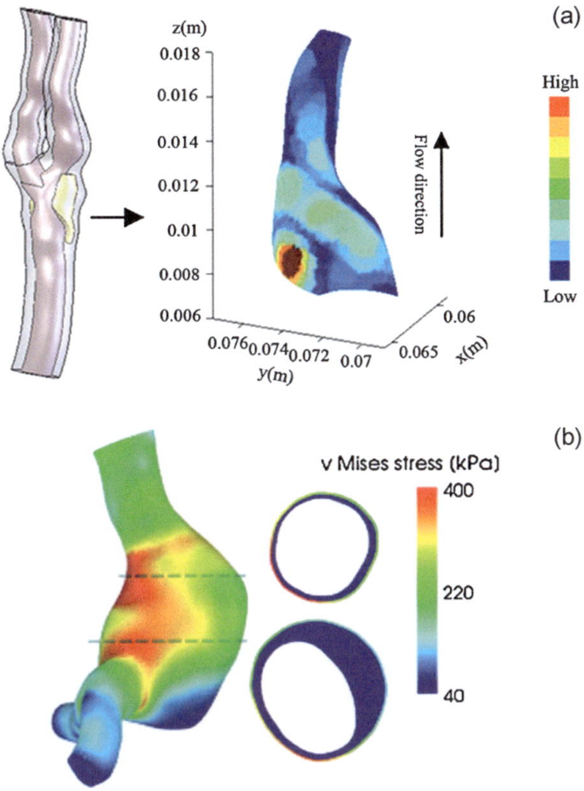

Fig. 3.1 Patient specific carotid plaque stress analysis (**a**) and patient specific AAA stress analysis (**b**) adapted from Gao et al. (2011) and Maier et al. (2010) respectively

Arteries are tethered to surrounding tissues and have residual stresses. Complex blood flow patterns exist in areas of complex geometry and disease sites which can produce complex and time varying pressures on the vessel walls. These factors all increase the complexity involved in accurately predicting the stress distribution within, and ultimately rupture of, plaques or aneurysms. A trade-off is therefore required between model complexity (and thus accuracy) and the availability and reliability of the necessary inputs, i.e. geometry and morphology, material characterization and the forces exerted *in vivo*.

Computational patient specific studies, aimed at identifying key rupture parameters, have focused mainly on two regions, atherosclerotic plaque in the carotid arteries and aneurysms of the abdominal aorta. This is due not only to the severity of the risks associated with rupture at these locations but also due to the size of the arteries. The carotid arteries and abdominal aorta are among the largest in the body. Thus sufficient resolution can be achieved using *in vivo* non-invasive imaging modalities (CT, MRI). Analysis of atherosclerosis in the coronary arteries and aneurysms in the cerebral arteries is more challenging as the resolution is limited using CT or MRI. Studies based on intravascular ultrasound (IVUS) provide a possible solution to this (Yang et al., 2009); however IVUS is an invasive modality and therefore may not be appropriate as a screening/diagnostic tool. This chapter will compare studies which have investigated carotid plaque and AAA.

Section 3.2 will review studies which are focused on technical challenges in patient specific studies which remain unresolved, including incorporating material anisotropy in complex geometries, modeling residual stresses and extracting true geometries from *in vivo* medical imaging. Section 3.3 will consider studies which have made a number of limiting assumptions in carrying out patient specific analyses and have aimed to use these studies to distinguish between symptomatic and asymptomatic patients using the finite element method. Finally, Sect. 3.4 will review studies which have developed simpler alternative indicators to finite element analyses based on observations found in these computational studies.

The methods used to-date, and the challenges to be overcome, in the development of new clinical indicators of plaque and aneurysm rupture are remarkably similar. By comparing investigations from both areas, therefore, new insights may be found in the development of non-invasive diagnostic tools for the detection of plaque and aneurysm rupture based on the use of computational patient specific models.

3.2 Current Technical Challenges

3.2.1 Anisotropic Response of the Arterial Wall

As stated above, the arterial wall is a heterogeneous structure, thus its mechanical response is complex. The orientation of wall constituents creates an anisotropic response (Rhodin, 1980). Anisotropic constitutive models of the arterial wall have been developed with a noteworthy example being that defined by Holzapfel et al. (2000). The arterial wall was modeled as an isotropic ground matrix with 2 families of embedded fibers providing anisotropy. In a straight vessel these fibers were assumed to be orientated helically based on experimental findings. Gasser et al. (2006) expanded this idea to also incorporate directional dispersion from the mean direction of each fiber family. They defined the strain energy density function as follows:

$$U = c_{10}(\overline{I}_1 - 3) + \sum_{fam=1,2} \frac{k_1}{2k_2}\left(\exp\left[k_2 \overline{E}_{fam}^2\right] - 1\right). \tag{3.1}$$

The first term represents the isotropic response of the ground matrix while the second term adds the anisotropic contribution of each family of fibers. $\overline{I}_1$, $\overline{E}_{fam\_1}$ and $\overline{E}_{fam\_2}$ are strain invariants and pseudo-invariants respectively while c_{10}, k_1, and k_2 are material constants. The pseudo-invariants $\overline{E}_{fam\_i}$ represent the strain component in a fiber direction and are defined by:

$$\overline{E}_{fam\_i} = H_{fam\_i} : \overline{C} - 1. \tag{3.2}$$

Here $\overline{C}$ is the deviatoric right Cauchy-Green deformation tensor. $H_{fam\_i=1,2}$ are second order structural tensors representing the configuration (mean direction, dispersion) of each family of fibers. The fibers are assumed to only contribute in tension. A number of different fiber dispersion schemes have been proposed, see Creane et al. (2011). A 2D fan splay dispersion was used in Creane et al. (2011) and defined by the following:

$$H_{fam\_i} = \kappa I + (1 - 2\kappa)(\overline{\mathbf{A}} \otimes \overline{\mathbf{A}}) - \kappa(\overline{\mathbf{B}} \otimes \overline{\mathbf{B}}) \tag{3.3}$$

where $\overline{\mathbf{A}}$ is a unit vector in the mean fiber direction, $\overline{\mathbf{B}}$ is a unit vector perpendicular to the plane of dispersion (dispersion occurs in only 1 plane, i.e. fan splay), κ controls the amount of dispersion and I is the identity matrix. In a straight vessel vectors $\overline{\mathbf{A}}$ and $\overline{\mathbf{B}}$ are easily set relative to the circumferential and axial directions (dispersion occurs in the circumferential–axial plane).

Plaque in the carotid arteries usually spans the carotid bifurcation while AAAs occur just proximal to the aortic bifurcation (Fig. 3.1). With both a distorted wall and bifurcation at these disease sites, circumferential and axial directions can become ambiguous and thus fiber directions are difficult to define. Many studies which attempt to create clinical indicators from FE results have therefore assumed the arterial wall behaves isotropically (Gao et al., 2011; Maier et al., 2010). This assumption may significantly alter the predicted stress distribution (Rodríguez et al., 2008; Vande Geest et al., 2008) and may therefore affect the diagnostic potential of the method used.

This limitation has been addressed by a number of studies, however most have not included anisotropy at a bifurcation. Kiousis et al. (2007) and Mortier et al. (2009) used geometric systems for defining fiber directions at a bifurcation with a local basis created in each element of the FE mesh with the fiber directions set at an angle from this basis. Similarly, Alastrué et al. (2010) set fiber directions at an angle to defined local bases, however these bases were instead created from the predicted principal strain directions using results from an initial isotropic simulation.

Hariton et al. (2007) and Creane et al. (2011) used fiber remodeling algorithms to define the fiber architecture at arterial bifurcations where the algorithm used was originally developed by Driessen et al. (2004). Driessen et al. (2004) used the observation that under normal physiological loads in a straight vessel, the maximum and intermediate principal strains (and stresses) coincided with the circumferential and axial directions, respectively. They developed a remodeling system in which fibers were allowed to reorientate towards a direction set at an angle between the maximum and intermediate principal strain directions. This angle was dependent on the ratio of the principal strain magnitudes. In Creane et al. (2011), the vectors $\overline{\mathbf{A}}$ and $\overline{\mathbf{B}}$ and dispersion parameter κ were made dependent on this algorithm via (3.4) and (3.5). Fiber dispersion was not considered in Hariton et al. (2007).

$$\theta = \tan^{-1}\frac{\upsilon_2}{\upsilon_1}; \quad \kappa = \frac{1}{2}\frac{\upsilon_2}{\upsilon_1}; \quad 0^\circ \leq \theta \leq 45^\circ; \; 0 \leq \kappa \leq \frac{1}{2}, \tag{3.4}$$

$$\begin{aligned} &\overline{\mathbf{A}}_{fam\_1} = \cos\theta\mathbf{e}_1 + \sin\theta\mathbf{e}_2; \qquad \overline{\mathbf{A}}_{fam\_2} = \cos\theta\mathbf{e}_1 - \sin\theta\mathbf{e}_2; \\ &\overline{\mathbf{B}}_{fam\_1} = \overline{\mathbf{B}}_{fam\_2} = e_3. \end{aligned} \tag{3.5}$$

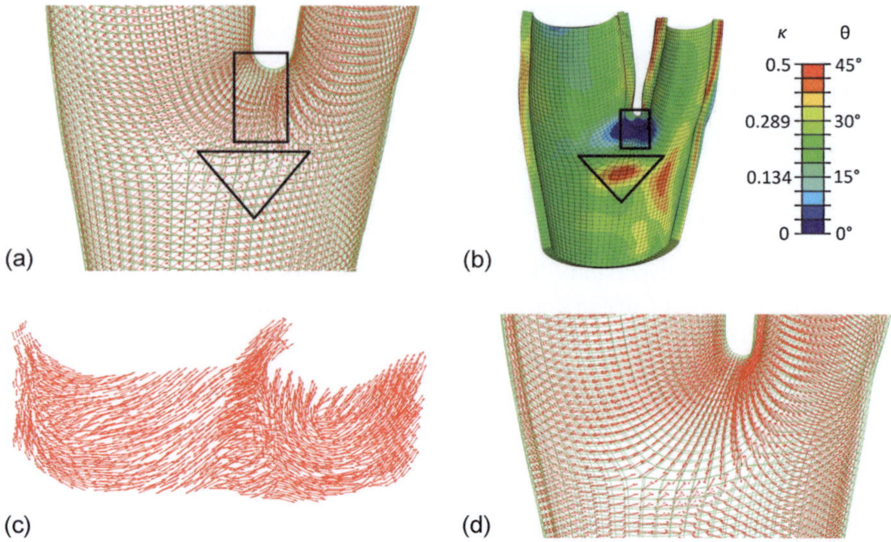

Fig. 3.2 Complex fiber architecture found at arterial bifurcations using strain based remodeling algorithms (**a**, **b**, **d**) and DT-MRI (**c**). Fiber family's mean orientation is seen in (**a**) while the directional dispersion parameter κ is shown in (**b**). Note that two interesting regions of architecture exist. The rectangular region highlights a unidirectional (uniaxial) region while the triangle represents the multidirectional (equibiaxial) region. The DT-MRI results in (**c**) can be compared to the total mean fiber directions (both families of fibers) from (**d**); there are considerable similarities between the two. (**a**) and (**b**) are adapted from Creane et al. (2011)

Here θ was the angle between the mean fiber directions $\overline{\mathbf{A}}_{fam\_1,2}$ and the maximum principal strain direction. $v_{1,2}$ are the maximum and intermediate principal values of the Green-Lagrangian strain tensor and $\mathbf{e}_{1,2}$ are their corresponding directions.

The fiber architecture predicted using the models in Hariton et al. (2007), Alastrué et al. (2010) and Creane et al. (2011) were all broadly similar and corresponded to experimental findings using polarizing light microscopy (Finlay et al., 1998; Rowe et al., 2003). Fibers were found to move from the typical helical pattern seen proximal and distal to the bifurcation into a more complex pattern. At the apex of the bifurcation, fibers were aligned in one direction along the flow divider (this was not observed in Alastrué et al. (2010) as the angle θ was fixed). This unidirectional region is a result of the high uniaxial strains and stresses experienced at that location (Figs. 3.2(a), (b)). The inclusion of a varying degree of fiber directional dispersion in Creane et al. (2011) gave further insight where below the apex of the bifurcation on either side of the arterial wall a multi-directional region with no consistent mean direction was predicted. The fiber dispersion in this location was at a maximum (Figs. 3.2(a), (b)). This multi-directional fiber pattern was created due to the equibiaxial strain experienced in this region.

Figure 3.2(c) presents preliminary results from *ex vivo* diffusion tensor magnetic resonance imaging (DT-MRI) of a bovine arterial bifurcation. DT-MRI has the capability of measuring the fiber architecture within arteries (Flamini et al., 2010) and other tissues including the myocardium (Wu et al., 2007; Zhang et al., 2010) and cartilage (Pierce et al., 2010). In this preliminary study only one mean fiber direction per pixel can be distinguished, however high angular resolution diffusion imaging (HARDI) techniques offer the potential to measure multiple directions. For comparison Fig. 3.2(d) plots the combined total mean fiber direction from both families of fibers at a bifurcation using the remodeling algorithm discussed above (Creane et al., 2011). There are considerable similarities between the architecture measured via DT-MRI and that predicted using the remodeling algorithm. DT-MRI is a non-invasive imaging modality and therefore may be useful in the measurement of the fiber architecture of complex arterial geometries *in vivo*. It may therefore provide information on key arterial material characteristics *in vivo* and consequently form the basis for a powerful diagnostic tool.

The above methods all investigated the mechanics of either healthy bifurcations or those affected by atherosclerosis. Studies which include anisotropy in AAAs are ambiguous as to how the local bases are defined at the aortic bifurcation (Rissland et al., 2009; Rodríguez et al., 2009; Vande Geest et al., 2008). The systems described above for carotid plaques could be easily translated to AAA studies to model the anisotropy in the aneurysm and at the aortic bifurcation. It can be seen in the AAA in Fig. 3.1(b) that areas of high stress occur close to the bifurcation and would therefore be affected by the fiber architecture at the bifurcation. Future studies which seek to accurately predict the stresses in an aneurysm wall or atherosclerotic plaque should incorporate an anisotropic constitutive model with realistic fiber directions; the methods discussed above provide a means to do so. The fiber architecture will also play a critical role in the local variation of material strength which is also crucial to predicting rupture.

3.2.2 Estimation of Residual Stress and the Stress Free State

Another consideration when modeling arteries is residual stress. A preload exists in arteries that can be observed by cutting an artery radially and noting that the artery springs open into a stress free state (Holzapfel et al., 2000). When the artery is intact the residual stress adds a circumferential compressive stress to the inner wall and a circumferential tensile stress to the outer wall. The effect promotes an equalization of the circumferential stress radially through the thickness of the wall when blood pressure is applied.

A limited number of studies have modeled this affect in a complex arterial geometry. Delfino et al. (1997) examined the opening behavior of human and porcine carotid bifurcations *ex vivo* by making specific cuts to a bifurcation and observing its opening behavior. From these experiments a representative geometric model of the stress free state at a bifurcation was generated. The residual stresses were taken into account in simulations by first deforming this stress free state into a corresponding unloaded state which was based on angiographic measurements (Fig. 3.3(a)). Results showed that the inclusion of residual stresses substantially changed the predicted stress distribution; the residually stressed simulation predicted a more uniform stress distribution through the thickness of the arterial wall.

Fig. 3.3 (**a**) The arterial stress free state (*top*) and the unloaded state (*bottom*); adapted from Delfino et al. (1997). (**b**) The predicted stress distribution on an AAA wall considering (*left*) and neglecting (*right*) the true unloaded configuration; adapted from Gee et al. (2010)

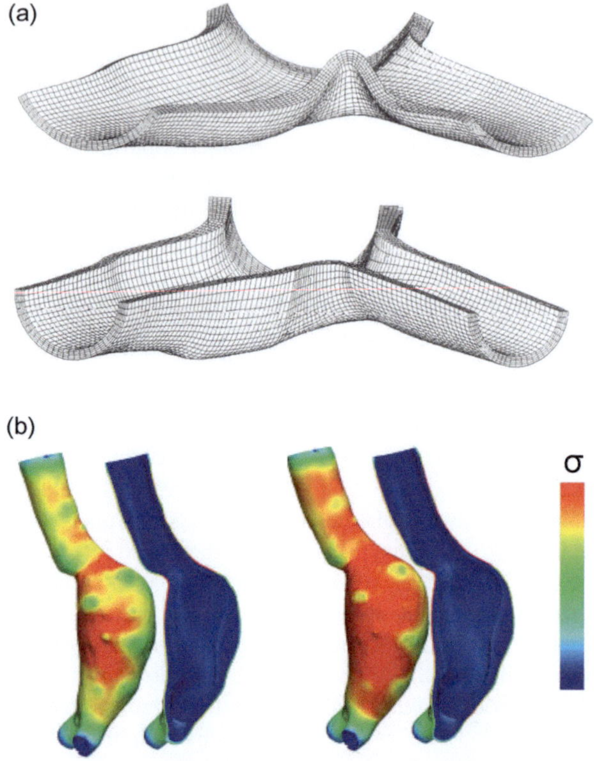

In a 2D histological investigation, Ohayon et al. (2007) studied the effect of residual stress on the stress distribution in coronary plaques. Similar to Delfino et al. (1997), residual stresses were included through deforming the artery's stress free state (found by cutting the artery open) into its intact unloaded state. Comparison of the predicted stress distributions with and without modeling residual stress found that the peak stresses and their locations were dramatically altered. Both Delfino et al. (1997) and Ohayon et al. (2007) show that the inclusion of residual stresses are necessary to accurately predict peak stresses and thus indicate rupture. However, these studies use knowledge of each artery's state *ex vivo*. This is not possible when considering *in vivo* patient specific analyses.

Alastrué et al. (2010) have produced a framework to incorporate residual stresses in patient specific models extracted from *in vivo* imaging. This is done by defining the preferred material orientations in the model as discussed in Sect. 3.2.1 and by then creating a pre-strain field. This pre-strain field can be incorporated into the model through the Kroner-Lee decomposition of the deformation gradient tensor. This method is applicable to both carotid plaque and AAA studies and may significantly increase the accuracy of the predicted stress distributions.

Arterial models extracted from *in vivo* imaging modalities have a number of forces acting upon them including blood pressure and axial tethering. Therefore the extracted geometry is not the artery's stress free state. The accuracy of the predicted stress distribution in the model would be diminished if this extracted geometry is assumed to be stress free. A number of both carotid plaque and AAA studies have accounted for this.

The simplest method is to use a trial and error basis where the model is shrunk by a chosen scaling factor, say 10 % which is used in Gao et al. (2011). A mean arterial pressure and axial tethering are then applied to the shrunken model to replicate *in vivo* conditions. The error associated with the shrinkage procedure can be measured through comparison of the originally extracted un-shrunk model and the predicted deformed state of the shrunken model after finite element analysis. The error can be calculated by the sum of the distances between corresponding nodes of the finite element meshes. If the error is within a specified limit the shrunken model is accepted as the stress free state of the vessel, whilst if the error is greater than this limit an adjustment is made to the scaling factors and the process is repeated. Variations of this method have been used in several studies (Huang et al., 2009; Raghavan et al., 2006; Tang et al., 2009). This process can take a considerable period of time since a number of finite element simulations may be required. Additionally, the shrinkage procedure of a multi-component model with differing material properties may be difficult to implement (Leach et al., 2010).

Inverse design analyses have been used to attempt to retrieve the stress free state of AAAs (Gee et al., 2010; Lu et al., 2007). Here the Cauchy stress is parameterized in terms of the inverse deformation gradient instead of the deformation gradient and thus the analysis can be solved for the initial stress free geometry. Gee et al. (2010) pointed out however that in a finite strain environment, there is no unique solution to this. They presented a second method which involves a multiplicative split of the deformation gradient where no displacement from the measured *in vivo* geometry is made but rather a pre-strain field is created in the model prior to forward analysis (Fig. 3.3(b)). Alastrué et al. (2010) use a similar approach to incorporate a pre-strain field at an arterial bifurcation. It is evident in Fig. 3.3(b) that the predicted stresses in the AAA wall are considerably higher in the model which assumes a stress free state during *in vivo* imaging. The above observations demonstrate that the inclusion of residual stresses and the use of stress-free geometries in patient specific models are pivotal to accurately predicting stress values and thus indicators of rupture. Methods discussed above can be implemented into patient specific models.

3.3 Comparison of Differing Clinical Groups Using Finite Element Analysis

Fillinger et al. (2002, 2003) were among the first to use finite element analysis to attempt to distinguish between different clinical groups. They succeeded whereby in both studies significant differences in predicted peak stress values were found between AAAs that ruptured and those that did not. Interestingly, a significant difference in diameter measurements was not found between the groups in Fillinger et al. (2002). This emphasizes the need for new clinical predictors of AAA rupture.

Vande Geest et al. (2008) also compared ruptured and unruptured AAA using finite element analysis. They found that the predicted stresses were higher in the ruptured group however this difference was not significant. They also compared results using two different constitutive models, one isotropic and one anisotropic. The resulting stresses were found to be significantly higher using the anisotropic model. This confirms that anisotropy can significantly affect the predicted stresses. In addition, peak stress results from the anisotropic model better distinguished the ruptured AAAs from the unruptured (although significance was again not reached). This therefore suggests that using an anisotropic model will provide a better indication of rupture.

Most recently Maier et al. (2010) compared symptomatic and asymptomatic AAAs using finite element analysis (Fig. 3.1(b)). They found a number of parameters which had significant differences between the groups; these included maximum values of wall displacement, strain, stress and rupture potential index (RPI). RPI had the most significant difference. RPI is defined as a ratio of local wall stress to local wall strength (Vande Geest et al., 2006); a locally varying wall strength measure is calculated through a combination of local thrombus thickness, local AAA diameter, AAA family history, and gender. Since material failure occurs when stress exceeds strength, it is logical that the inclusion of material strength in an indicator will enhance its predictive capacity. A measure similar to RPI could also be a useful tool in carotid plaque studies, however to the authors' knowledge one has yet to be created. The RPI could be further enhanced if locally varying structural information on the wall was available. As discussed in Sect. 3.2.1, the use of arterial DT-MRI in *in vivo* studies may provide this (Flamini et al., 2010).

Li et al. (2007, 2008) compared symptomatic and asymptomatic carotid plaques. Using cross-sectional 2D simulations they found that the predicted stresses were significantly higher in the symptomatic group. By comparing histological results with finite element analyses they also confirmed that rupture occurred at regions of peak stress, this usually occurred in a region known as the plaque shoulders. The shoulders of the plaque are the plaque edges, where there is a sharp reduction in plaque thickness. Li et al. (2008) observed that there was high lumen curvature at this location. This led them to the interesting finding that the maximum values of curvature in each model were significantly higher in the symptomatic group. Teng et al. (2010, 2011) confirmed using similar 2D analyses that the location of maximum plaque stress and maximum lumen curvature were likely to coincide in the plaque shoulder region.

Sadat et al. (2010, 2011) were also able to distinguish between clinical groups using 2D analyses. They found that peak stresses were higher in symptomatic plaques compared to asymptomatic. Within the symptomatic group, patients who experienced recurrent transient ischemic attacks had higher predicted peak stresses compared to those who had just one single event (Sadat et al., 2011). Gao et al. (2011) used 3D fluid structure interaction simulations to compare symptomatic and asymptomatic carotid plaques (Fig. 3.1(a)). While the simulations were considerably more complex than those in Li et al. (2007, 2008) or Sadat et al. (2010, 2011), results were similar to those observed therein. Peak stress was found to be significantly higher in symptomatic plaque and in 85 % of models peak stress occurred at the plaque shoulders.

The above studies all have considerable limitations. The arterial residual stresses discussed in Sect. 3.2.2 are neglected in each of them. Li et al. (2007, 2008) and Sadat et al. (2010, 2011) presented 2D studies. All but one of the studies assumed isotropic material properties. Every additional level of complexity (e.g. material anisotropy, residual stresses, fluid structure interaction, RPI) requires additional inputs into the model. Each of these inputs has a varying degree of accuracy. Consider for example, the use of an anisotropic material model. This requires the definition of preferred material orientations (fiber directions). While the schemes discussed in Sect. 3.2.1 can give a good estimate of these fiber directions *in vivo* they are by no means 100 % accurate. Therefore a balance needs to be found, where the inclusion of an additional input will increase the accuracy and thus predictive capacity of a model without significantly undermining its precision or reproducibility. The above models have stuck such a balance. Their predicted values of stress (and RPI) may have varying degrees of accuracy from the true values *in vivo* however they contain the required precision to differentiate between clinical groups and thus provide useful indicators of plaque or aneurysm disruption.

3.4 Geometric Clinical Indicators

While the finite element method can provide an excellent predictive tool as discussed above, it requires a considerable degree of complexity. Automation of the processes required to predict stresses from patient specific imaging is a difficult challenge. For this reason it has yet to be fully incorporated into a clinical environment. It may be more beneficial, therefore, to use results from current patient specific finite element studies to create simpler alternatives to the indicators used in these studies. These analogues could then be more easily introduced into a clinical setting. Since it has been observed that areas of peak stress coincide with areas of high curvature, specific measures of curvature may provide these alternative indicators.

Several studies have defined measures of AAA curvature (Doyle et al., 2009; Georgakarakos et al., 2010; Giannoglou et al., 2006; Martufi et al., 2009). Giannoglou et al. (2006) found that mean centerline curvature was a significant predictor of peak wall stress in a study of 39 patients while Georgakarakos et al. (2010) reported that centerline tortuosity was found to be significantly correlated with peak wall stress in 19 AAAs. As discussed above, high peak stresses can cause plaque disruption and aneurysm rupture. Thus the measures of curvature reported in the above studies may provide indications of vulnerability in patients, however this was not specifically considered in these studies.

Shum et al. (2010b) used curvature measures defined by Martufi et al. (2009) to study the differences between ruptured and unruptured AAA. They found that two measures of surface irregularity (GLN and MLN, the L_2 norms of Gaussian and mean curvature respectively) were found to be significantly higher in the ruptured group and thus could be used as an indication of rupture. These measures gave a total figure of surface irregularity for the entire AAA rather than giving a maximum value. The link, therefore, between locations of peak stress and maximum curvature were not studied. Since high stresses occur in regions of high curvature (Sacks et al., 1999; Vorp et al., 1998) a measure of maximum curvature may too provide a useful indicator of rupture.

As discussed in Sect. 3.3, a number of carotid studies have shown that the shoulder region of a plaque is prone to rupture due to the high stresses which occur there (Li et al., 2008; Sadat et al., 2010; Teng et al., 2011). The shoulder occurs at the plaque edges where the thickness of the plaque reduces sharply, there is therefore a mismatch in the curvature of the lumen and that of the plaque artery interface. In a perfectly symmetrical plaque the difference in curvature between lumen and outer plaque boundary is constant (dependent on the ratio of radii), however in a typical asymmetric plaque this difference will spike at the plaque shoulders. This measure was defined in Creane et al. (2010) as $k_\delta = k_l - k_o$, a 2D measure of lumen curvature, k_l, minus that of the outer plaque boundary, k_o. The curvature at each mesh node on the lumen is calculated and can be compared with a corresponding mesh node on the outer plaque boundary through the use of a structured mesh (Fig. 3.4). This measure differs from that defined by Li et al. (2008) or Teng et al. (2010) simply by the inclusion of the outer plaque boundary curvature, k_o. Through outward remodeling of the vessel wall during plaque growth it is possible that the lumen cross-section will remain relatively circular—in this case a measure of lumen curvature alone will not detect the plaque shoulders yet stress concentrations will remain due to the asymmetry. This is not the case when using k_δ as the asymmetry of the plaque will cause k_l to differ from k_o at the plaque shoulders and cause a spike in k_δ (Fig. 3.4). k_δ was calculated at each cross-section of finite element meshes from 12 plaques. Creane et al. (2010) found that regions of peak stress and maximum k_δ coincided. The maximum value of k_δ was also significantly higher in symptomatic plaques compared to asymptomatic plaques.

Li et al. (2008), Teng et al. (2010) and Creane et al. (2010) all used 2D measures of curvature. A diseased carotid bifurcation is a complex 3D geometry and therefore axial curvature will also have an effect on the stress distribution and risk of rupture. We present here a 3D analog of the k_δ measure defined in Creane et al. (2010). To study its utility 16 patient specific finite element models of stenosed carotid bifurcations were extracted from CTA imaging data of eight patients using the same methods described in Creane et al. (2010). Each patient had a symptomatic carotid plaque and a contralateral asymptomatic carotid plaque. The maximum principal curvature at each node on the lumen and outer plaque surfaces was calculated as follows.

Firstly the surface normal was estimated at each surface node. This is achieved by finding the unit normal which best fits each surface quadrilateral connected to the node (using orthogonal distance regression). The nodal surface normal is then given by a weighted average of each quadrilateral normal where the weight is the reciprocal of each quadrilateral's area. The normal curvature κ_n of a discrete surface at a node P in the direction of a neighboring node Q can be estimated by (3.6) where N is the unit surface normal.

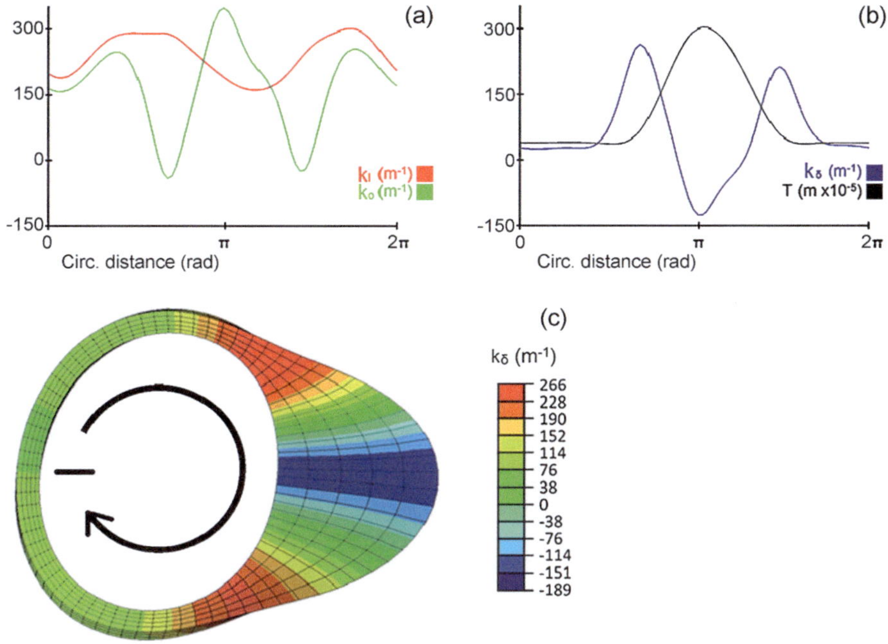

Fig. 3.4 Inner (*red*) and outer (*green*) plaque curvature k_I and k_o respectively. (**b**) The curvature measure $k_\delta = k_I - k_o$ (*blue*) and the thickness of the plaque T (*black*). (**c**) Contour of k_δ on circumferential cross-section—note k_δ is radially constant. See Creane et al. (2010) for further details

$$\kappa_n = \frac{2N \cdot (Q - P)}{\|(Q - P)\|^2} \tag{3.6}$$

There is a normal surface curvature κ_n in any tangential direction to the surface at node P. Thus on a discrete surface, the normal curvature can be estimated in the direction of any neighboring node. Using these normal curvatures, the Weingarten map at P can be calculated and thus the principal curvatures and invariants (mean and Gaussian curvature) can be estimated. There have been many schemes proposed to calculate these variables, we follow that originally proposed by Chen and Schmitt (1992) and adapted in Hameiri and Shimshoni (2003).

We define an arbitrary tangent T that creates an angle $\widehat{\theta}$ with the maximum principal curvature direction T_1. The principal curvatures κ_1 and κ_2 can then be related to any normal curvature κ_n measured at an angle θ from the arbitrary tangent T using Euler's formula:

$$\kappa_n = \kappa_1 \cos^2(\theta + \widehat{\theta}) + \kappa_2 \sin^2(\theta + \widehat{\theta}). \tag{3.7}$$

By manipulating (3.7) we can show that:

$$\kappa_n = A\cos^2\theta - 2B\cos\theta\sin\theta + C\sin^2\theta \tag{3.8}$$

where A, B and C are defined by:

$$A = \kappa_1 \cos^2\widehat{\theta} + \kappa_2 \sin^2\widehat{\theta}, \quad (3.9)$$

$$B = (\kappa_1 - \kappa_2)\cos\widehat{\theta}\sin\widehat{\theta}, \quad (3.10)$$

$$C = \kappa_1 \sin^2\widehat{\theta} + \kappa_2 \cos^2\widehat{\theta}. \quad (3.11)$$

Since we can estimate a normal curvature κ_n for each neighboring node on the surface, we can use (3.8) to solve for A, B and C through a least squares solution (typically κ_n is calculated for 8 neighboring nodes). The principal curvatures and $\widehat{\theta}$ are then calculated using:

$$\kappa_{1,2} = \frac{1}{2}\left(A + C \pm \sqrt{(A-C)^2 + 4B^2}\right), \quad (3.12)$$

$$\widehat{\theta} = \frac{1}{2}\tan^{-1}\left(\frac{2B}{A-C}\right). \quad (3.13)$$

The Mean H and Gaussian K curvatures are the trace/2 and determinant of the Weingarten map respectively and thus can be defined in terms of the principal curvatures by:

$$H = \frac{(\kappa_1 + \kappa_2)}{2}; \qquad K = \kappa_1 \kappa_2. \quad (3.14)$$

A number of AAA studies have used measures based on mean or Gaussian curvature to describe wall irregularity (Martufi et al., 2009; Shum et al., 2010a). However we contend that the maximum principal curvature is a more suitable variable for defining such irregularity or asymmetry. Consider for example, a carotid plaque with a high circumferential normal curvature at its shoulders yet with little or no axial curvature in that region. Gaussian curvature K (equation 3.14(b)) would be near zero at this point due to one principal curvature being near zero yet high stresses would remain due to the high circumferential curvature. In the case of mean curvature (equation 3.14(a)), consider a saddle point on an AAA lumen surface. While both principal curvatures may have high magnitudes, the mean curvature may not have a large magnitude as κ_1 and κ_2 have opposite signs. Therefore we propose to use κ_1, the maximum principal curvature of the surface. To create an analogue of the 2D measure k_δ, we calculate κ_1 on both the lumen κ_l and outer plaque surface κ_o of the FE mesh and then define the 3D measure $\kappa_\delta = \kappa_l - \kappa_o$.

If this curvature measure κ_δ is to be used as a simpler alternative to mechanical stress and thus as an indicator of rupture, it needs to fulfill two key criterion. Firstly, it should have peaks in the same location as stress (regions likely to rupture) and second have a higher maximum magnitude in symptomatic/ruptured plaque compared to asymptomatic/unruptured plaque. Figure 3.5 displays contour plots of κ_δ and maximum principal stress σ_1 at 2 symptomatic and 2 asymptomatic carotid bifurcations. It is evident that in each model locations of high κ_δ and high σ_1 coincide. This is replicated in each of the 16 vessels considered, both symptomatic

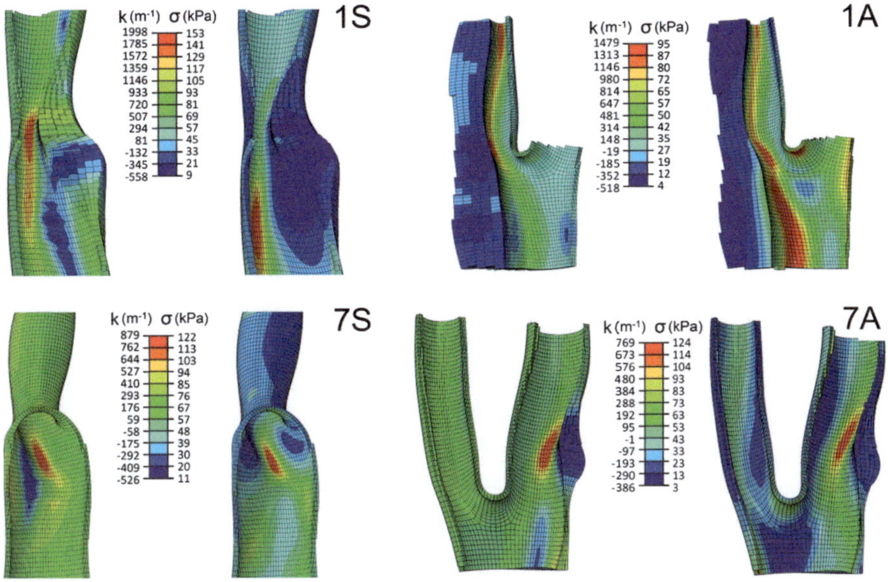

Fig. 3.5 Contours of the 3D curvature measure κ_δ (*left*) and maximum principal stress (*right*) in selected regions of the symptomatic (S) and asymptomatic (A) bifurcation of patients 1 and 7

and asymptomatic. Figure 3.6 plots a bar chart of the maximum κ_δ in each patient's symptomatic and (contralateral) asymptomatic bifurcation. In each patient, the symptomatic plaque has a higher value of κ_δ compared with the asymptomatic plaque. A paired sample Wilcoxon signed rank test establishes that there is a significant difference between the groups.

Interestingly, the predicted values of maximum principal stress σ_1 cannot be distinguished as being higher in the symptomatic group. This is most likely due to a number of limitations in the finite element analysis. The most significant of which is most likely the assumption of a homogeneous plaque. The finite element models were extracted from CTA scans of patients prior to endarterectomy procedures. It is not possible to distinguish individual plaque components using CTA unlike MRI. However, CTA has advantages over MRI. A higher resolution scan can be taken in a shorter period of time which is important when dealing with symptomatic patients. This therefore suggests that in a clinical environment, the measure κ_δ, while only considering geometric properties, may currently be a more practical indicator of plaque vulnerability than predicted stress values from complex finite element analyses derived from longer high-resolution MRI scans.

3.5 Conclusion

Patient specific finite element models of atherosclerotic plaques and aneurysms have provided important insights into their biomechanics, including identification of vul-

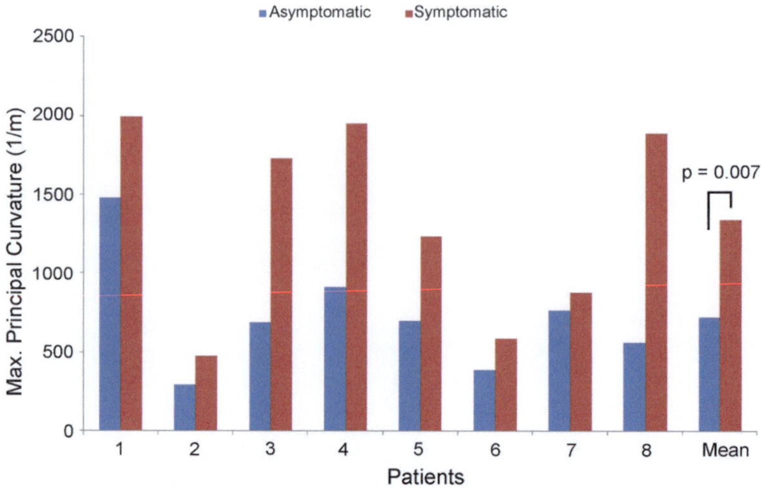

Fig. 3.6 Bar chart of maximum κ_δ in each model. Maximum κ_δ is significantly higher in the symptomatic group than the asymptomatic group ($p = 0.007$)

nerable characteristics. Considerable technical challenges remain in the accurate prediction of *in vivo* stress distributions. These challenges are similar in plaque and aneurysm studies and thus methods used in one category can be transferable to the other. Using the methods discussed in Sect. 3.2 further insights into the mechanics of rupture can be found.

Several studies have been able to distinguish between differing clinical groups (symptomatic, asymptomatic) using finite element analyses. These studies require a trade-off between model complexity and the accuracy of available inputs. These studies show that the finite element method is an excellent predictive tool, however developing patient specific models remains a complex task and has yet to be fully automated. This currently inhibits their use in a clinical environment. We propose that simpler analogues such as measures of curvature may provide more practical indicators in a clinical environment.

3.6 Future Directions

Whilst techniques in patient specific modeling in cardiovascular mechanics have clearly advanced considerably in the last few years, the ultimate aim of such studies is to predict the risk posed by atherosclerotic plaques or AAAs following assessment using non-invasive imaging techniques. The real power of these models will only be fully realized when inter-patient variability can be incorporated into the models, thereby generating similar data to clinical trials where the probability of rupture can be pre-determined. This can be achieved using patient-specific geometry and material properties obtained from non-invasive imaging but also by incorporating variations in patient growth responses, risk factors based on patient history and even genetic information. Ultimately, clinicians may be in a position to not only diagnose vulnerable plaques and AAAs at risk of rupture but to prescribe the optimum pharmacological or interventional technique for these patients and to preclinically test interventional devices such as stents in the patient specific models. By using preclinical patient specific predictive models to obtain the probability of plaque or AAA rupture, based on established rupture indicators such as vessel curvature, stresses and material strength, the long term outcomes for patients may be significantly improved.

Acknowledgements This publication has emanated from research conducted with the financial support of Science Foundation Ireland under Research Frontiers Grant 07/RFP/ENMF660 and grant 07/RFP/ENMF660 TIDA Feasibility 10.

References

Alastrué V, Garía A, Peña E, Rodríguez JF, Martínez MA, Doblaré M (2010) Numerical framework for patient-specific computational modeling of vascular tissue. Int J Numer Methods Biomed Eng 26(1):35–51

Chen X, Schmitt F (1992) Intrinsic surface properties from surface triangulation. In: ECCV'92 proceedings of the second European conference on computer vision. Springer, Berlin, pp 739–743

Creane A, Maher E, Sultan S, Hynes N, Kelly DJ, Lally C (2010) Finite element modeling of diseased carotid bifurcations generated from in vivo computerised tomographic angiography. Comput Biol Med 40(4):419–429

Creane A, Maher E, Sultan S, Hynes N, Kelly DJ, Lally C (2011) Prediction of fiber architecture and adaptation in diseased carotid bifurcations. Biomech Model Mechanobiol 10(6):831–843

Delfino A, Stergiopulos N, Moore J, Meister JJ (1997) Residual strain effects on the stress field in a thick wall finite element model of the human carotid bifurcation. J Biomech 30(8):777–786

Doyle BJ, Callanan A, Burke PE, Grace PA, Walsh MT, Vorp DA, McGloughlin TM (2009) Vessel asymmetry as an additional diagnostic tool in the assessment of abdominal aortic aneurysms. J Vasc Surg 49(2):443–454

Driessen NJB, Wilson W, Bouten CVC, Baaijens FPT (2004) A computational model for collagen fiber remodeling in the arterial wall. J Theor Biol 226(1):53–64

Fillinger MF, Marra SP, Raghavan ML, Kennedy FE (2003) Prediction of rupture risk in abdominal aortic aneurysm during observation: wall stress versus diameter. J Vasc Surg 37(4):724–732

Fillinger MF, Raghavan ML, Marra SP, Cronenwett JL, Kennedy FE (2002) In vivo analysis of mechanical wall stress and abdominal aortic aneurysm rupture risk. J Vasc Surg 36(3):589–597

Finlay HM, Whittaker P, Canham PB (1998) Collagen organization in the branching region of human brain arteries. Stroke 29(8):1595

Flamini V, Kerskens C, Moerman KM, Simms CK, Lally C (2010) Imaging arterial fibers using diffusion tensor imaging—feasibility study and preliminary results. EURASIP J Adv Signal Process 2010:1–14

Gao H, Long Q, Kumar Das S, Halls J, Graves M, Gillard JH, Li Z-Y (2011) Study of carotid arterial plaque stress for symptomatic and asymptomatic patients. J Biomech 44(14):2551–2557

Gasser TC, Ogden RW, Holzapfel GA (2006) Hyperelastic modeling of arterial layers with distributed collagen fiber orientations. J R Soc Interface 3(6):15–35

Gee MW, Förster C, Wall WA (2010) A computational strategy for prestressing patient-specific biomechanical problems under finite deformation. Int J Numer Methods Biomed Eng 26(1):52–72

Georgakarakos E, Ioannou CV, Kamarianakis Y, Papaharilaou Y, Kostas T, Manousaki E, Katsamouris AN (2010) The role of geometric parameters in the prediction of abdominal aortic aneurysm wall stress. Eur J Vasc Endovasc Surg 39(1):42–48

Giannoglou G, Giannakoulas G, Soulis J, Chatzizisis Y, Perdikides T, Melas N, Parcharidis G, Louridas G (2006) Predicting the risk of rupture of abdominal aortic aneurysms by utilizing various geometrical parameters: revisiting the diameter criterion. Angiology 57(4):487–494

Golledge J, Greenhalgh RM, Davies AH (2000) The symptomatic carotid plaque. Stroke 31(3):774–781

Hameiri E, Shimshoni I (2003) Estimating the principal curvatures and the Darboux frame from real 3-d range data. IEEE Trans Syst Man Cybern, Part B, Cybern 33(4):626–637

Hariton I, deBotton G, Gasser TC, Holzapfel GA (2007) Stress-modulated collagen fiber remodeling in a human carotid bifurcation. J Theor Biol 248(3):460–470

Holzapfel GA, Gasser TC, Ogden RW (2000) A new constitutive framework for arterial wall mechanics and a comparative study of material models. J Elast 61(1):1–48

Huang X, Yang C, Yuan C, Liu F, Canton G, Zheng J, Woodard PK, Sicard GA, Tang D (2009) Patient-specific artery shrinkage and 3D zero-stress state in multi-component 3D FSI models for carotid atherosclerotic plaques based on in vivo MRI data. Mol Cell Biomech 6(2):121

Kiousis DE, Gasser TC, Holzapfel GA (2007) A numerical model to study the interaction of vascular stents with human atherosclerotic lesions. Ann Biomed Eng 35(11):1857–1869

Leach JR, Rayz VL, Soares B, Wintermark M, Mofrad MRK, Saloner D (2010) Carotid atheroma rupture observed in vivo and FSI-predicted stress distribution based on pre-rupture imaging. Ann Biomed Eng 38(8):2748–2765

Li Z-Y, Howarth SPS, Tang T, Graves MJ, U-King-Im J, Trivedi RA, Kirkpatrick PJ, Gillard JH (2007) Structural analysis and magnetic resonance imaging predict plaque vulnerability: a study comparing symptomatic and asymptomatic individuals. J Vasc Surg 45(4):768–775

Li ZY, Tang T, U-King-Im J, Graves M, Sutcliffe M, Gillard JH (2008) Assessment of carotid plaque vulnerability using structural and geometrical determinants. Circ J 72(7):1092–1099

Lu J, Zhou X, Raghavan ML (2007) Inverse elastostatic stress analysis in pre-deformed biological structures: demonstration using abdominal aortic aneurysms. J Biomech 40(3):693–696

Ma B, Harbaugh RE, Raghavan ML (2004) Three-dimensional geometrical characterization of cerebral aneurysms. Ann Biomed Eng 32(2):264–273

Maier A, Gee MW, Reeps C, Pongratz J, Eckstein HH, Wall WA (2010) A comparison of diameter, wall stress, and rupture potential index for abdominal aortic aneurysm rupture risk prediction. Ann Biomed Eng 38(10):3124–3134

Martufi G, Di Martino ES, Amon CH, Muluk SC, Finol EA (2009) Three-dimensional geometrical characterization of abdominal aortic aneurysms: image-based wall thickness distribution. J Biomech Eng 131(6):061015

Mortier P, Holzapfel GA, Beule M, Loo D, Taeymans Y, Segers P, Verdonck P, Verhegghe B (2009) A novel simulation strategy for stent insertion and deployment in curved coronary bifurcations: comparison of three drug-eluting stents. Ann Biomed Eng 38(1):88–99

Naghavi M (2003) From vulnerable plaque to vulnerable patient: A call for new definitions and risk assessment strategies: part I. Circulation 108(14):1664–1672

Ohayon J, Dubreuil O, Tracqui P, Le Floc'h S, Rioufol G, Chalabreysse L, Thivolet F, Pettigrew RI, Finet G (2007) Influence of residual stress/strain on the biomechanical stability of vulnerable coronary plaques: potential impact for evaluating the risk of plaque rupture. Am J Physiol, Heart Circ Physiol 293(3):H1987–H1996

Pierce DM, Trobin W, Raya JG, Trattnig S, Bischof H, Glaser C, Holzapfel GA (2010) DT-MRI based computation of collagen fiber deformation in human articular cartilage: a feasibility study. Ann Biomed Eng 38(7):2447–2463

Raghavan M, Ma B, Fillinger MF (2006) Non-invasive determination of zero-pressure geometry of arterial aneurysms. Ann Biomed Eng 34(9):1414–1419

Rhodin JAG (1980) Architecture of the vessel wall. In: Bohr DF, Somlyo AD, Sparks HV (eds) The cardiovascular system. Handbook of physiology, vol 2. Am Physiol Soc, Bethesda, pp 1–31

Rissland P, Alemu Y, Einav S, Ricotta J, Bluestein D (2009) Abdominal aortic aneurysm risk of rupture: patient-specific FSI simulations using anisotropic model. J Biomech Eng 131(3):031001

Rodríguez JF, Martufi G, Doblaré M, Finol EA (2009) The effect of material model formulation in the stress analysis of abdominal aortic aneurysms. Ann Biomed Eng 37(11):2218–2221

Rodríguez JF, Ruiz C, Doblaré M, Holzapfel GA (2008) Mechanical stresses in abdominal aortic aneurysms: influence of diameter, asymmetry, and material anisotropy. J Biomech Eng 130(2):021023

Rowe AJ, Finlay HM, Canham PB (2003) Collagen biomechanics in cerebral arteries and bifurcations assessed by polarizing microscopy. J Vasc Res 40(4):406–415

Sacks MS, Vorp DA, Raghavan M, Federle MP, Webster MW (1999) In vivo three-dimensional surface geometry of abdominal aortic aneurysms. Ann Biomed Eng 27(4):469–479

Sadat U, Teng Z, Young VE, Graves MJ, Gaunt ME, Gillard JH (2011) High-resolution magnetic resonance imaging-based biomechanical stress analysis of carotid atheroma: a comparison of single transient ischaemic attack, recurrent transient ischaemic attacks, non-disabling stroke and asymptomatic patient groups. Eur J Vasc Endovasc Surg 41(1):83–90

Sadat U, Teng Z, Young VE, Walsh SR, Li ZY, Graves MJ, Varty K, Gillard JH (2010) Association between biomechanical structural stresses of atherosclerotic carotid plaques and subsequent ischaemic cerebrovascular events—a longitudinal in vivo magnetic resonance imaging-based finite element study. Eur J Vasc Endovasc Surg 40(4):485–491

Schaar JA, Muller JE, Falk E, Virmani R, Fuster V, Serruys PW, Colombo A, Stefanadis C, Ward Casscells S, Moreno PR (2004) Terminology for high-risk and vulnerable coronary artery plaques. Eur Heart J 25(12):1077

Shum J, DiMartino ES, Goldhammer A, Goldman DH, Acker LC, Patel G, Ng JH, Martufi G, Finol EA (2010a) Semiautomatic vessel wall detection and quantification of wall thickness in computed tomography images of human abdominal aortic aneurysms. Med Phys 37(2):638

Shum J, Xu A, Chatnuntawech I, Finol EA (2010b) A framework for the automatic generation of surface topologies for abdominal aortic aneurysm models. Ann Biomed Eng 39(1):249–259

Tang D, Teng Z, Canton G, Hatsukami TS, Dong L, Huang X, Yuan C (2009) Local critical stress correlates better than global maximum stress with plaque morphological features linked to atherosclerotic plaque vulnerability: an in vivo multi-patient study. Biomed Eng 8(1):15

Teng Z, Sadat U, Ji G, Zhu C, Young VE, Graves MJ, Gillard JH (2011) Lumen irregularity dominates the relationship between mechanical stress condition, fibrous-cap thickness, and lumen curvature in carotid atherosclerotic plaque. J Biomech Eng 133(3):034501

Teng Z, Sadat U, Li Z, Huang X, Zhu C, Young VE, Graves MJ, Gillard JH (2010) Arterial luminal curvature and fibrous-cap thickness affect critical stress conditions within atherosclerotic plaque: an in vivo MRI-based 2D finite-element study. Ann Biomed Eng 38(10):3096–3101

Vande Geest JP, Schmidt DE, Sacks MS, Vorp DA (2008) The effects of anisotropy on the stress analyses of patient-specific abdominal aortic aneurysms. Ann Biomed Eng 36(6):921–932

Vande Geest JP, Wang DHJ, Wisniewski SR, Makaroun MS, Vorp DA (2006) Towards a noninvasive method for determination of patient-specific wall strength distribution in abdominal aortic aneurysms. Ann Biomed Eng 34(7):1098–1106

Vorp DA (2007) Biomechanics of abdominal aortic aneurysm. J Biomech 40(9):1887–1902

Vorp DA, Raghavan M, Webster MW (1998) Mechanical wall stress in abdominal aortic aneurysm: influence of diameter and asymmetry. J Vasc Surg 27(4):632–639

Wu EX, Wu Y, Nicholls JM, Wang J, Liao S, Zhu S, Lau C-P, Tse H-F (2007) MR diffusion tensor imaging study of postinfarct myocardium structural remodeling in a porcine model. Magn Reson Med 58(4):687–695

Yang C, Bach RG, Zheng J, Ei Naqa I, Woodard PK, Teng Z, Billiar K, Tang D (2009) In vivo IVUS-based 3-D fluid–structure interaction models with cyclic bending and anisotropic vessel properties for human atherosclerotic coronary plaque mechanical analysis. IEEE Trans Biomed Eng 56(10):2420–2428

Zhang S, Crow JA, Yang X, Chen J, Borazjani A, Mullins KB, Chen W, Cooper RC, McLaughlin RM, Liao J (2010) The correlation of 3D DT-MRI fiber disruption with structural and mechanical degeneration in porcine myocardium. Ann Biomed Eng 38(10):3084–3095

Chapter 4
Modeling the Human Heart Under Acute Ischemia

E.A. Heidenreich, J.M. Ferrero, and J.F. Rodríguez

Abstract Ventricular tachycardia and ventricular fibrillation are known to be two types of cardiac arrhythmias that usually take place during acute ischemia and frequently lead to sudden death. In this work, a methodology for the in-silico study of the regionally acute ischemic heart is presented. The chapter describes the mathematical formulation of the electrophysiology of the heart. A numerical scheme for the efficient numerical solution of the mathematical problem is also given. Along with the mathematical basis for the solution of the electrophysiology problem, the highly electrophysiological detailed action potential model for human proposed by ten Tusscher (Am J Physiol Heart Circ Physiol 291:1088–1100, 2006) has been adapted to make it suitable for modeling ischemic conditions (hyperkalemia, hipoxia, and acidic conditions). At this step, a formulation of the ATP-sensitive K^+ current has been introduced into the existing model and the resulting model has been subjected to ischemic conditions. The results show that the three components of ischemia decrease the action potential duration (APD) as well as the conduction velocity, while effective refractory period (ERP) depicts a non-monotonic behavior. The modified action potential model was implemented on a 3-D geometrically and anatomically accurate regionally ischemic human heart. The ischemic region was located in the anterior side of the left ventricle mimicking the occlusion of the circumflex artery. Realistic heterogeneity and fiber anisotropy were considered in the model. The model predicts the generation of figure-of-eight re-entries which cross the central ischemic zone formed in the epicardial surface due to the longer refractory period of the midmyocardial layers. Also, focal activity experimentally

J.F. Rodríguez (✉)
Aragón Institute of Engineering Research (I3A), University of Zaragoza, María de Luna s/n, Edif. Betancourt, 50018 Zaragoza, Spain
e-mail: jfrodrig@unizar.es

E.A. Heidenreich
Engineering School, Universidad Lomas de Zamora, Ruta 4, Km 2. Lomas de Zamora, CP 1832, Buenos Aires, Argentina

J.M. Ferrero
Departmento de Ingeniería Electrónica, Universidad Politécnica de Valencia, Camino de Vera S/N, 46022 Valencia, Spain

B. Calvo, E. Peña (eds.), *Patient-Specific Computational Modeling*,
Lecture Notes in Computational Vision and Biomechanics 5,
DOI 10.1007/978-94-007-4552-0_4, © Springer Science+Business Media Dordrecht 2012

observed in the epicardium caused by re-entrant wavefronts propagating in the mid-myocardium that re-emerge in the heart surface was found in the simulations.

4.1 Introduction

The study of the electrical activity of the heart has interested the scientific community for more than hundred years, since Einthoven introduced, in 1903, the dipole model to explain the electrocardiogram (ECG), helping, therefore, to understand the origin of myocardial activation. This seminal work inspired important research as the ground breaking work by Hodgkin and Huxley (1952). In their work Hodking and Huxley proposed the first mathematical model to explain the action potential of an excitable cell giving origin to a the new discipline of cellular electrophysiology modeling. The original model proposed by Hodking and Huxley has been extended to a number of species (Beeler and Reuter, 1977; Carro et al., 2011; DiFrancesco and Noble, 1985; Grandi et al., 2010; Luo and Rudy, 1994, 1991; O'Hara et al., 2011; ten Tusscher et al., 2004). These complex models of action potential can be incorporated to models of the cardiac tissue used to build a mathematical model of the whole heart. In this regard, the tissue model proposed by Tung (1978) assumes that at any point of the cardiac tissue the intracellular and extracellular space coexist. This assumption leads to the well known bidomain model of the cardiac tissue which relates the extracellular potential with the transmembrane potential responsible for the action potential of the cell. Therefore, coupling the electrical activity at cellular level with the propagation of the electrical signal at tissue level. The bidomain equation considers the tissue as orthotropic, in which the conduction velocity along the fiber direction is faster than the velocity in the transversal direction to the fiber. It is important to point out however, that the bidomain model is costly to solve numerically. This characteristic have lead to proposed simplified models of the tissue that assume the extracellular medium to have infinity conductivity in what is known as the mono-domain model (Keener and Sneyd, 1998). Therefore, the electrophysiology problem consist of the coupled solution of a linear partial differential equation, describing electric conduction, with a nonlinear stiff system of ordinary differential equations describing the cellular ionic currents. The multiscale nature of the ionic current (time constants for the different kinetics ranging from 0.1 to 500 msec) makes difficult the solution of the reaction-diffusion problem, requiring temporal resolution of 0.01 ms and a spatial resolution of 0.2 mm for highly accurate simulations (Colli Franzone et al., 2006; Qu and Garfinkel, 1999; ten Tusscher and Panfilov, 2006). These requirements lead to models with more than 2.0×10^7 degrees of freedom and more than 8×10^4 time steps for simulating a single heart beat of normal activity.

Ventricular tachycardia and fibrillation are among the major cause of sudden cardiac death (Rubart and Zipes, 2005). Even though these arrhythmias arise from different clinical conditions, ischemic heart disease is the foremost perpetrator among them. During ischemia, the delivery of substrates, primarily oxygen, to the myocardium stops, resulting in a progressive deterioration of the electric activity in

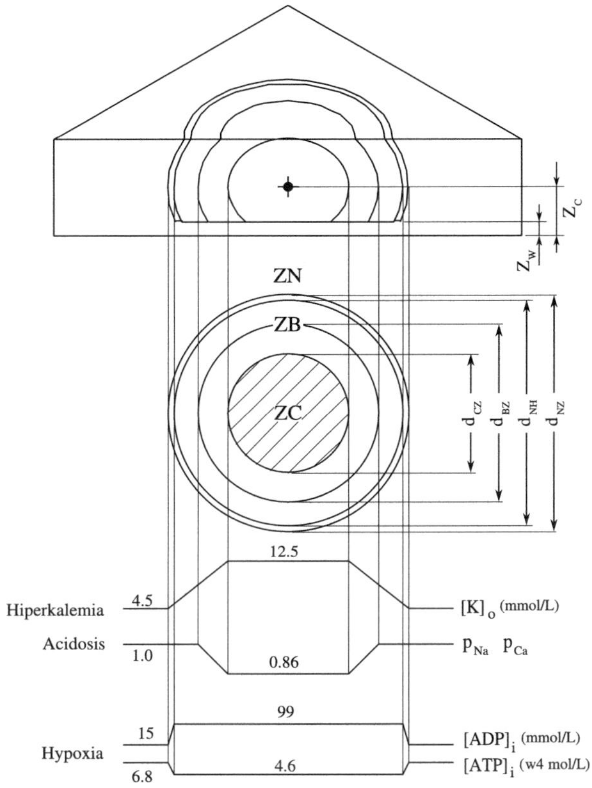

Fig. 4.1 A 3D representation of an acute ischemic tissue: central zone (CZ), border zone (BZ) and normal zone (NZ), along with the most relevant electrophysiological parameters

the injured region and subsequently to a loss of function and ultimately pump failure (Katz, 2005). Occlusion of the coronary artery, which causes ischemia, is followed by profound metabolic changes in the intracellular and extracellular space of the cardiac tissue. This metabolic changes are mainly hypoxia, increased concentrations of the extracellular, $[K^+]_o$ (hyperkalemia), increased concentrations of intracellular $[Na^+]_i$, and $[Ca^{2+}]_i$, decreased concentration of extracellular $[Na^+]_o$, decrease of intracellular $[ATP]_i$, and acidosis (Carmeliet, 1999; Rodriguez et al., 2006). In addition, the impact of ischemia in the myocardium is characterized with a high degree of heterogeneity. Due to diffusion of ions and metabolites, the core of the tissue suffering from the lack of blood (the central ischemic zone, (CIZ) is surrounded by a border zone (BZ) which comprises changes in electrophysiological properties between the healthy and ischemic regions (Coronel et al., 1988; Coronel, 1994; Janse et al., 1979). These heterogeneities are produced not only intramurally, but also transmurally, in the depth of the ventricular wall (see Fig. 4.1).

From an electrophysiologic point of view, these changes imply alterations in action potential configurations, excitability, conduction velocities, refractive period among others, which enormously favor reentrant activity, and therefore arrhythmias and fibrillation (Ferrero et al., 2003; Janse and Kleber, 1981; Rodriguez et al., 2004). Over the last years, mathematical modeling and computer simulations have been a useful tool in analyzing electrophysiological phenomena. In this particular, one of the major contributions of computer electrophysiology has been in understanding important relations between electrophysiological parameters (Rodriguez et al., 2006). For the ischemic heart, computer models have allowed to address the role of ischemic abnormalities in cardiac electrophysiological behavior (Ferrero et al., 2003). However, most of these simulations have been restricted to 2D (Ferrero et al., 2003; Tice et al., 2005) simulations or 3D simulations of total ischemic heart (Rodriguez et al., 2004). Little work has been carried out in modeling the entire heart subjected to acute ischemic conditions (Weiss et al., 2009). However, in the work by Weiss et al., even though they have accounted for heterogeneities caused by ischemia, their characterization of the action potential under acute ischemic conditions has mostly relied on the model characterized for guinea pigs (Ferrero et al., 1996).

In this work we develop a methodology for in-silico studies of acute regional ischemia in the heart. The proposed framework will be based on the mono domain model for simulating the electrical activity of the heart. The action potential model proposed by ten Tusscher and Panfilov (2006), TP06, will be modified to account for ischemia by incorporating an ATP sensitive Potassium, $I_{K(ATP)}$, current. The ventricular model used in this study was segmented from a diffusion tensor magnetic resonance imaging (DTMRI) dataset acquired at John Hopkins University, Baltimore, MD (Helm, 2005). The ventricle model also includes realistic fiber orientation and transmural, apico-basal, and interventricular electrophysiological heterogeneities.

4.2 Mathematical Model of Heart Electrophysiology

The mathematical model describing the variation of the intracellular potential, V_i, extracellular potential, V_e, and the transmembrane potential, $V = V_e - V_i$, is given by the well known bi-domain model (Tung, 1978)

$$\nabla \cdot (D_i \nabla V) + \nabla \cdot (D_i \nabla V_e) = C_m \frac{\partial V}{\partial t} + J_{ion}(V, \mathbf{u}), \tag{4.1}$$

$$\nabla \cdot (D_i \nabla V) + \nabla \cdot \big((D_i + D_e) \nabla V_e\big) = 0, \tag{4.2}$$

$$\frac{\partial \mathbf{u}}{\partial t} = \mathbf{f}(\mathbf{u}, V, t), \tag{4.3}$$

where D_i and D_e are the intracellular and extracellular symmetric and positive definite conductivity tensors, $J_{ion}(V, \mathbf{u})$ the transmembrane ionic current, $\mathbf{u}(\mathbf{x}, t)$ is a vector of gating variables and concentrations, $\mathbf{f}$ is a vector valued function, and t refers to time. Both, J_{ion} and $\mathbf{f}$ depend on the cellular model used. The boundary conditions associated with this model are

$$\mathbf{n} \cdot (D_i \nabla V + D_i \nabla V_e) = 0, \tag{4.4}$$

$$\mathbf{n} \cdot \nabla (D_e \nabla V_e) = 0, \tag{4.5}$$

where $\mathbf{n}$ is the outward normal.

The bi-domain model is in general difficult to solve and analyze. However, it can be simplified to a single PDE by making assumptions in the conductivity tensors. If equal anisotropy ratios are assumed for D_i and D_e, i.e. $D_e = \lambda D_i$, the bidomain model reduces to what is called the mono-domain model

$$\nabla \cdot (\mathbf{D}\,\nabla V) = C_m \frac{\partial V}{\partial t} + J_{ion}(V, \mathbf{u}), \tag{4.6}$$

$$\frac{\partial \mathbf{u}}{\partial t} = \mathbf{f}(\mathbf{u}, V, t) \tag{4.7}$$

with boundary conditions

$$\mathbf{n} \cdot \nabla(\mathbf{D}\,\nabla V) = 0. \tag{4.8}$$

The monodomain model represents an important simplification of the bi-domain model with important advantages for mathematical analysis and computation, resulting adequate for studying the onset of ischemia in the electric behavior of the heart.

From a mathematical and computational point of view, the electrophysiology problem is the couple solution of a linear partial differential equation, describing electric conduction, with a nonlinear stiff system of ordinary differential equations describing the cellular ionic currents which leads to a nonlinear reaction-diffusion problem. An efficient way of solving (4.6)–(4.8) is by applying the operator splitting technique (Strang, 1968). The operator splitting technique was applied to the monodomain equations in Qu and Garfinkel (1999). The basic steps are summarized in the following.

- **Step 1:** Using $V(t)$ as the initial condition to integrate equation

$$C_m \frac{\partial V}{\partial t} = \nabla \cdot (\mathbf{D}\nabla V), \qquad \text{for } t \in [t, t + \Delta t/2]. \tag{4.9}$$

- **Step 2:** Use the result obtained in Step 1 as the initial conditions to integrate

$$\left.\begin{aligned} C_m \frac{\partial V}{\partial t} &= -I_{ion}(V, \mathbf{u}), \\ \frac{\partial \mathbf{u}}{\partial t} &= \mathbf{f}(\mathbf{u}, V, t), \end{aligned}\right\} \qquad \text{for } t \in [t, t + \Delta t]. \tag{4.10}$$

- **Step 3:** Use the result obtained in Step 2 as the initial condition to integrate

$$C_m \frac{\partial V}{\partial t} = \nabla \cdot (\mathbf{D}\nabla V), \qquad \text{for } t \in [t + \Delta t/2, t + \Delta t]. \tag{4.11}$$

In practice, Steps 1 and 3 can be combined in one, except for the very first increment. Hence, after the first increment, the algorithm only has two steps, Step I corresponding to the integration of the ODEs (Step 2) and Step II corresponding to the integration of the homogeneous parabolic equation (Step 1 and 3).

When performing Step II, the computational domain must be discretized in space by a mesh of either finite elements or finite differences to approximate the dependent variables of the problem, V and $\mathbf{u}$. Hence, after the spatial discretization, the system of partial differential equations (4.9) or (4.11), can be written in matrix notation as

$$\mathbf{M}\dot{\mathbf{V}} + \mathbf{K}\mathbf{V} = \mathbf{0}, \tag{4.12}$$

where $\mathbf{M}$ is the mass matrix associated with $C_m \partial V/\partial t$, and $\mathbf{K}$ is the stiffness matrix associated with $\nabla \cdot (\mathbf{D}\nabla V)$. These matrices are obtained by assembling individual element matrices. Equation (4.12) is called a semidiscrete equation because time is left continuous.

The implicit Euler algorithm can be used to integrate (4.12) in time. Let $\mathbf{V}^k$ denote a vector of the transmembrane potential at each nodal point of the discretized domain (mesh) at time t^k, where k is index of the time step, then at time t^{k+1} we can write

$$\mathbf{M}\frac{\mathbf{V}^{k+1} - \mathbf{V}^k}{\Delta t} + \mathbf{K}\mathbf{V}^{k+1} = \mathbf{0}. \tag{4.13}$$

When using the operator splitting algorithm for solving the monodomain model, (4.6)–(4.8) are solved in two steps. First, the electrophysiological cellular model

$$\mathbf{V}^* = \mathbf{V}^k - \Delta t\, J_{ion}\left(\mathbf{V}^k, \mathbf{u}\right) \tag{4.14}$$

is solved at each mesh point to obtain an intermediate transmembrane potential vector $\mathbf{V}^*$ (Step I). Even though an explicit integration scheme has been used in (4.14), any ODE solver, either implicit or explicit, can be used to calculate $\mathbf{V}^*$. With this intermediate solution at hand, (4.13) becomes

$$\mathbf{M}\frac{\mathbf{V}^{k+1} - \mathbf{V}^*}{\Delta t} = -\mathbf{K}\,\mathbf{V}^{k+1}, \tag{4.15}$$

or alternatively

$$\hat{\mathbf{K}}\mathbf{V}^{k+1} = \hat{\mathbf{b}}, \tag{4.16}$$

where $\hat{\mathbf{K}}$ is everything that multiplies onto $\mathbf{V}^{k+1}$, and $\hat{\mathbf{b}}$ contains the other terms in (4.15). Equation (4.16) is solved for the entire domain to obtained $\mathbf{V}^{k+1}$ (Step II).

Hence, the basic algorithm at time t^{k+1} can be summarized, as:

- **Step I:** Use $\mathbf{V}^k$ as the initial condition to integrate equation (4.14) to obtain $\mathbf{V}^*$.
- **Step II:** Use the result obtained in Step I to solve (4.16) for $\mathbf{V}^{k+1}$.

4.3 Cell Model of Acute Ischemia

Simulation of the ischemic heart requires both, an accurate description of the organ that incorporates its muscular structure and heterogeneity (described in the following sections), and an appropriate model of its electrophysiology. This section is dedicated to the characterization of the mathematical model of action potential (AP) used to performed the numerical simulations of the regional acute ischemic heart. All simulations were performed with a modified version of the ten Tusscher and Panfilov (TP06) model of action potential (ten Tusscher and Panfilov, 2006).

4.3.1 Action Potential Model Characterization Under Ischemic Conditions

A modified version of the ten Tusscher cardiac action potential model (ten Tusscher and Panfilov, 2006) was used in the simulations. The model describes the principal ionic currents through the cardiac cell membrane with high degree of electrophysiological detail for the three types of cardiac cells. The basic model was completed with the formulation of the ATP-sensitive K^+ current ($I_{K(ATP)}$) described by Ferrero et al. (1996). Heterogeneities in the $I_{K(ATP)}$ current were not considered in this study.

The influence of Action potential generation and propagation in one dimension version of the mono domain model (4.6)

$$C_m \frac{\partial V}{\partial t} = -(J_{ion} + J_{stim}) + \frac{\partial}{\partial x}\left(\sigma \frac{\partial V}{\partial x}\right), \tag{4.17}$$

where J_{stim} is the externally applied transmembrane current, and σ is de conductivity of the fiber. A multicellular fiber 4 cm long was considered in the numerical study. For the simulations, the operator splitting technique previously described was implemented. Forward Euler integration with a time step $\Delta t = 0.02$ ms was used for integrating the single cell equation. Implicit Euler with a time step $\Delta t = 0.02$ ms and with a space discretization of $\Delta x = 0.01$ cm was used to integrate the parabolic equation. The conductivity of the tissue was set to $\sigma = 0.0013$ cm^2/s which yields a conduction velocity of 71 cm/s under normal conditions.

Hyperkalemic conditions were simulated by increasing the extracellular K^+ concentration ($[K^+]_o$) from 4.0 mmol/L to different values depending on the degree of hyperkalemia. Hypoxia was simulated by activating $I_{K(ATP)}$ to 0.55 % of its maximum activation value which produced a 50 % reduction of the APD, corresponding to 10 minutes of ischemia (Venkatesh et al., 1992). Acidosis was simulated by varying the maximum conductances of I_{Na} and $I_{\mathrm{Ca}(L)}$ over a wide range, depending on the severity of acidosis (Shaw and Rudy, 1997). No shifting in the potential of the I_{Na} kinetics was considered in this study.

The stimulation protocol consisted on a train of ten basic stimulations (S1) with a cyclic length of 1 s following an extrasystole stimulus (S2) in 1 millisecond steps in order to determine ERP. The APD was measured at the tenth stimulus, and was defined as 90 % of depolarization time and was taken as the average of three cells located at the 50 %, 75 % and 95 % of the length of the strang. The ERP was defined as the shortest S1S2 interval such that the S2 propagated successfully through the

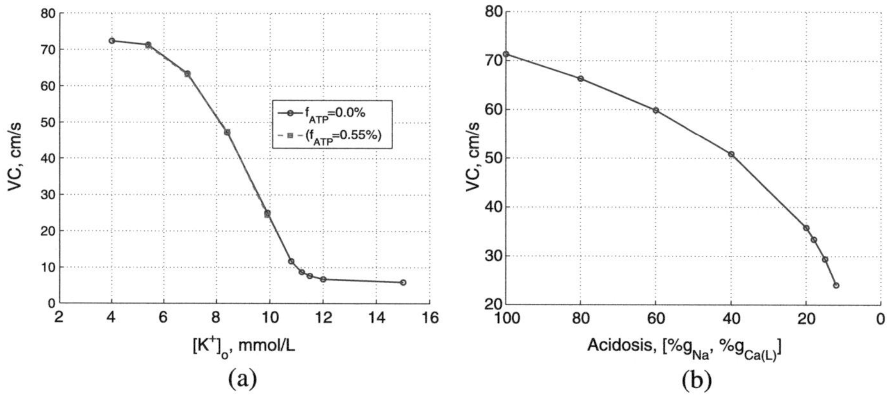

Fig. 4.2 Effect of ischemic conditions on conduction velocity. The three conditions of ischemia were applied with different levels of severity, except for anoxia where only one condition was considered for different levels of hyperkalemia. No supernormal conduction is observed under hyperkalemic conditions. While hyperkalemia and acidosis very much change the conduction velocity, anoxia seems to have no influence on conduction velocity under hyperkalemic conditions

fiber. The basic and test stimuli consisted on rectangular pulses 3 ms in duration and 1.5 times the diastolic threshold in amplitude. Diastolic threshold was determined as follows. For a given $[K^+]_o$ value, the model was first stabilized until when the product of the gates $h \cdot j$ reached the 99 % of the steady state value $h_\infty \cdot j_\infty$. Once the model had reached steady-state conditions, an stimulation current was applied at the left end of the cable. Diastolic threshold was defined as the minimum stimulation current required in order to propagate an action potential in the cable.

Figure 4.2 shows the computed conduction velocity for the condition of elevated $[K^+]_o$, elevated $[K^+]_o$ and anoxia (Fig. 4.2a), and acidosis (Fig. 4.2b). The figure demonstrates that the three components of ischemia decrease the conduction velocity. Elevated concentrations of $[K^+]_o$ has the greatest influence on reducing conduction. However, the model does not show "supernormal conduction" near physiologic values as has been observed in other cardiac cell models (Shaw and Rudy, 1997). The results also show that anoxia does not very much affect the conduction velocity under hyperkalemic conditions, but blocking occurs at lower $[K^+]_o$ values ($[K^+]_o > 10$ mmol/L). Under hyperkalemic conditions, conduction block occurred at $[K^+]_o > 15$ mmol/L. Acidosis monotonically decreases conduction. At a 60 % reduction of I_{Na} and $I_{\mathrm{Ca}(L)}$, conduction velocity decreases 28.7 % from 71.3 cm/s to 50.9 cm/s, causing conduction block at 90 % reduction of both I_{Na} and $I_{\mathrm{Ca}(L)}$.

Figure 4.3 shows the results for the APD and ERP for the epicardial cell only (a similar behavior was observed for endocardial and midyocardial cells). Figure 4.3(a) shows the APD of the last basic beat and ERP as hyperkalemia increases. Solid lines correspond to conditions of increasing hyperkalemia only ($I_{K(ATP)} = 0$), while dashed lines correspond to conditions of hyperkalemia + hypoxia. When considering hypoxia, the fraction of open $I_{K(ATP)}$ channels, f_{ATP}, was set to 0.55 % which causes a 50 % reduction in the APD. Figure 4.3(b) shows the APD and ERP under acidic conditions.

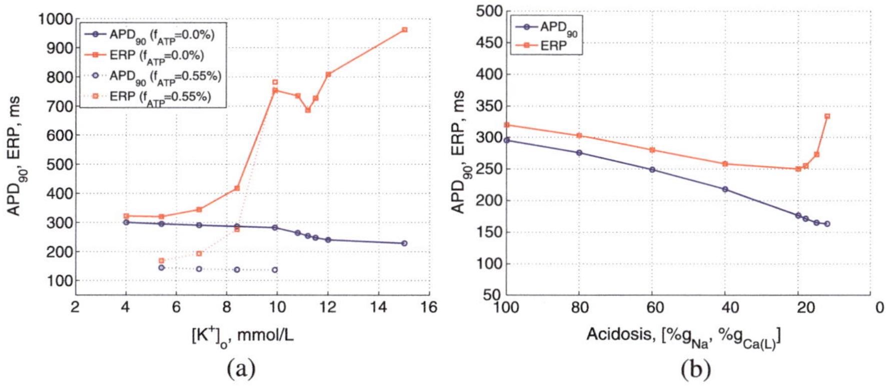

Fig. 4.3 (**a**) Action potential duration (APD) of the last basic beat and effective refractory period (ERP) for different $[K^+]_o$ values and different cell types. *Solid lines* correspond to normoxia and *dashed lines* correspond to hypoxia. (**b**) Action potential duration (APD) of the last basic beat and effective refractory period (ERP) for different acidic conditions

Results demonstrate that all components of ischemia cause postrepolarization refractoriness in the TP06 model. For hyperkalemic and hyperkalemic+hypoxic conditions, the difference between ERP and APD remains almost constant for $[K^+]_o \leq 7$ mmol/L, with this difference increasing rapidly for $[K^+]_o > 7$ mmol/L. For values of $[K^+]_o < 8.4$ mmol/L, the absolute difference between ERP and APD is not significantly different in hyperkalemia and hyperkalemia + hypoxia. However, for $[K^+]_o$ close to 10.0 mmol/L, the ERP value for hyperkalemia + hypoxia overtakes the value in hyperkalemia, with total block occurring in the hypoxic tissue for $[K^+]_o > 10$ mmol/L. For the hyperkalemic tissue, a highly nonlinear behavior is observed for $[K^+]_o > 10$ mmol/L. For acidic conditions, the results show an important influence of acidosis on ERP for reductions in I_{Na} and $I_{\mathrm{Ca}(L)}$ above 60 %, from which the absolute difference between ERP and APD increases monotonically until reaching the blocking value of 90 % reduction.

4.3.2 *Adapting the Action Potential Model to Ischemic Conditions. The $I_{K(ATP)}$ Current*

One of the most important aspects in simulating the ischemic heart is to incorporate the ATP sensitive potassium current $I_{K(ATP)}$, a dormant depolarization current under physiological conditions that is activated under ischemic condition (Ferrero et al., 1996). K_{ATP} ion channels have been investigated in different regions of the heart, i.e., atria and ventricle, the sinoatrial (SA) and the atrioventricular (AV) node, on different species (Furukawa et al., 1991; Light et al., 1999; Nichols et al., 1991; Venkatesh et al., 1992). However, very little experimental data regarding the $I_{K(ATP)}$ current for different tissue layers within the ventricle is available. Furukawa et al.

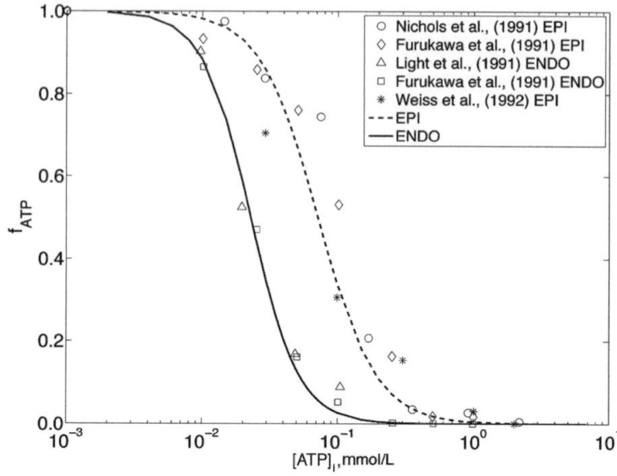

Fig. 4.4 Fraction of K_{ATP} channels for different cell models and different animal species. Lines have been added to facilitate visualization

(1991) has characterized K_{ATP} channels in isolated endocardial and epicardial cells of cats. Experiments by Furukawa et al. suggest that the open probability of K_{ATP} channels reduces with the intracellular ATP concentration, $[ATP]_i$, for both cell types. However, $[ATP]_i$ concentration responsible for a 50 % block of K_{ATP} channels is approximately 4 times less for endocardial cells than for epicardial cells. Similar observations have been done by Light et al. (1999) in rabbit, and by Nichols et al. (1991) and Venkatesh et al. (1992) in epicardial cells of guinea pig.

Figure 4.4 shows experimental results corresponding to the open probability of K_{ATP} channels, f_{ATP}, for different cell types and different animal species. This figure shows a greater correlation between data corresponding to the same cell type independent of the animal specie. In other words, data suggests a low specificity to animal specie but a high specificity to cell type. We have adopted this hypothesis to incorporate the $I_{K(ATP)}$ model by Ferrero et al. (1996) originally formulated for guinea pig, to the TP06 model for human. A similar hypothesis has also been adopted by Michailova et al. (2007) in developing an heterogeneous model of $I_{K(ATP)}$ for rabbit.

The procedure followed consisted on modifying the original formulation for the f_{ATP} proposed by Ferrero et al. (1996) in order to fit the data from Fig. 4.4 for different cell types. The maximal conductance for the $I_{K(ATP)}$ was modified on order to adjust the experimental observations on the action potential duration by Furukawa et al. (1991). In words, a 50 % reduction in the APD under conditions of hypoxia and hyperkalemia for the epicardium, and a 10 % reduction under the same conditions for the endocardium. For the mid-miocardium, there are no experimental data available regarding the behavior of K_{ATP} channels. For this case, we have adjusted the value of f_{ATP} such that the same reduction in APD as for epicardial cells was obtained without modifying the maximal conductance of the channel. Gima and Rudy (2002) and Michailova et al. (2007) have assumed that the midmyocardium half-maximal saturation constant (K_m in (4.19)) is $\approx$50 % that in epicardial cells. Finally, for all cell models, for physiological values of $[ATP]_i$ and $[ADP]_i$, the APD

Table 4.1 Extracellular potassium and intracellular ADP and ATP concentrations defining physiologic and ischemic conditions for the simulations

Condition	$[K^+]_o$ mmol/L	$[ATP]_i$ mmol/L	$[ADP]_i$ µmol/L
Normoxia	5.4	6.8	15.0
Ischemia	9.9	4.6	99.0

and the resting potential should not be affected by the presence of the $I_{K(ATP)}$ current in the AP model.

The $I_{K(ATP)}$ current has been formulated as (Ferrero et al., 1996)

$$I_{K(ATP)} = g_0 \left(\frac{[K^+]_o}{5.4} \right)^{0.24} f_M f_N f_T f_{ATP}(V - E_K), \tag{4.18}$$

where g_0 is the maximum channel conductance in the absence of Na^+, Mg^{2+} and ATP, f_M, f_N, f_T are correction factors, f_{ATP} is the fraction of opened channels, V the transmembrane potential, and E_K is the inversion potential of the channel. The maximum channel conductance and the fraction of opened channels, f_{ATP}, have been modified with respect to its original formulation

$$f_{ATP} = \frac{1}{1 + ([ATP]_i / K_m)^H}, \tag{4.19}$$

where $[ATP]_i$ is the intracellular concentration of ATP, and K_m (in mmol/L) and H (–) are given as

$$K_m = \alpha\left(35.8 + 17.9[ADP]_i^{0.256}\right), \tag{4.20}$$

$$H = 1.3 + 0.74\beta \exp\left(-0.09[ADP]_i\right), \tag{4.21}$$

where $[ADP]_i$ is the intracellular concentration of ADP in µmol/L, and α, β fitting parameters that account for the cellular heterogeneity. Parameters α and β where identified by fitting experimental data available for different animal models from Fig. 4.4. To adjust g_0, 10 stimuli at a basic cycle length (BCL) of 1000 ms were applied to an isolated cell. The APD at the last stimulus was measured under physiological and pathological conditions. The variation in APD obtained between the pathological and physiological conditions was used to adjusted g_0. Table 4.1 shows the adopted $[K^+]_o$, $[ATP]_i$ and $[ADP]_i$ values to define physiologic and ischemic conditions for fitting g_0.

Table 4.2 summarizes the parameters identified in the fitting process. The table also shows the obtained APD value under physiologic and ischemic conditions defined in Table 4.1, in addition to the APD value obtained when the $I_{K(ATP)}$ current remains inactive. The APD variation between normal and hypoxic conditions given in Table 4.2 are in good agreement with experimental observations by Furukawa et al. (1991).

Figure 4.5 shows the variation of f_{ATP} with $[ATP]_i$ for $[ADP]_i = 15.0$ µmol/L for different cell types along with experimental values obtained in different animal species.

Table 4.2 Value of the parameters for the $I_{K(ATP)}$ current adapted to the ten Tusscher model for different cell types. Also shown, the APD under physiologic and ischemic conditions

Cell type	Parameter			$I_{K(ATP)}$ active		$I_{K(ATP)}$ inactive
	g_0 mS	α –	β –	APD_{90}^{Nor} ms	APD_{90}^{Isq} ms	APD_{90}^{Nor} ms
EPI	2.01	1.0	6.0	294.2	148.6	294.6
ENDO	1.92	0.32	6.0	294.0	257.4	294.0
MID	2.01	0.86	6.0	374.8	189.2	375.2

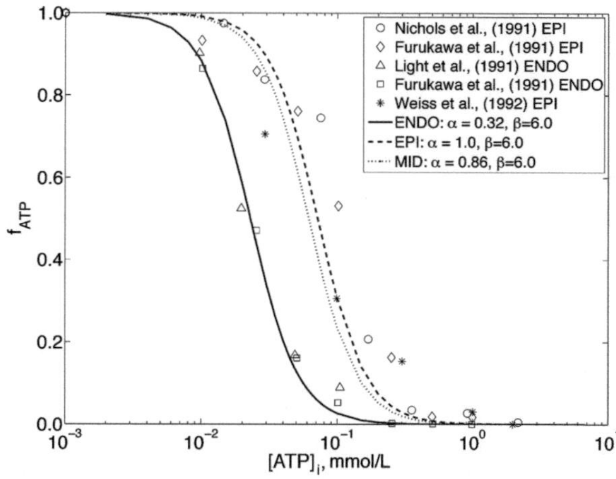

Fig. 4.5 Fraction of open channels for different cell types for the adjusted model (*solid lines*). *Symbols* represent experimental values for different cell types in different species

4.4 A Model of the Heart

This section is dedicated to describe an accurate model of a bi-ventricular heart considering the muscular structure and electrophysiological heterogeneity under physiologic and acute ischemic conditions.

4.4.1 Geometry and Fiber Directions

The geometry of the bi-ventricular heart (the atria has not been considered in the model) and the orientation of the muscle fibers were obtained from diffusion tensor magnetic resonance imaging (DT-MRI), from images acquire at John Hopkins University (Helm, 2005). From the segmented image, a regular volumetric mesh was constructed with hexahedral elements and a resolution of 0.5 mm × 0.5 mm × 0.5 mm, which gave rise to 1.43 million nodes and 1.29 million hexahedra.

The structure of the myocardium plays an important roll in the electrical and mechanical activity of the heart. The distribution of the fiber orientation of the cardiac muscle dictates the correct activation patterns in the healthy heart (Roberts et al.,

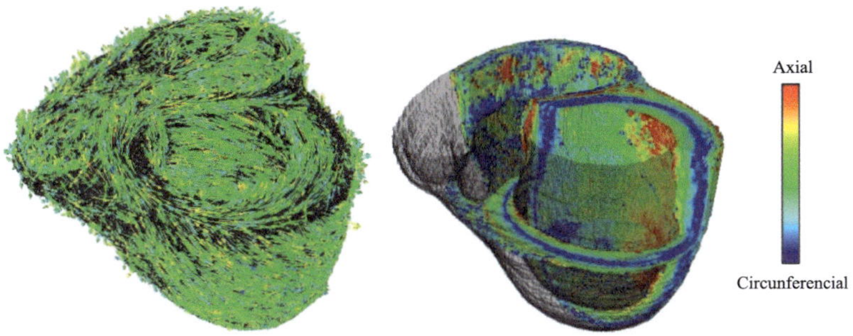

(a) (b)

Fig. 4.6 Fiber orientation in the model. (**a**) Three dimensional view of the fiber orientation on the epicardial surface. (**b**) Distribution of the z component of the fiber direction

1979; Taccardi et al., 1994). The fiber direction in the model were obtained directly from the DTMRI images, since this technique permits rapid non-invasive estimation of tissue structure. DTMRI is based on the principle that proton diffusion in the presence of a magnetic field gradient causes signal attenuation. Hence, a symmetric tensor representing the mean path of water diffusion may be estimated from multiple images obtained with different gradient weighting (Basser et al., 1994). It has been shown by correlation of two-dimensional (2D) DTMRI and histology that the principle direction of water diffusion in cardiac tissue is parallel to the fiber long-axis (Hsu et al., 1998). Therefore, the principle axis of the tissue microstructure for each voxel may then be inferred from the principle component of this diffusion tensor. From the available DTMRI images, only information regarding the fiber direction was taken into consideration, therefore considering the cardiac tissue as transversally isotropic. Figure 4.6 shows the fiber orientation in the epicardium of the heart and the z component of the fiber direction for the heart model. The angle of the fiber with respect to the circumferential direction is found to vary from approximately $-60°$ on the epicardium to $+40°$, $+60°$ on the endocardium.

4.4.2 Cell Type Heterogeneity

Recent studies have demonstrated the ventricular myocardium to be formed of three distinctive cells: epicardial, M and endocardial (Antzelevitch and Fish, 2001). These three types of cardiac cells have a different morphology of the action potential, particularly in regard to the spike and dome shape present in the M and epicardial cells and absent in the endocardial cells, or the longer Action Potential Duration (APD) of the M-cells in comparison to the endocardial and epicardial cells. This regional difference has been demonstrated in ventricular myocites of different species (dog (Liu et al., 1993), cat (Furukawa et al., 1990), rabbit (Fedida and Giles, 1991), rat (Clark et al., 1993) and human (Nabauer et al., 1996; Wettwer et al., 1994)). From a

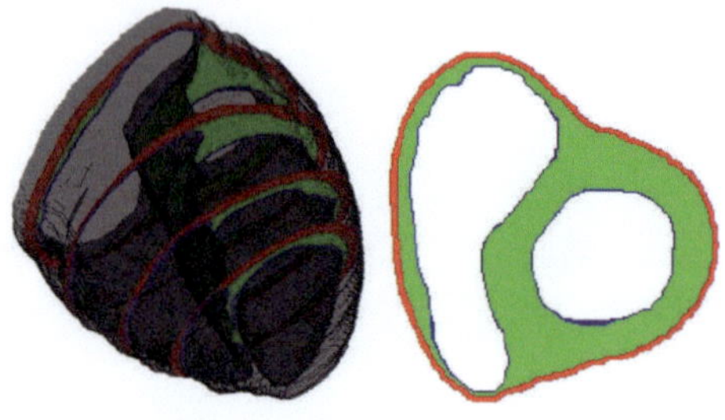

(a) (b)

Fig. 4.7 Transmural heterogeneity considered in the model. (**a**) 3D view with different cuts along the myocardium. (**b**) Sagital view cut at a distance of 81 mm from the apex

histologic point of view, all three cell types are similar. However, M-cells show electrophysiological features intermediate between those of myocardial and Purkinje cells and pharmacological responsiveness different from that of either epicardium or endocardium (Antzelevitch et al., 1991). In addition, differently to Purkinje cells, M-cells are located in the deep sub-epicardial layers. M cells can be distinguished from other cell types by the presence of a slow component of the delayed rectifying potassium current, I_{Ks}, and strong transient outward current, I_{to}, and electrogenic Sodium-Calcium exchanger current, I_{NaCa}. On the contrary, the rapid component of the delayed rectifying potassium current, I_{Kr} and the inward rectifying current, I_{K1} are similar for all three cell types (Antzelevitch et al., 1991).

The heterogeneity of the myocardium has been quantified by Drouin et al. (1995) using micro electrodes in portions of the human ventricle; their findings show that the epicardium accounts for approximately 15 % of the ventricular wall. M-cells have been found to be distributed in the form of vertical layers (discrete patches) in the lateral wall, after the sub-epicardium (Sicouri and Antzelevitch, 1991). In dogs, M-cells have been found in the subendocardium of the anterior wall (Yan et al., 1998). The distribution in layers of M-cells is quite variable ranging from a 20 % up to a 70 % of the myocardial volume (Antzelevitch et al., 1999). A posterior study in dog hearts by Poelzing et al. (2004) suggests that approximately a 20 % of the myocardial wall corresponds to epicardial cells, the endocardium accounts for another 50 %, with the remaining 30 % being occupied by M-cells distributed between the endocardial and epicardial layers. A recent study based on optical mapping of left-ventricular free wall preparations of human hearts by Glukhov et al. (2010) has identified islands of M-cells located at the sub-endocardium.

At the moment, the existence of M-cells is generally accepted and their importance in heart repolarization recognized. However, their actual distribution along the myocardium is unknown. In this work, myocardium heterogeneity has been defined assuming a distribution in layers (Sicouri and Antzelevitch, 1991; Yan et al., 1998), with a proportion in volume of: 7 % for endocardium, 71 % for M-cells, and 22 % for epicardium. Figure 4.7 shows the resulting distribution of myocardial cells.

Table 4.3 Value of parameters used to define acute regional ischemia in the simulations

Parameter	Normal	Ischemic
$[K^+]_o$, [mmol/L]	5.4	9.9
g_{Na}, [μA]	14.84	11.13
g_{CaL}, [μA]	3.98×10^{-5}	2.92×10^{-5}
ATP_i, [μmol/L]	6.80	4.60
ADP_i, [mmol/L]	1.50	99

4.4.3 Electrophysiologic Heterogeneity Under Acute Ischemia

In order to simulate a human heart under acute regional ischemia, an ischemic zone corresponding to an occlusion of the circumflex coronary artery. The structure of the ischemic zone was defined according to the representation in Fig. 4.1 distinguishing between a central zone and a normal zone separated by a border zone. The geometry of the ischemic zone was defined as the solution of the following equation:

$$\frac{\partial u}{\partial t} = \nabla(\mathbf{D} \cdot \nabla u) - Au(u - 1.0)\left(u - \frac{u_{th}}{u_p}\right), \tag{4.22}$$

where, $0 \leq u \leq 1$, $\mathbf{D}$ is a second order diffusion tensores, and A, u_{th}, and u_p are constant parameters. Equation (4.22) is subjected to zero-flux boundary conditions (homogeneous Neumann boundary conditions). The solution corresponds to a propagating front in time, with the solution varying between 0 and 1. Parameters in (4.22) were set to: $A = 5.764$ 1/min, $u_{th} = 0.13$, $u_p = 1.0$, and the diffusion tensor $\mathbf{D}$ was defined as transversally isotropic with a conductivity along the fiber, $D_L = 0.1$ cm^2/min, and a conductivity transverse to the fibers, $D_T = 0.025$ cm^2/min. The ratio between conductivities was kept the same as for the electrophysiology simulations. These parameters lead to a propagating velocity of 0.35 cm/min. Under this conditions it was defined an ischemic zone of approximately 7.5 cm in diameter after 10 minutes of the occlusion, in agreement to results reported by Coronel (1994).

Results from the solution of (4.22) have been used to define the different zones present in regional acute ischemia: (i) $u = 1$ defines the central zone (CZ), (ii) $u = 0$ indicates the normal zone (NZ), whereas intermediate values are used to define the border zone (BZ). Table 4.3 summarizes the electrophysiologic parameters modified in ischemic zone. Extracellular potassium concentration, $[K^+]_o$, in the CZ correspond to values reported by Coronel (1994) in pig hearts after 10 minutes of ischemia. Values for the maximal conductance of sodium, g_{Na}, and L type calcium, g_{CaL}, currents correspond to a 25 % reduction with respect to their normal values, whereas values for $[ATP]_i$ and $[ADP]_i$ have been taken from previous works on guinea-pigs (Ferrero et al., 2003).

Figure 4.8 shows a detail of the ischemic zone defined from the solution of (4.22). The distribution of $[ADP]_i$ is not shown but it is quite similar to the corresponding distribution of $[ATP]_i$. In addition to the heterogeneities shown in the figure,

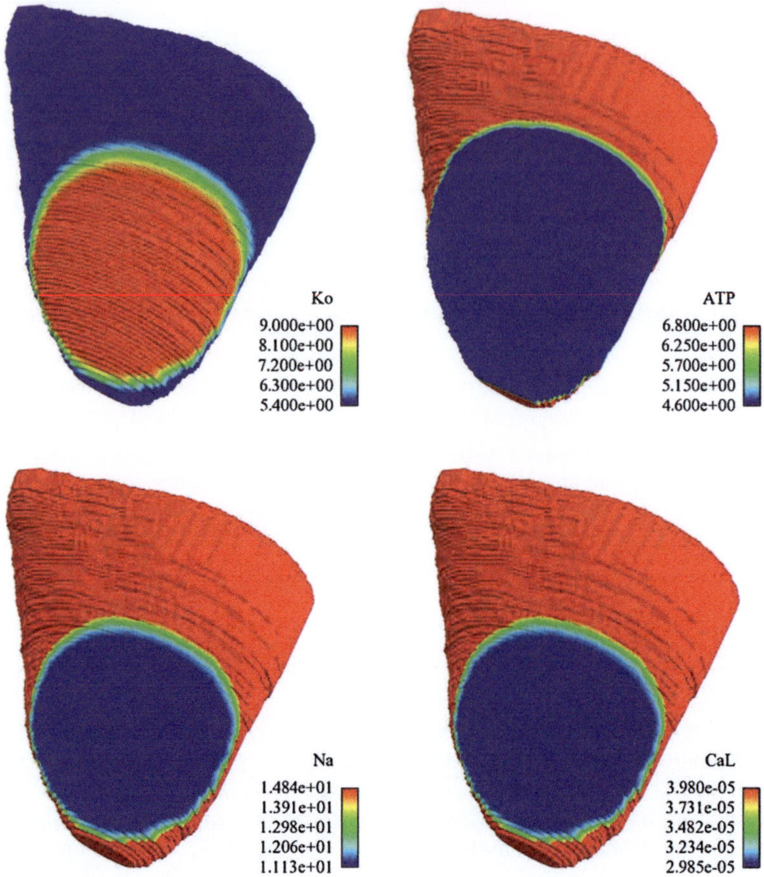

Fig. 4.8 Electrophysiologic heterogeneity in the acute regional ischemic heart

a 1.0 mm thick wash out zone was introduced in the endocardium to simulate the effect of the interaction of the endocardial tissue with the blood in the ventricular cavities (Wilensky et al., 1986).

4.4.4 Stimulation Points

This work does not incorporate the specialized conduction system to stimulate the heart. Discrete stimulation zones have been defined according to the work performed by Freud et al. (1970). According to this work endocardial stimulation in the left ventricle starts at three well defined locations within a time window of 5 ms:

1. an area high on the anterior paraseptal wall just below the attachment of the mitral valve,

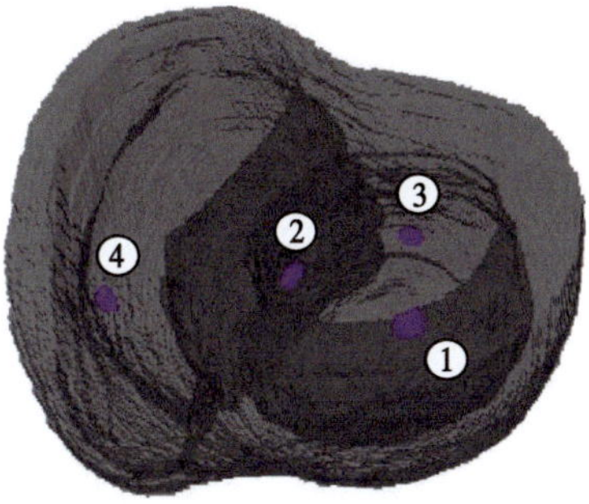

Fig. 4.9 The four stimulation zones during normal activity

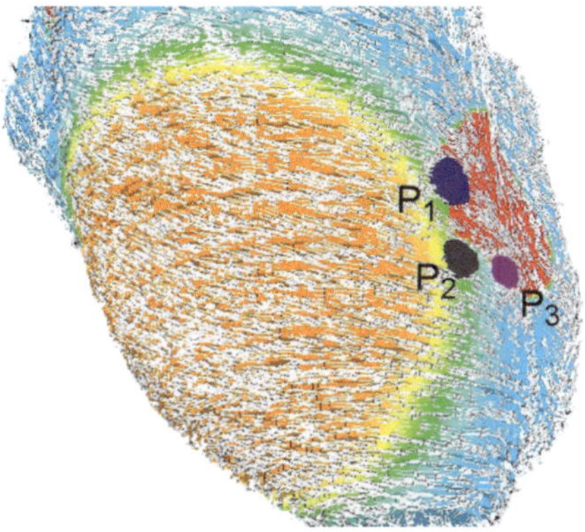

Fig. 4.10 Location of ectopic stimulation points for the simulation of the acute regional ischemic heart

2. a central area on the left surface of the interventricular septum,
3. the posterior paraseptal area at about one third of the distance from apex tobase.

For the right ventricle we have defined an stimulation area near the insertion of the anterior papillary muscle. In the right ventricle stimulation start 5 ms after the onset of the left ventricular potential. Figure 4.9 shows the location for the four stimulation areas.

For the ischemic simulations, the stimulation protocol consisted on the delivering five stimulation pulses at normal excitation position in the endocardium of the heart (at the four positions shown in Fig. 4.9) at a frequency of 1.25 Hz, for preconditioning the tissue, followed by an extra-stimulus located in the border zone with different coupling intervals (CI). Figure 4.10 depicts the location of the extra-stimulation points. P1 and P2 are located in the border zone, whereas P3 is located just outside the ischemic zone. The location of the ectopic focal activity obeys to experimental observations by Janse et al. (1980).

4.5 Electrical Activity in the Ischemic Heart

The finite element methodology described in the first section has been implemented in Fortran using the Message Passing Interface (MPI) for parallel computations

(Heidenreich et al., 2010). Domain decomposition for parallel computations has been carried out using the METIS library (Karypis and Kumar, 1998). The linear system of equations was solved using the Conjugate Gradient (CG) method with an ILU preconditioner from the PSBLAS library (Buttari and Filippone, 2008). The resulting code has been used to solve the numerical model of ischemic heart described in the previous section.

Our simulations have shown spatial heterogeneities in the propagated action potential, as reported experimentally, throughout the regional ischemic tissue, such as resting membrane potential (−86.1 mV in NZ, and −70.3 mV in the CZ, with potentials varying between these values in the BZ). Secondly, different patterns of activation were found depending on the CI. For CIs in the range 418–428 ms, reentry occurred at the epicardium whereas the mid-myocardium remained in refractory period. The reentrant front quickly aligned and propagated along the fiber direction on the epicardium as shown in Fig. 4.11 for two CI.

Whereas for a CI = 418 ms, the reentrant front was able to exit the ischemic zone propagating through the normal tissue of the heart, for larger CI, i.e., CI = 428 ms, the re-entrant front is not able to abandon the ischemic zone generating a an spiral pattern that cease activity within the central zone with no further propagation into the normal cardiac tissue. Figure 4.12 shows a snapshot of the re-entrant front leaving the ischemic zone and completing an eight shape figure for CI = 418 ms, and the spiral pattern for the CI = 428 ms.

After the first re-entrant circuit, mid-myocardial layers were excited by the reentrant wavefront causing rather complicated patterns within the ischemic zone in the epicardium due to the re-entrant wavefront coming from the mid-myocardium. On the other hand, the faster propagation of the electrical activity through the endocardium, due to the wash-out zone prevented the perpetuation of the re-entrant activity in the ischemic zone. These re-entrant patterns generate a pathway within the central ischemic zone through which reentrant circuits can be sustained in the epicardium for high enough CIs as shown in Fig. 4.13.

The main results of the performed simulations can be summarized as follows: (i) As a consequence of the applied extra-stimulus that originates an ectopic beat, reentrant activity is generated in all cases considered. This activity corresponds to an eight shape figure in some cases (CI = 418 ms) whereas in other cases it corresponds to a spiral like shape (CI = 428 ms). (ii) The reentrant activity generated as a consequence of the extra-stimulus ceases in all cases as a consequence of the interaction between wavefronts emerging from the from the wash-out zone into the ischemic zone.

For the eight shape reentrant pattern, the mechanisms governing the reentrant activity is similar to that obtained in 2D. The propagating wavefront is blocked when trying to invade the ischemic zone since the tissue is still in the refractory period. The electric wave then bypasses the zone of block propagating through the normal tissue and later reentering the ischemic zone retrogradely. However, this pattern of excitation only occurs at the epicardium in the ischemic heart since the mid-myocardium tissue remains in the refractory period.

In other cases, the reentry pattern corresponds to a single spiral. In this case, the reentrant front is not able to re-excite the normal tissue since it finds the tissue in

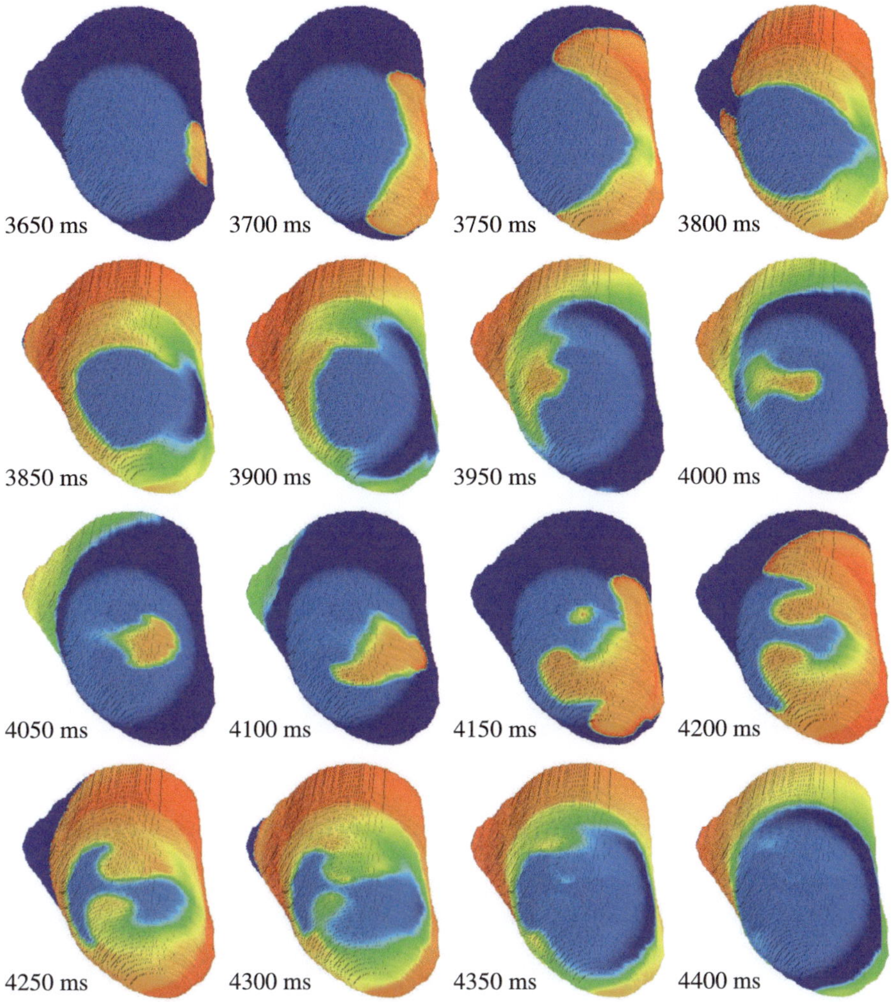

Fig. 4.11 Reentrant pattern for CI = 418 ms

the border zone within the refractory period forcing the wavefront to initiate a rotor that does not perpetuates within the ischemic zone.

Both described patterns from the simulations have been reported in the experimental work by Janse et al. (1980, 1981) in pig and dog hearts. For instance, Fig. 3, panels A and B in Janse and Kleber (1981) shows the eight shape reentrant pattern also obtained in our simulations, whereas panel D in the same figure shows the spiral pattern obtained for the larger CI. However, differently to the experimental studies by Janse et al., none of the cases studied lead to self perpetuating reentrant activity. In all our simulations the reentrant activity did not last more than three cycles. The main reason for this behavior was the existence of the wash-out zone. In our sim-

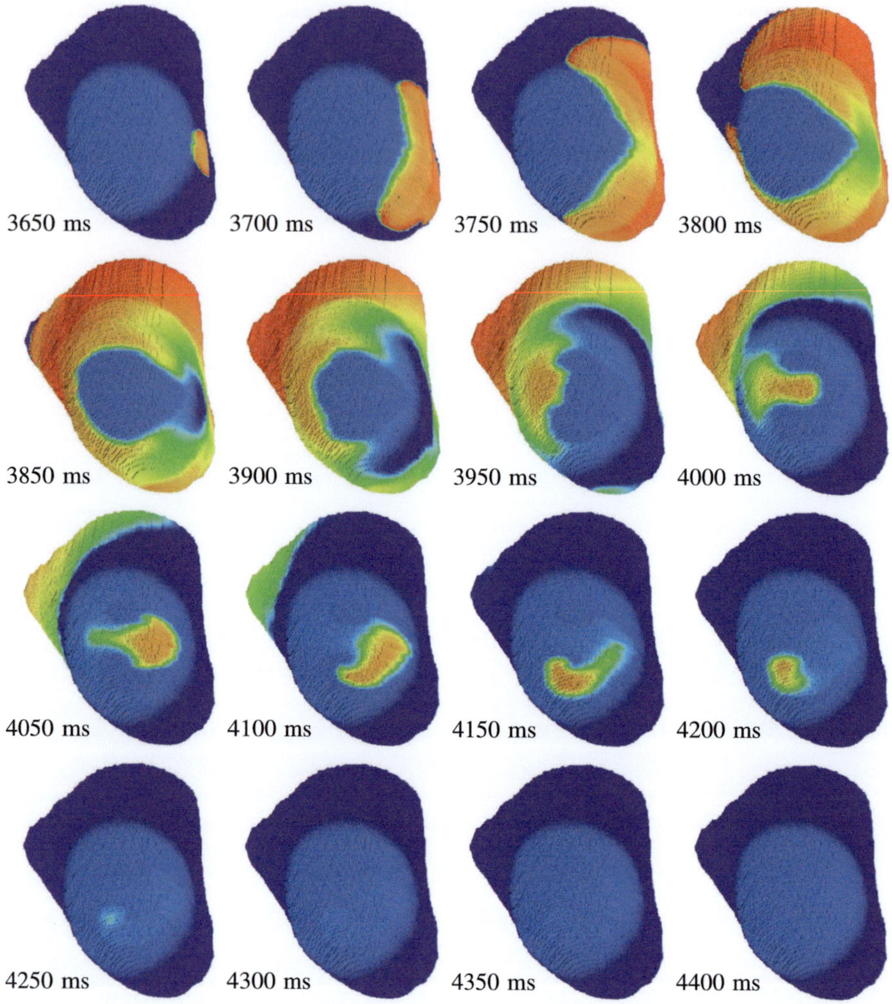

Fig. 4.12 Reentrant pattern for CI = 428 ms

ulations, the interaction of epicardial wavefronts coming from the subendocardial wash-out zone with reentrant wave fronts caused the last to disappear preventing the perpetuation of reentrant activity in the ischemic heart. Additional studies on larger ischemic zones are required in order to determine if this effect is reduced as the area affected by ischemia becomes larger.

In conclusion, the model predicts the generation of figure-of-eight re-entries which cross the central ischemic zone formed in the epicardial surface due to the longer refractory period of the midmyocardial layers. Also, focal activity experimentally observed in the epicardium could be caused by re-entrant wavefronts propagating in the mid-myocardium that re-emerge in the heart surface.

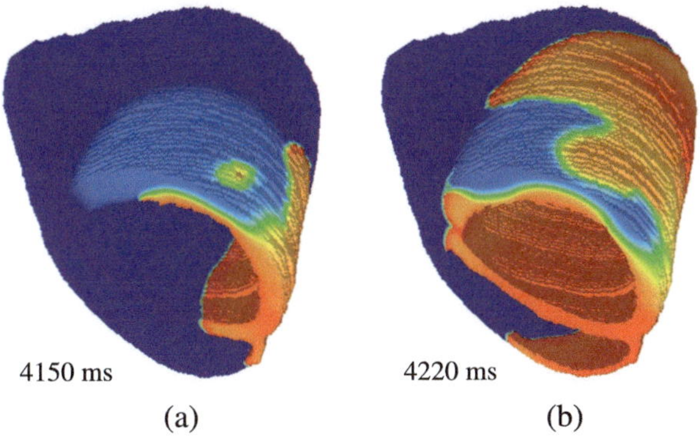

Fig. 4.13 Detailed of the re-entrant activity for CI = 418 ms (**a**) Reentrant wave front coming form the mid-myocardium. (**b**) Premature completion of the re-entrant circuit through the endocardium

Acknowledgements The authors gratefully acknowledge the research support of the Spanish Ministry of Education and Science through the research projects TEC2008-0290 and DPI2007-63254, and the Aragon Government through the project PI113-2005.

References

Antzelevitch C, Sicouri S, Litovsky SH, Lukas A, Krishnan SC, Di Diego JM, Gintant GA, Liu DW (1991) Heterogeneity within the ventricular wall. electrophysiology and pharmacology of epicardial, endocardial, and m cells. Circ Res 69(6):1427–1449

Antzelevitch C, Shimizu W, Yan GX, Sicouri S, Weissenburger J, Nesterenko VV, Burashnikov A, Diego J, Saffitz J, Thomas GP (1999) The M cell: its contribution to the ECG and to normal and abnormal electrical function of the heart. J Cardiovasc Electrophysiol 10(8):1124–1152

Antzelevitch C, Fish J (2001) Electrical heterogeneity within the ventricular wall. Basic Res Cardiol 96(6):517–527

Beeler GW, Reuter H (1977) Reconstruction of the action potential of ventricular myocardial fibres. J Physiol 268(1):177–210

Basser PJ, Mattiello J, LeBihan D (1994) Estimation of the effective self-diffusion tensor from the NMR spin echo. J Magn Reson B 103(3):247–254

Buttari A, Filippone S (2008) PSBLAS 2.3 user's guide. University of Rome and Tor Vergata, Rome

Carmeliet E (1999) Cardiac ionic currents and acute ischemia: from channels to arrhythmias. Physiol Rev 79(3):917–1017

Carro J, Rodríguez JF, Laguna P, Pueyo E (2011) A human ventricular cell model for investigation of cardiac arrhythmias under hyperkalemic conditions. Philos Trans R Soc, Math Phys Eng Sci 369(1954):472–480

Clark RB, Bouchard RA, Salinas-Stefanon E, Sanchez-Chapula J, Giles WR (1993) Heterogeneity of action potential waveforms and potassium currents in rat ventricle. Cardiovasc Res 27(10):1795–1799

Colli Franzone P, Deuflhard P, Erdmann B, Lang J, Pavarino LF (2006) Adaptivity in space and time for reaction-diffusion systems in electrocardiology. SIAM J Sci Comput 28(3):942–962

Coronel R, Fiolet JW, Wilms-Schopman FJ, Schaapherder AF, Johnson TA, Gettes LS, Janse MJ (1988) Distribution of extracellular potassium and its relation to electrophysiologic changes during acute myocardial ischemia in the isolated perfused porcine heart. Circulation 77(5):1125–1138

Coronel R (1994) Heterogeneity in extracellular potassium concentration during early myocardial ischaemia and reperfusion: implications for arrhythmogenesis. Cardiovasc Res 28(6):770–777

DiFrancesco D, Noble D (1985) A model of cardiac electrical activity incorporating ionic pumps and concentration changes. Philos Trans R Soc Lond B, Biol Sci 307(1133):353–398

Drouin E, Charpentier F, Gauthier C, Laurent K, Le-Marec H (1995) Electrophysiologic characteristics of cells spanning the left ventricular wall of human heart: evidence for presence of M cells. J Am Coll Cardiol 26(1):185–192

Fedida D, Giles WR (1991) Regional variations in action potentials and transient outward current in myocytes isolated from rabbit left ventricle. J Physiol 442(1):191–209

Ferrero JM Jr, Saiz J, Ferrero JM, Thakor NV (1996) Simulation of action potentials from metabolically impaired cardiac myocytes: role of ATP-sensitive K+ current. Circ Res 79(2):208–221

Ferrero JM Jr, Rodriguez B TB, Saiz J (2003) Electrical activity and reentry during acute regional myocardial ischemia: insights from simulations. Int J Bifurc Chaos Appl Sci Eng 13:3703–3715

Freud G, Janse M, Meijler F, Arzbaecher R, Durrer D, Van Dam R (1970) Total excitation of the isolated human heart. Circulation 41:899–912

Furukawa T, Kimura S, Furukawa N, Bassett AL, Myerburg RJ (1991) Role of cardiac ATP-regulated potassium channels in differential responses of endocardial and epicardial cells to ischemia. Circ Res 68(6):1693–1702

Furukawa T, Myerburg RJ, Furukawa N, Bassett AL, Kimura S (1990) Differences in transient outward currents of feline endocardial and epicardial myocytes. Circ Res 67(5):1287–1291

Gima K, Rudy Y (2002) Ionic current basis of electrocardiographic waveforms: a model study. Circ Res 90(8):889–896

Glukhov AV, Fedorov VV, Lou Q, Ravikumar VK, Kalish PW, Schuessler RB, Moazami N, Efimov IR (2010) Transmural dispersion of depolarization in failing and non failing human ventricle. Circ Res 106:981–991

Grandi E, Pasqualini FS, Bers DM (2010) A novel computational model of the human ventricular action potential and ca transient. J Mol Cell Cardiol 48(1):112–121

Heidenreich EA, Ferrero JM, Doblare M, Rodriguez JF (2010) Adaptive macro finite elements for the numerical solution of monodomain equations in cardiac electrophysiology. Ann Biomed Eng 38(7):2331–2345

Helm PA (2005) A novel technique for quantifying variability of cardiac anatomy application to the dyssynchronous failing heart. PhD thesis, Johns Hopkins University

Hodgkin AL, Huxley AF (1952) A quantitative description of membrane current and its application to conduction and excitation in nerve. J Physiol 117(4):500–544

Hsu EW, Muzikant, AL, Matulevicius SA, Penland RC, Henriquez CS (1998) Magnetic resonance myocardial fiber-orientation mapping with direct histological correlation. Am J Physiol 274(5 Pt 2):H1627–H1634

Janse MJ, Cinca J, Morena H, Fiolet JW, Kleber AG, de-Vries GP, Becker AE, Durrer D (1979) The "border zone" in myocardial ischemia. An electrophysiological, metabolic, and histochemical correlation in the pig heart. Circ Res 44(4):576–588

Janse MJ, van Capelle FJ, Morsink H, Kleber AG, Wilms-Schopman F, Cardinal R, d'Alnoncourt CN, Durrer D (1980) Flow of "injury" current and patterns of excitation during early ventricular arrhythmias in acute regional myocardial ischemia in isolated porcine and canine hearts. Evidence for two different arrhythmogenic mechanisms. Circ Res 47(2):151–165

Janse MJ, Kleber AG (1981) Electrophysiological changes and ventricular arrhythmias in the early phase of regional myocardial ischemia. Circ Res 49:1069–1081

Karypis G, Kumar V (1998) METIS. A software package for partitioning unstructured graphs, partitioning meshes, and computing fill-reducing orderings of sparse matrices, 4th edn. University of Minnesota, Department of Computer Science/Army HPC Research Center, Minneapolis

Katz AM (2005) Physiology of the heart. Lippincott Williams & Wilkins, Philadelphia

Keener J, Sneyd J (1998) Mathematical physiology. Springer, Berlin

Light PE, Cordeiro JM, French RJ (1999) Identification and properties of ATP-sensitive potassium channels in myocytes from rabbit purkinje fibres. Cardiovasc Res 44(2):356–369

Liu DW, Gintant GA, Antzelevitch C (1993) Ionic bases for electrophysiological distinctions among epicardial, midmyocardial, and endocardial myocytes from the free wall of the canine left ventricle. Circ Res 72(3):671–687

Luo CH, Rudy Y (1994) A dynamic model of the cardiac ventricular action potential. II. Afterdepolarizations, triggered activity, and potentiation. Circ Res 74(6):1097–1113
Luo CH, Rudy Y (1991) A model of the ventricular cardiac action potential. Depolarization, repolarization, and their interaction. Circ Res 68(6):1501–1526
Michailova A, Lorentz W, McCulloch A (2007) Modeling transmural heterogeneity of KATP current in rabbit ventricular myocytes. Am J Physiol, Cell Physiol 293(2):542–557
Nabauer M, Beuckelmann DJ, Uberfuhr P, Steinbeck G (1996) Regional differences in current density and rate-dependent properties of the transient outward current in subepicardial and subendocardial myocytes of human left ventricle. Circulation 93(1):168–177
Nichols CG, Ripoll C, Lederer WJ (1991) ATP-sensitive potassium channel modulation of the guinea pig ventricular action potential and contraction. Circ Res 68(1):280–287
O'Hara T, Virag L, Varro A, Rudy Y (2011) Simulation of the undiseased human cardiac ventricular action potential: model formulation and experimental validation. PLoS Comput Biol 7(5):e1002061
Poelzing S, Akar FG, Baron E, Rosenbaum DS (2004) Heterogeneous connexin43 expression produces electrophysiological heterogeneities across ventricular wall. Am J Physiol, Heart Circ Physiol 286(5):H2001–2009
Qu Z, Garfinkel A (1999) An advanced algorithm for solving partial differential equation in cardiac conduction. IEEE Trans Biomed Eng 46(9):1166–1168
Roberts DE, Hersh LT, Scher AM (1979) Influence of cardiac fiber orientation on wavefront voltage, conduction velocity, and tissue resistivity in the dog. Circ Res 44(5):701–712
Rodriguez B, Tice BM, Eason JC, Aguel F, Trayanova N (2004) Cardiac vulnerability to electric shocks during phase 1a of acute global ischemia. Heart Rhythm 1(6):695–703
Rodriguez B, Trayanova N, Noble D (2006) Modeling cardiac ischemia. Ann NY Acad Sci 1080:395–414
Rubart M, Zipes DP (2005) Mechanisms of sudden cardiac death. J Clin Invest 115(9):2305–2315
Shaw RM, Rudy Y (1997) Electrophysiologic effects of acute myocardial ischemia: a mechanistic investigation of action potential conduction and conduction failure. Circ Res 80(1):124–138
Sicouri S, Antzelevitch C (1991) A subpopulation of cells with unique electrophysiological properties in the deep subepicardium of the canine ventricle. The M cell. Circ Res 68(6):1729–1741
Strang G (1968) On the construction and comparison of difference schemes. SIAM J Numer Anal 5(3):506–517
Taccardi B, Macchi E, Lux RL, Ershler PR, Spaggiari S, Baruffi S, Vyhmeister Y (1994) Effect of myocardial fiber direction on epicardial potentials. Circulation 90(6):3076–3090
ten Tusscher KHWJ, Noble D, Noble PJ, Panfilov AV (2004) A model for human ventricular tissue. Am J Physiol, Heart Circ Physiol 286(4):1573–1589
ten Tusscher KHWJ, Panfilov AV (2006) Alternans and spiral breakup in a human ventricular tissue model. Am J Physiol, Heart Circ Physiol 291(3):1088–1100
Tice B, Rodriguez B, Trayanova N (2005) Arrthythmogenicity of transmural heterogeneities in a realistic model of regional ischemia. Heart Rhythm 2(5):S261
Tung L (1978) A bi-domain model for describing ischemic myocardial d-c potentials. PhD thesis, Dept of Electrical Engineering and Computer Science, Massachusetts Institute of Technology
Weiss DL, Ifland M, Sachse FB, Seemann G, Dossel O (2009) Modeling of cardiac ischemia in human myocytes and tissue including spatiotemporal electrophysiological variations. Biomed Tech 54(3):107–125
Venkatesh N, Weiss JN, Lamp ST (1992) ATP-sensitive K channels and cellular K loss in hypoxic and ischaemic mammalian ventricle. J Physiol 447:649–673
Wettwer E, Amos GJ, Posival H, Ravens U (1994) Transient outward current in human ventricular myocytes of subepicardial and subendocardial origin. Circ Res 75(3):473–482
Wilensky RL, Tranum-Jensen J, Coronel R, Wilde AAM, Fiolet JWT, Janse MJ (1986) The subendocardial border zone during acute ischemia of the rabbit heart: an electrophysiologic, metabolic, and morphologic correlative study. Circulation 74:1137
Yan GX, Shimizu W, Antzelevitch C (1998) Characteristics and distribution of m cells in arterially perfused canine left ventricular wedge preparations. Circulation 98(18):1921–1927

Chapter 5
Detailing Patient Specific Modeling to Aid Clinical Decision-Making

S. Richmond, A.M. Al Ali, L. Beldie, Y.T. Chong, A. Cronin, J. Djordjevic, N.A. Drage, D.M. Evans, D. Jones, Y. Lu, D. Marshall, J. Middleton, G. Parker, L. Paternoster, R.A. Playle, H. Popat, P.L. Rosin, K. Sidorov, A.M. Toma, B. Walker, C. Wilson, and A.I. Zhurov

Abstract The anatomy of the craniofacial skeleton has been described through the aid of dissection identifying hard and soft tissue structures. Although the macro and microscopic investigation of internal facial tissues have provided invaluable information on constitution of the tissues it is important to inspect and model facial tissues in the living individual. Detailing the form and function of facial tissues will be invaluable in clinical diagnoses and planned corrective surgical interventions such as management of facial palsies and craniofacial disharmony/anomalies.

S. Richmond (✉) · A.M. Al Ali · Y.T. Chong · J. Djordjevic · R.A. Playle · H. Popat · A.M. Toma · C. Wilson · A.I. Zhurov
Applied Clinical Research and Public Health, Dental School, Cardiff University, Cardiff, Wales CF14 4XY, UK
e-mail: richmonds@cardiff.ac.uk

L. Beldie · B. Walker
Ove Arup & Partners, The Arup Campus, Blythe Gate, Blythe Valley Park, Solihull B90 1TG, UK

A. Cronin
Dental and Maxillofacial Surgery, University Dental Hospital, Heath Park, Cardiff, Wales CF14 4XY, UK

N.A. Drage
Dental and Maxillofacial Radiology, University Dental Hospital, Heath Park, Cardiff, Wales CF14 4XY, UK

D.M. Evans · L. Paternoster
Biostatistical Genetics, MRC Centre for Causal Analyses in Translational Epidemiology, School of Social and Community Medicine, University of Bristol, Oakfield House, Oakfield Grove, Bristol BS8 2BN, UK

D. Jones
Cardiff University Brain Research Imaging Centre (CUBRIC), School of Psychology, Cardiff University, Park Place, Cardiff CF10 3AT, UK

Y. Lu
Institute of Biomechanics, Hamburg University of Technology, Denickestraße 15, 21073 Hamburg, Germany

B. Calvo, E. Peña (eds.), *Patient-Specific Computational Modeling*, Lecture Notes in Computational Vision and Biomechanics 5,
DOI 10.1007/978-94-007-4552-0_5,

Recent advances in lower-cost, non-invasive imaging and computing power (surface scanning, Cone Beam Computerized Tomography (CBCT) and Magnetic Resonance (MRI)) has enabled the ability to capture and process surface and internal structures to a high resolution. The three-dimensional surface facial capture has enabled characterization of facial features all of which will influence subtleties in facial movement and surgical planning.

This chapter will describe the factors that influence facial morphology in terms of gender and age differences, facial movement—surface and underlying structures, modeling based on average structures, orientation of facial muscle fibers, biomechanics of movement—proof of principle and surgical intervention.

5.1 Introduction

Subtle facial differences make an individual unique and it is this uniqueness that needs to be recognized, defined, categorized and incorporated into a computerized patient specific model. The craniofacial structures are complex and there are many clinical and non-clinical specialties that have a specific interest in the dental and oro-facial region. Although there have been significant investments in research to explain development and facial variation, the mechanisms of how normal and abnormal growth/facial development occurs still remains unclear and subject to many theories. Improving knowledge in how the facial tissues arise and function will enhance the validity of computerized models. The aim of this chapter is to highlight advancements that have led to characterization of facial tissues and how these can be utilized and refined for computerized models to aid clinical decision-making.

This chapter will address the progress made so far in determining a patient specific model in terms of:

1. Acquisition of facial data
2. Genetic and non-genetic factors contributing to facial variation
3. Modeling facial structures based on average estimates for surgical planning and simulation
4. Methods to determine facial movement pre- and post-surgical intervention
5. On-going refinement of techniques:
    5.1. Registration
    5.2. Determination of the orientation of facial muscle fibers

D. Marshall · G. Parker · P.L. Rosin · K. Sidorov
Cardiff School of Computer Science and Informatics, Cardiff University, Queens Buildings, 5 The Parade, Roath, Cardiff CF24 3AA, UK

J. Middleton
Biomaterials and Biomechanics Research Centre, Cardiff University, Cardiff, Wales CF14 4XY, UK

5.2 Acquiring Facial Data

To model or visualize living anatomical structures it is important to capture clinical data in a non-destructive way. Over the last 40 years there have been significant advances in imaging techniques, which have enabled visualization and reconstruction of the living internal organs, which previously were only visible by operation or by dissection. Static images of structures have been invaluable but more recently it has been realized that observing structures during function has added benefit, for example, cardiac magnetic resonance imaging to evaluate cardiac function (Hundley et al., 2010) and videofluoroscopy to study swallowing impairment in patients with neurological impairment (Kang et al., 2011).

Therefore to develop a patient specific model to aid clinical decision making for the head and neck we need not only information on the constitutive components on the head and neck but we also need imaging techniques to record and model the internal structures during rest and also undergoing a range of functions. In addition it is important to diagnose craniofacial anomalies based on normal variation and plan the surgery necessary to normalize any facial disharmony if required.

Every person has a unique soft tissue and skeletal facial structure and these structures are complex and require a variety of techniques to capture the full depth of facial tissues. For surface scanning, static or video-imaging techniques are used (laser or photogrammetric techniques) (Kau, 2010). To capture the detail of the skeletal framework computed tomography (CT), Cone Beam Computed Tomography (CBCT) and Magnetic Resonance Imaging (MRI) can be applied (Drage and Rout, 2010). To capture the detail of the underlying soft tissues (e.g. muscle and brain) techniques such as MRI, CT and ultrasound are required. Examples of the images obtained from the image capture machines are shown later in the text. Specialized techniques have been developed to identify muscle fiber orientation such as diffusion weighted imaging. Capturing any facial data is complex and the data requires validation as certain capture techniques are subject to distortion due to variation in image uniformity (Bryant et al., 2008) and relative spatial position of these structures that make up the face (e.g. surface air interface in CT and MRI).

5.3 Genetic and Non-genetic Factors Contributing to Facial Variation

The relative proportions of genetic and non-genetic factors contributing to dentofacial variation has evoked strong debate (Lundström, 1984). Quantifying the heritability of craniofacial features is a prerequisite for understanding normal craniofacial development and elucidating how abnormal pathology arises. Evidence from twin, family and animal studies has suggested that much of the variation in craniofacial features is heritable (Kohn, 1991; Saunders et al., 1980), although the majority of studies have involved small sample sizes, and/or less than ideal study designs. For example, most of the larger studies in craniofacial development have involved parent-offspring designs, which cannot distinguish between common environmen-

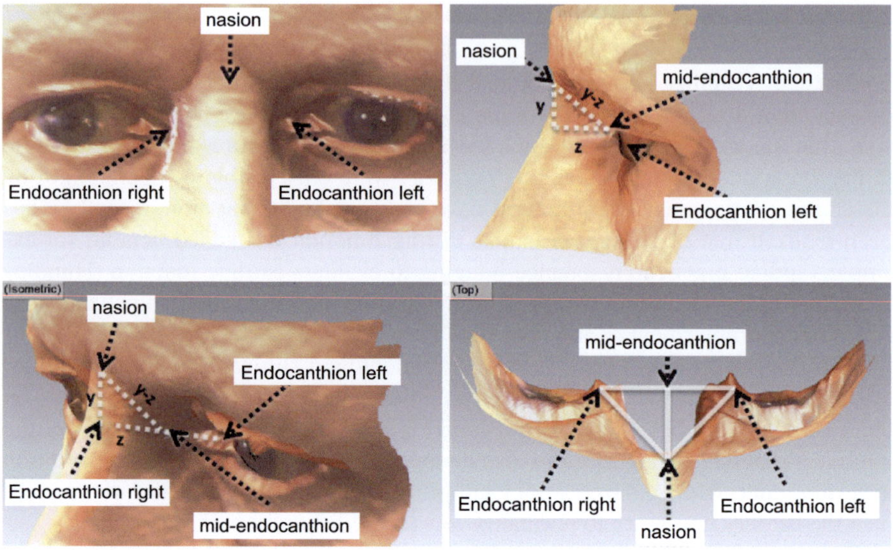

Fig. 5.1 Showing construction of the nasion to mid-endocanthion distance associated with the PAX3 gene

tal and genetic sources of variation, and thus may produce inflated estimates of the underlying heritability.

With the advent of molecular genetic techniques over the past thirty years, attention has now turned to identifying the individual genes influencing craniofacial development. In this respect, mutation bearing genes have been identified for over 340 syndromes associated with oral facial clefts, and numerous candidate genes have been implicated by allelic association and linkage analyses (Cohen, 2002). Whilst considerable advances have been made in elucidating the genetic basis of pathological conditions, the identity of individual genetic variants which affect normal craniofacial development in population based samples are largely unknown. However, a recent genome-wide association study of normal facial morphology in 2185 15-year-old children found a robustly replicated association between a SNP in PAX3 (rs7559271) and the nasion to mid-endocanthion distance (n-men) (Paternoster et al., 2012), see Fig. 5.1. Although genetic studies of normal craniofacial variation are in their infancy, it is hoped that the insights they provide will inform clinicians on how the face develops and reacts to surgical interventions.

There are many other factors that can affect facial variation such as the age of the individual, ethnicity, gender and environment. In a study of facial variation in 4747 children of the same age (15-years-old), 82 percent of variation could be explained by 14 principal components (Toma et al., 2011). The first 3 components explained 46 % of variation. These components were face height (28.8 %), inter eye distance (10.4 %) and nose prominence (6.7 %) (Fig. 5.2).

Significant facial variations have been highlighted between five different ethnic populations for example similarities in facial shapes were identified between females in Wales and Hungary but less concordance with females in Wales and the

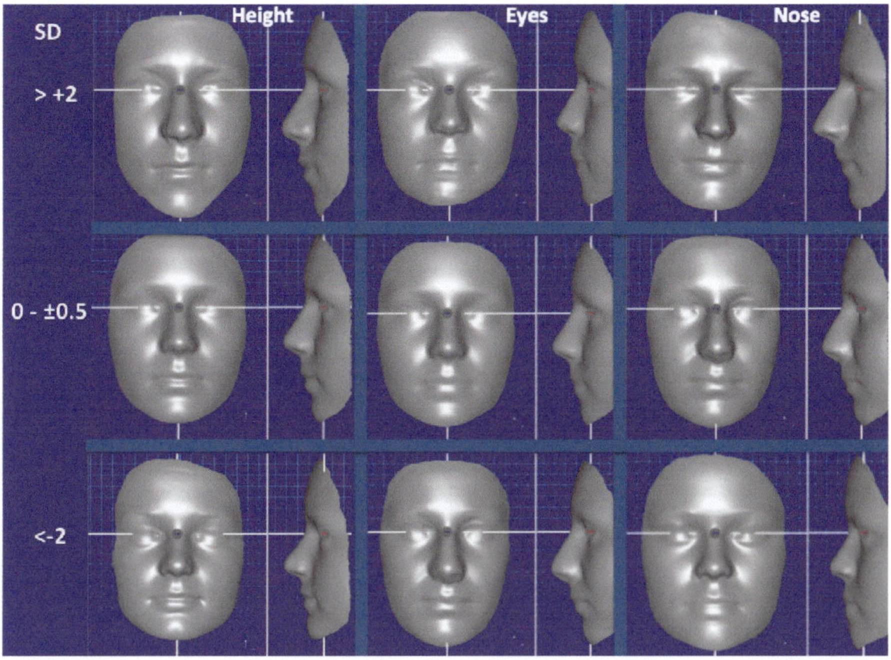

Fig. 5.2 Facial variation: *Left column* showing variation from long face (*top*) to short face (*bottom*); *middle column* eyes further apart (*top*) and eyes closer together (*bottom*) and *right column* large nose (*top*) to small nose (*bottom*)

USA (Kau et al., 2010). The face changes throughout life, increasing in size and changing shape. Puberty is when key facial differences between the sexes become defined (Fig. 5.3). Males tend to develop prominent noses and chins, with flatter infra-orbital regions than females between 12 and 17 years of age. Females tend to reach puberty 12 to 14 years of age and males 14 to 16 years of age. Subtle facial changes occur throughout life as the individual ages.

There have been a few studies assessing the influence of medical conditions on facial variation. In a study of insulin sensitivity in 2181 white 15-year-old children (1027 males, 1154 females) the first two principal components (facial height and inter-eye distance) were significantly, though weakly, associated with insulin sensitivity. The average face of males with low insulin sensitivity was wider (up to 3.24 mm) with a shorter nose and less protrusive lips (up to 2.26 mm) compared with the average face of males with high insulin sensitivity. The average face of females with low insulin sensitivity was also wider, with a more protrusive chin (up to 1.71 mm), shorter nose and less protrusive lips (up to 1.28 mm) compared with the average face of females with high insulin sensitivity (Djordjevic et al., 2010).

A further study of the influence of asthma on facial development was conducted in 471 children who had been diagnosed as asthmatic at 91 months of age (Henderson et al., 2008). The facial parameters were assessed against a control of 1637 healthy children. The inter ala distance (width of the nose) was 0.4 mm wider

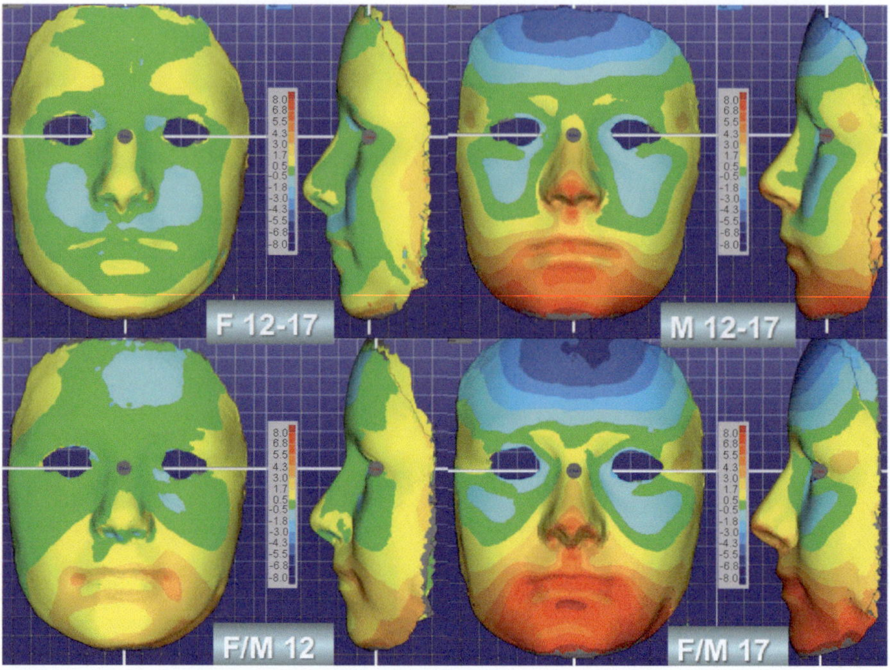

Fig. 5.3 Color maps showing differences between females and males between 12 and 17 years of age: Females (*top left*), males (*top right*), females and males aged 12 (*bottom left*) and females and males at 12 years of age (*bottom left*) and at 17 years of age (*bottom right*). Cooler colors (*light and dark blues*) show negative distances and warmer colors (*oranges and reds*) positive distances. Male chins and noses grow significantly forward from age 12 to 17 years of age

and mid-face height was 0.4 mm shorter in asthmatic females compared with non-asthmatic females. No facial differences were detected in males.

These few examples have shown that facial size and shape can be influenced by genetic and environmental influences. There are a wide variety of shapes and sizes of cheeks, chins, noses and lips and as a consequence will grow differently and respond differently to surgical interventions.

5.4 Modeling Facial Structures Based on Average Estimates for Surgical Planning and Surgical Simulations

It has been traditional for the assessment of facial discrepancies to be compared with average estimates for the normal population. This is undertaken on relatively small population groups usually between the ages 12 to 18 years of age (Bhatia and Leighton, 1993; Riolo et al., 1979). There are relatively few repositories for 3D facial analyses. A significant proportion of facial evaluations have been dependent on 2D cephalometric analyses and out-dated subjective assessments. Although these assessments are helpful they do not characterize the numerous permutations and associations of facial characteristics.

To date it is possible to acquire an accurate 3D facial shell (static and dynamic) using laser scanners or by photogrammetric techniques and skeletal topography using CBCT. It has been challenging to acquire detail of the underlying tissues (fascia, fat, nerves, blood vessels and muscles) lying between the facial surfaces and underlying bone. One possible solution is to apply average data acquired from forensic reconstruction (Richmond et al., 2010). The muscles can be fashioned and placed in the approximate anatomical positions (Fig. 5.4).

A finite element model was created using Simpleware® (Simpleware Ltd, 2006) and (Oasys.PRIMER, 2009). The material properties for different components were given as: the skeletal structure—rigid; subcutaneous—Neo-Hookean; facial skin, nose cartilage and eyeballs—linear elastic; facial muscles—user defined materials or linear elastic (Fig. 5.4) (Beldie et al., 2010). For the finite element model to produce valid predictions, an accurate constitutive model of the muscles is critical (Richmond et al., 2010). The constitutive muscle model was formulated based on Hill's one-dimensional model and can be described as active, quasi-incompressible, fiber reinforced and hyperelastic (Hill, 1938). The model was validated against experimental data under passive and active elongation simulations and was proved to be capable of simulating active and passive behavior (Lu et al., 2011). The constitutive model was implemented into LS-DYNA (LSTC, 2007) through user-defined material (UMAT) and utilized to simulate facial expressions. Facial expressions were achieved by activating the facial muscle groups. For example disgust was achieved by stimulating the levator labii superioris alaeque nasi, orbicularis oculi and depressor anguli oris muscles simultaneously and smiling was achieved by activating the orbicularis oculi, zygomaticus minor and zygomaticus major muscles simultaneously (Fig. 5.5).

5.4.1 Surgical Planning and Simulation

A 20-year-old patient expressed an interest in improving his appearance by reducing the prominence of his chin. At his first appointment full records were taken and the plan was to align his teeth prior to surgery. Once his teeth were aligned a surface facial laser scan (with color texture) and a CBCT was performed. The surface scan was fitted to the surface of the CBCT 3D construction. An average facial template for an 18 to 22-year-old male was fitted to the patients facial shell using best-fit with both shells aligned to the mid-intercanthal line (Zhurov et al., 2010). A color deviation map was used to highlight differences between the individual and the average face (Fig. 5.6). The patient's cheeks showed a deficiency of 5 mm although the chin was in a similar anterior-posterior position and the facial height was 3 to 4 mm longer than the average male. Analyzing these data it was decided to move the maxilla upwards by 4 mm and forwards by 5 mm. The movement of the maxilla will correct the mid-face discrepancy. The mandible was moved to the best-fit of the upper and lower teeth. Achieving the best occlusal interdigitation was a priority although by doing this it was recognized that the position of the chin would

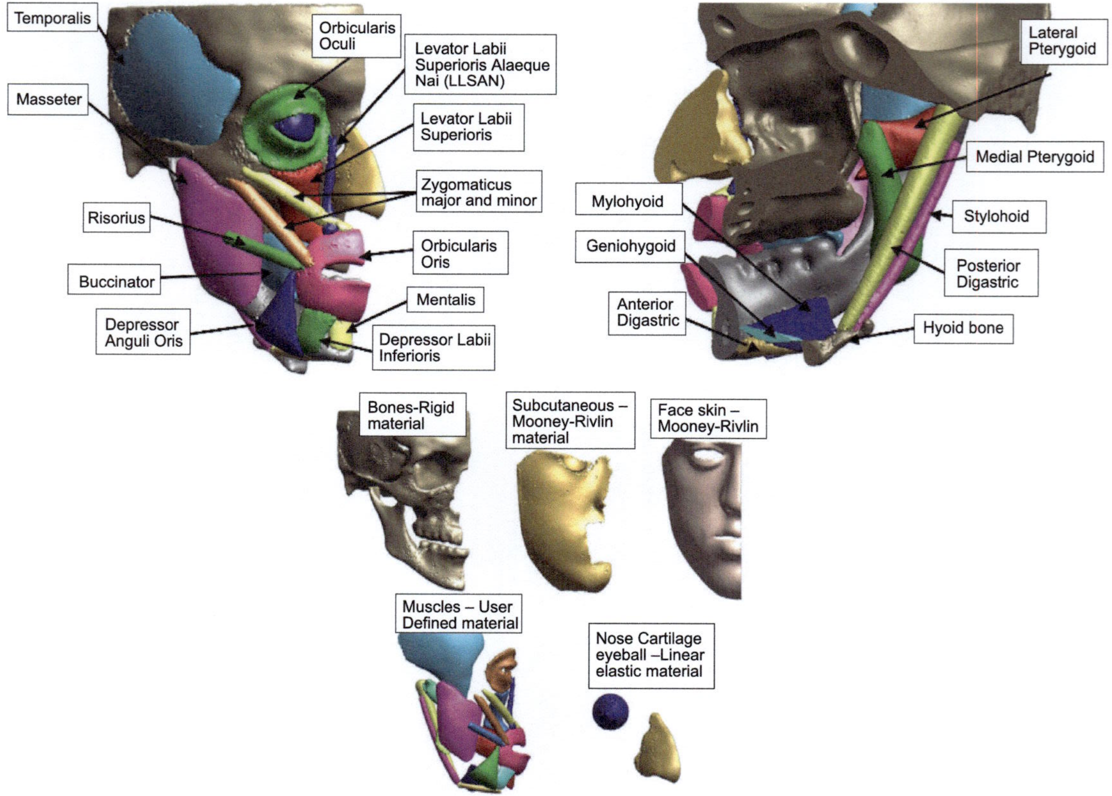

Fig. 5.4 The positioning of muscles on a segmented facial skeleton obtained from a CBCT (*left and middle*). The facial tissues can be modeled: bone—rigid; subcutaneous fat and skin—Mooney/Rivlin; muscles—user defined; nose cartilage/eyeball—linear elastic (*right*)

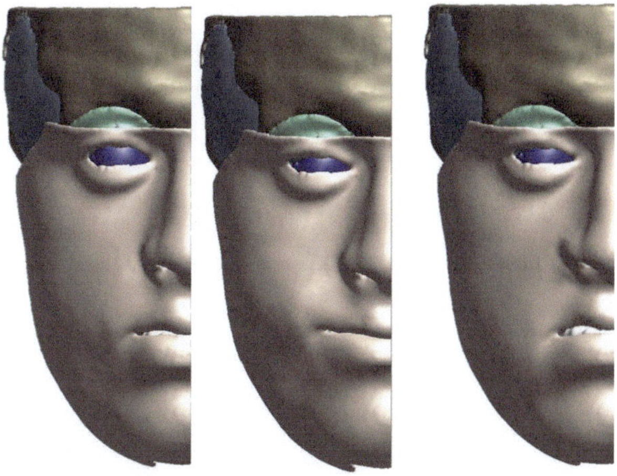

Fig. 5.5 Facial expressions rest (*left*), smiling (*middle*) and disgust (*right*)

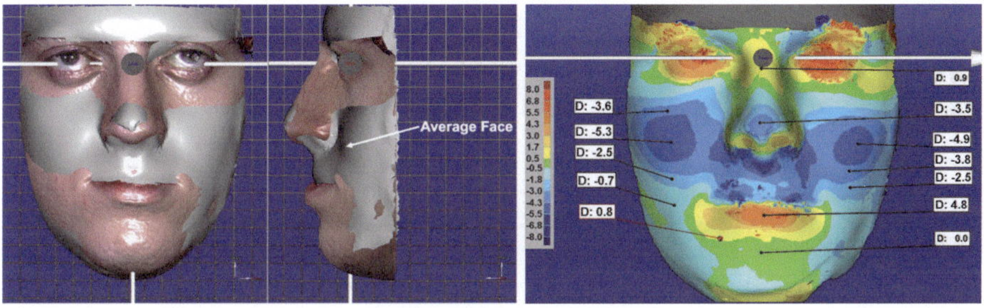

Fig. 5.6 Color textured image overlaid on average face for males 18 to 22 years of age (*left*); color deviation map of patient compared with a facial average highlighting a deficiency in the middle part of the face by 5 mm (*right*)

be less prominent than the average face. The relationship of the soft tissues to the hard tissues have changed substantially pre- and post-operatively (Fig. 5.7). The finite element predictions showed a very similar outcome to that achieved with small areas of discrepancy at 3 and 6 months. The green areas indicate that the surgical prediction was generally within 0.8 mm of the actual surgical correction (Fig. 5.7).

5.5 Methods to Determine Facial Movement Pre- and Post-surgical Intervention

Our facial appearance and expressive behaviors have a major impact on how we are perceived and how others in society perceive us. The inability to express oneself via facial movement can have serious social consequences as both verbal and non-verbal movements communicate our emotional state of mind to others. Such patients who may be affected include those with facial nerve paralysis, those with

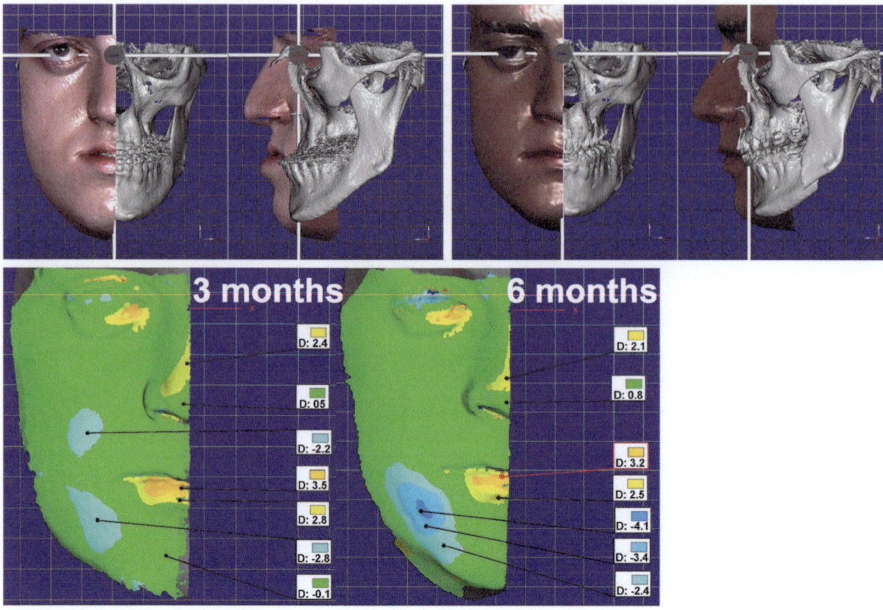

Fig. 5.7 Pre-surgical (*top left*) and post-surgical plan (*top right*). 3 month and 6 month post surgical evaluation of the surgical plan and actual outcome. There is a high level of concordance between the surgical plan and surgical outcome at 3 and 6 months (*green* represents difference of less than 0.8 mm). Greater errors were particularly associated with the lower lip (3.5 mm). This reconstruction was undertaken on static images but it is also important to evaluate facial changes during normal function (speech, expressions and mastication)

dentofacial deformities and patients with cleft lip. Many of these patients will opt to have reconstructive or orthognathic surgery to correct their aesthetic and functional deficits. It is important that there are adequate measures for objectively quantifying pre- and post-operative function for these patients as this will help in diagnosing the severity of the impairment and aid in outcome assessment (Mishima et al., 2009; Nooreyazdan et al., 2004; Okudaira et al., 2008).

The first consideration in facial movement analysis pre- and post-operation is what facial gesture is most appropriate to use to measure movement. The choice of action can broadly be classified into verbal and non-verbal facial gestures (Popat et al., 2011). In principle, any facial gestures can be employed for the assessment of facial movement. However facial gestures that may be appropriate for use in psychology assessments for example may not be so for assessment in pre- and post-operation. One must therefore consider the application carefully.

In addition, when monitoring facial movement over time or through intervention the measure of facial movement used should be repeatable. If this is not the case, then individual variation or difference in the performed facial gesture between two time points will induce error into the assessment. Verbal facial gestures tend to exhibit higher reproducibility when compared to facial expressions (Popat et al., 2010).

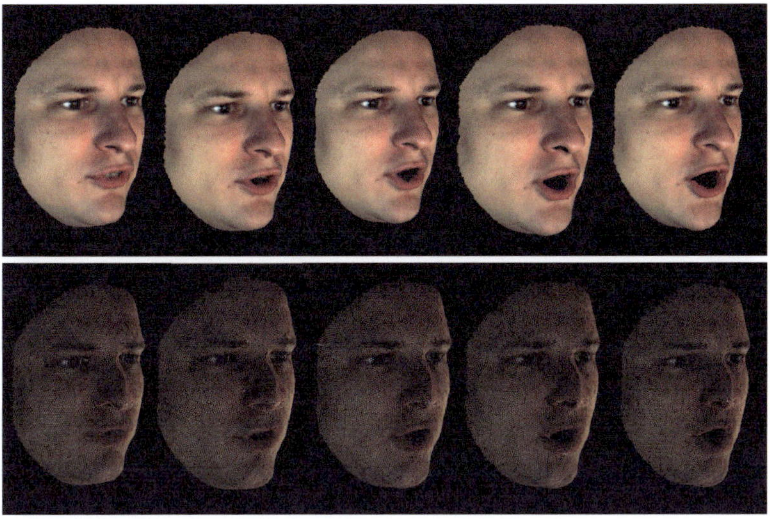

Fig. 5.8 Selected sequential frames of a patient saying the word /rope/

5.5.1 Data Analysis

Research into facial movement utilizes statistical modeling techniques to analyze the dynamic 3D data acquired. A sequence of facial movement may typically contain a set of 3D images at 30–60 frames per second (Fig. 5.8).

Images from the sequence must be registered within the same 3D space. This allows valid comparison of facial movement between frames from within a sequence but also between different groups and time points. Using 3D facial landmarks, the coordinates of interest can then extracted from images along the timeline to form the dataset. Landmark trajectories can be plotted and inter-landmark distances measured to give information on facial movement pre- and post-operation to assess functional change. To explore variability in facial shape however and isolate patterns/relationships between the areas of facial movement more sophisticated methods of modeling are required such as Principal Component analysis (PCA).

Here we illustrate a patient with a prominent chin who was part of a cohort that underwent orthognathic surgery to both upper and lower jaws. The change in lip movement pre- and post-operation is statistically modeled using the x, y and z coordinates of 6 anthropometric landmarks: labiale superius (ls)—the midpoint of the upper vermilion line, labiale inferius (li)—the midpoint of the lower vermilion line, crista philtri (cph L/R)—the point on the left and right elevated margins of the philtrum above the vermilion line and cheilion (ch L/R)—the point located at the left and right labial commissure (Farkas, 1993). Data of the patient saying several words were acquired immediately pre- and 6 months post-operation using a 3D motion capture system (Fig. 5.9).

The 3D facial shells at rest and at maximum displacement for each word both pre- and post operation were registered (aligned) in space using Generalised Procrustes

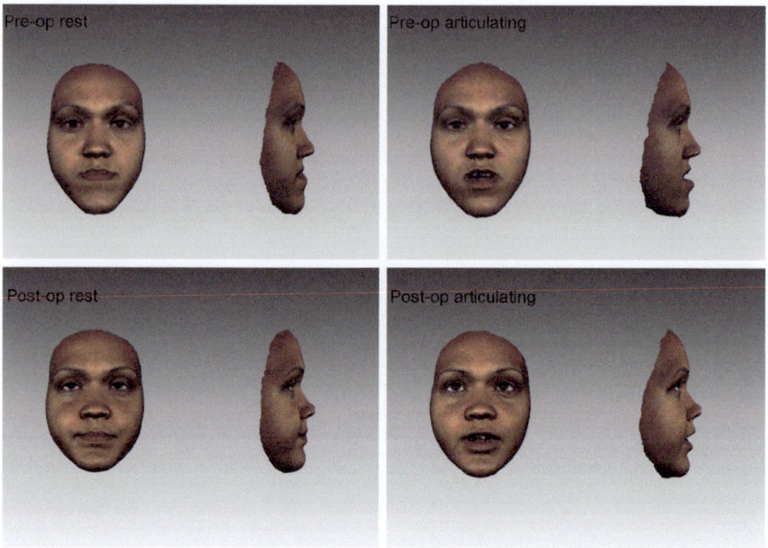

Fig. 5.9 Patient with a severe Class 3 dentofacial deformity pre- and post-operation at rest and articulating the word /rope/

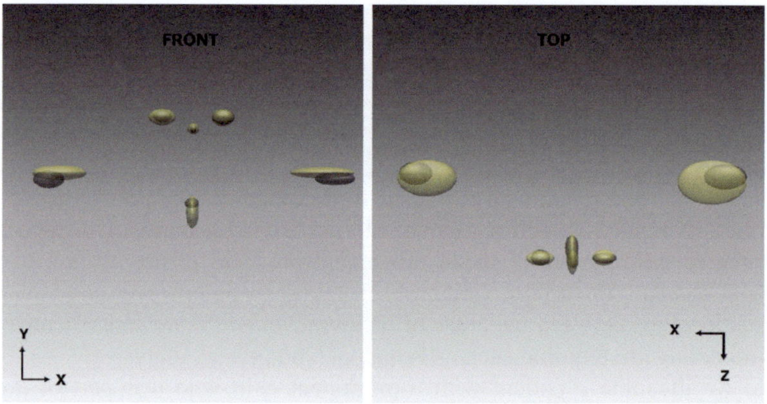

Fig. 5.10 3D ellipsoid plot (mean ± 2 SD) showing the difference in lip shape pre- and post-operation (pre—*yellow*, post—*black*)

Analysis by removing translation and rotation (Dryden and Mardia, 1998). Scaling was not incorporated to preserve lip size and shape. The mean position of each landmark (centroid) was plotted with 2 standard deviations to give a 3D ellipsoid representing 95 percent of the variation in lip shape for each time point. Figure 5.10 shows the difference in lip shape for the group from pre- to post-operation. Post-operation the mean lip height has been reduced and the mean lip width increased.

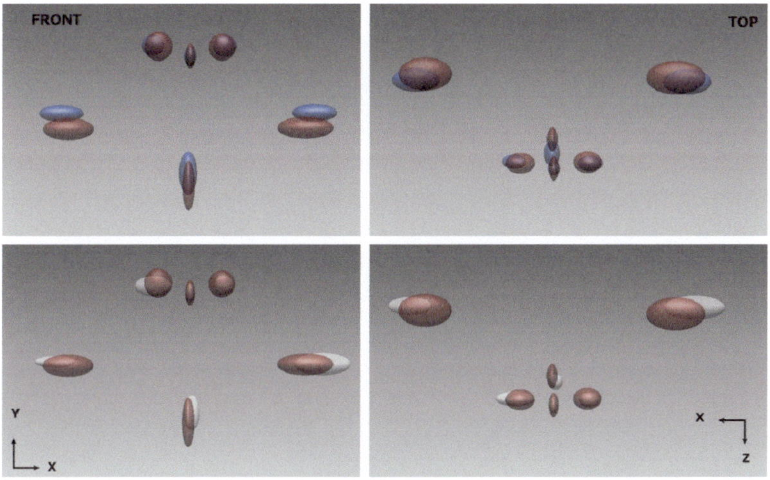

Fig. 5.11 3D ellipsoid plot (mean ± 2 SD) showing lip shape for maximum articulation of the word /rope/ comparing normal movement (*red*) to pre-operation (*blue*) and post-operation (*white*)

The effect of this on lip movement can be visualized in Fig. 5.11 where 3D ellipsoids have been used to plot pre- and post-operation movement for the word /rope/ against a control or average group. Post-operation, there is less protrusion and more downward movement of the corners of the mouth, which when compared with the control group shows that both the dentofacial aesthetics and function have been normalized (Fig. 5.12).

Although treatment aims for patients have always been to restore aesthetics and function, traditionally methods to monitor facial function has lacked precision and objectivity. With 3D motion capture systems, statistical modeling techniques are a valuable technique in processing large volumes of data resulting in a concise and meaningful interpretation of facial function.

5.5.2 Tracking Movement of the Mandible

Although surface movement is important for daily interactions it is also necessary to reliably record movement of the mandible also during function and especially prior to surgical planning. There have been several methods employed in the past such as photography (Wood, 1979), Kinesiograph (Martin et al., 2000) and radiographic (Kim et al., 2010). However any motion capture system should also incorporate mandible movement. An example is shown in Fig. 5.13 whereby 4 spheres have been attached to an upper and lower framework, which is then attached to upper and lower teeth using two orthodontic brackets. Movement of the spheres in space will determine the trajectory of mandibular movement. Documenting this movement will be useful to plan the path of opening and closure of the jaw during surgery for

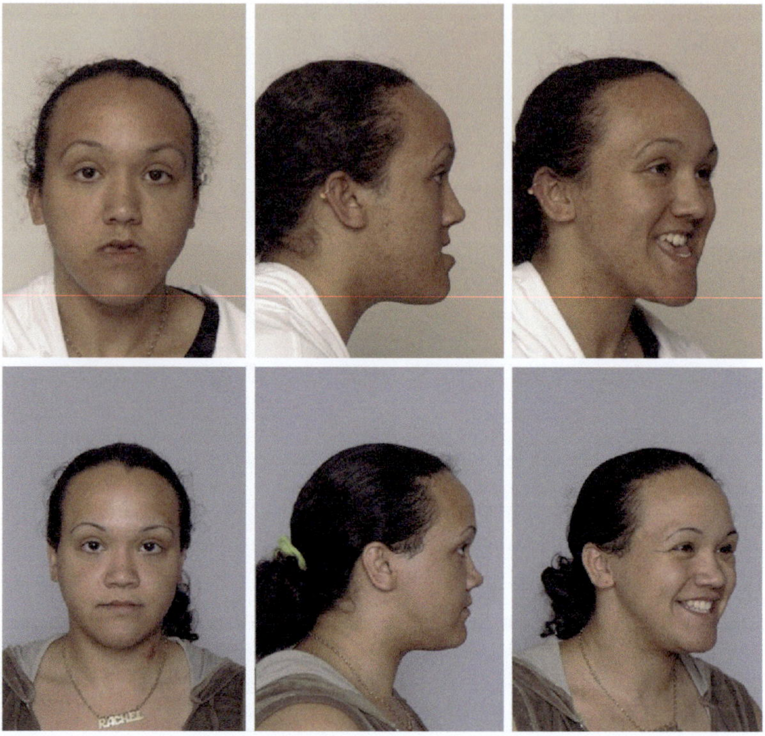

Fig. 5.12 Pre- and post-operation facial appearance. Surgery has brought the maxilla forwards and moved the mandible backwards enabling an excellent interdigitation of the upper an lower dentitions

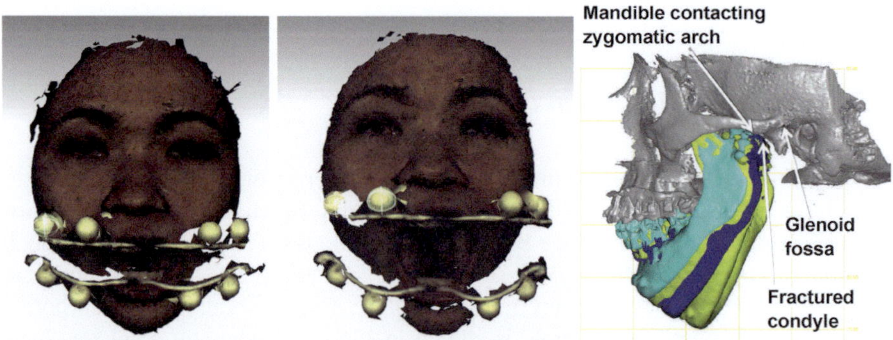

Fig. 5.13 Tracking movement of the mandible using 4 spheres on a frame attached to upper and lower teeth (*left* 18 mm opening; *middle* 42 mm opening). The image on the *right* tracks mandibular movement for an individual with bilateral fractures of the condyle whereby the mandible pivots on the zygomatic arch as oppose to the condyle articulating with the glenoid fossa (*right*)

individuals presenting with facial, trauma, oro-facial cancer and facial disharmony. All that is needed is a CBCT and at least 3 spheres located to the upper and lower dentition. The reliability of this system is generally within 1 mm. An example is shown of an individual with bilateral fractures of the condyle and instead of the condyle articulating in the glenoid fossa the broken fragment is seen articulating with the zygomatic arch (Fig. 5.13).

5.6 Refinement of Techniques

5.6.1 Registration

It is often the case in medical imaging that important information is contained in more than one image (ensemble). A practical example of this would be latitudinal or longitudinal ensembles of facial 3D surface scans, obtained with surface scanners which are becoming a common and a valuable diagnostic tool. It is convenient to refer to 2D and 3D images, as well as surface scans, henceforth as simply "images".

Typically, analysis of image ensembles involves construction of some statistical model. In contrast to hand-crafted models, which are inevitably inflexible and often inaccurate, modern statistical modeling methods allow for automatic construction of models directly from data. Before any meaningful analysis, statistical or otherwise, can be performed on an ensemble of images, correspondences between analogous parts of the images, across the entire ensemble, must first be established. This is accomplished by a procedure called *registration*. In other words, registration is a necessary prerequisite to extracting and aggregating useful information from an ensemble of images.

The methods for registration are classified according to the nature and modality of imagery to which they are applicable, according to the separation of samples (spatial, temporal, or both), by interactivity (manual, semi-automatic, automatic), by feature understanding (sparse, or feature-based, as opposed to dense, or area-based), by the model of admissible deformations, by multiplicity paradigm (pairwise or groupwise), and other properties (Sidorov, 2010).

Manual registration of large ensembles of images is tedious and error prone—while humans can easily determine correspondences between salient features (e.g. eyes), they fail to establish correspondences between points in featureless regions (e.g. cheeks). Further, while manual annotation of 2D imagery is easily possible, in three dimensions it becomes prohibitively difficult for practical reasons. Hence, advances of computer vision are employed to perform registration tasks automatically.

Here, we briefly address automatic dense non-rigid groupwise registration applied to craniofacial 3D surface scans. Principal registration problems are: to register an ensemble of temporally separated images of the same subject (over various lengths of time: e.g. video of a person speaking; longitudinal study of growth over several years), and to register ensembles of images of several subjects, termed intra- and inter- subject registration accordingly.

Let us call what is actually observed by the imaging device (or the eye) the *appearance* of an image. Changes in appearance result from variations in the shape of the object e.g. deformation of the face during function, and from variations in the *texture* of the object e.g. blushing, shadows and facial hair. Both factors are usually present when images are obtained from different subjects.

Changes in appearance due to variations in shape are typically highly non-linear and a priori unpredictable—simple changes in shape may cause complicated changes in appearance.

The purpose of registration is to determine the underlying deformation process that leads to the observed changes in appearance, and so determine how every point in one image is transformed into the analogous point in another image.

Depending on the range of admissible deformations, registration methods are roughly subdivided into *rigid* and *non-rigid*. Rigid methods crudely align the samples together, by computing global rigid transformations that bring all samples into alignment. Non-rigid methods allow for more general, local deformations to be recovered; this, however, comes at a much higher computational cost, as a substantially larger search space has to be explored. Some modern algorithms (Sidorov et al., 2009, 2011) explore the space of all possible deformation models in addition to exploring the space of parameters of a particular model, when searching for optimal correspondences.

Traditionally, when registering an ensemble of images, one image would be chosen as a "reference" and a pairwise registration method would be applied repeatedly to establish correspondences between the reference image and every other image in the ensemble, so establishing the correspondences between all pairs of images via the intermediate reference (the problem of registering a *pair* of images has been well-researched; Zitova and Flusser, 2003). However, it has been recently shown (Cootes et al., 2010; Sidorov et al., 2009, 2011) that this approach is sub-optimal. Indeed, in such approaches the results is inevitably biased to the choice of the reference image; and an unfortunate choice of the reference, for example one that is uncharacteristic of the rest of the ensemble, complicates matters further. More importantly, it has been shown (Cootes et al., 2010; Sidorov et al., 2009, 2011) that a superior paradigm is to utilize as much information from the *entire* ensemble, rather than from only a pair at a time. Only by considering multiple examples simultaneously can corresponding structures be reliably identified. Registration methods that operate on this principle are called *groupwise*. Typically (Cootes et al., 2010; Sidorov et al., 2009, 2011), groupwise registration amounts to constructing a common reference model of texture (to account for the variation in texture) and computing a set of models of deformation such that variation in the ensemble can be parsimoniously explained in terms of applying computed deformations to the model of texture. Accuracy and reliability of modern groupwise registration methods is typically higher than that of the pairwise registration, and higher than that of manual annotation (especially for relatively featureless imagery).

The problem of registration is ill-defined in the sense that there is no obvious criterion for optimality of registration results. Typically, the aim is to find a model of the underlying deformation process such that it best explains the changes of appearance in the *simplest* possible way.

Having registered the samples (that is, having found, for every point in each sample, the corresponding positions of the analogous points in every other sample), one can perform statistical analysis on the corresponding features.

To illustrate the usefulness of inter-subject registration, we took a corpus of 32 facial scans of different individuals, applied our registration algorithm to it (the evolution of the reference model is illustrated in Fig. 5.14) and, having found the dense correspondences, computed a generative appearance model (Cootes et al., 1998). The principal modes of variation, automatically found by registration and statistical modeling, are shown. We can use these registration techniques to explore facial expressions and speech.

5.6.2 Determination of the Orientation of Facial Muscle Fibers

Previously we used average estimates for facial muscle positioning, however each individual has different muscle masses and different origins and insertions. The manner in which a muscle delivers mechanical force is strongly dependent on its fibrous architecture has been understood for some time (Bovendeerd et al., 1994). Thus, to improve the understanding of subject-specific muscle mechanics, accurate estimations of fiber orientation must first be obtained *in vivo*. Some of the first successful non-invasive techniques worked by inspection of muscle fiber striation patterns visible through high-resolution structural MRI (Engstrom et al., 1991). Unfortunately, within MRI, not all muscles produce visible striations at feasible image resolutions and so, with the lack of any other inherent orientational information within structural MRI, such approaches were limited to the study of large muscles. It was not until the introduction of diffusion-weighted MRI (DW-MRI) (Stjeskal and Tanner, 1965) that we could begin to probe tissue microstructure and begin to retrieve voxel-wise orientational information.

In principle, DW-MRI measures the rate of diffusion of water along a given orientation within a volume of interest. At first glance this appears disconnected from the retrieval of *in vivo* muscle fiber orientations; however, it was noticed that the particular cellular organizations (i.e. regularly arranged elongated fibrous cells) would produce distinct variations in the rate of diffusion of water relative to their macroscopic orientation. In other words, water may diffuse faster along a fiber than across fibers because it will encounter fewer hydrophobic cellular boundaries per unit length; in doing so this produces a measurable, modelable, diffusion anisotropy. From these observations various techniques were developed to turn raw directionally encoded 4D DW-MRI images into voxel-wise estimates of fiber orientation (Fig. 5.15).

One of the earliest, and potentially still the most popular of such techniques is Diffusion Tensor MRI (DT-MRI) (Basser et al., 1994a, 1994b). DT-MRI model as-

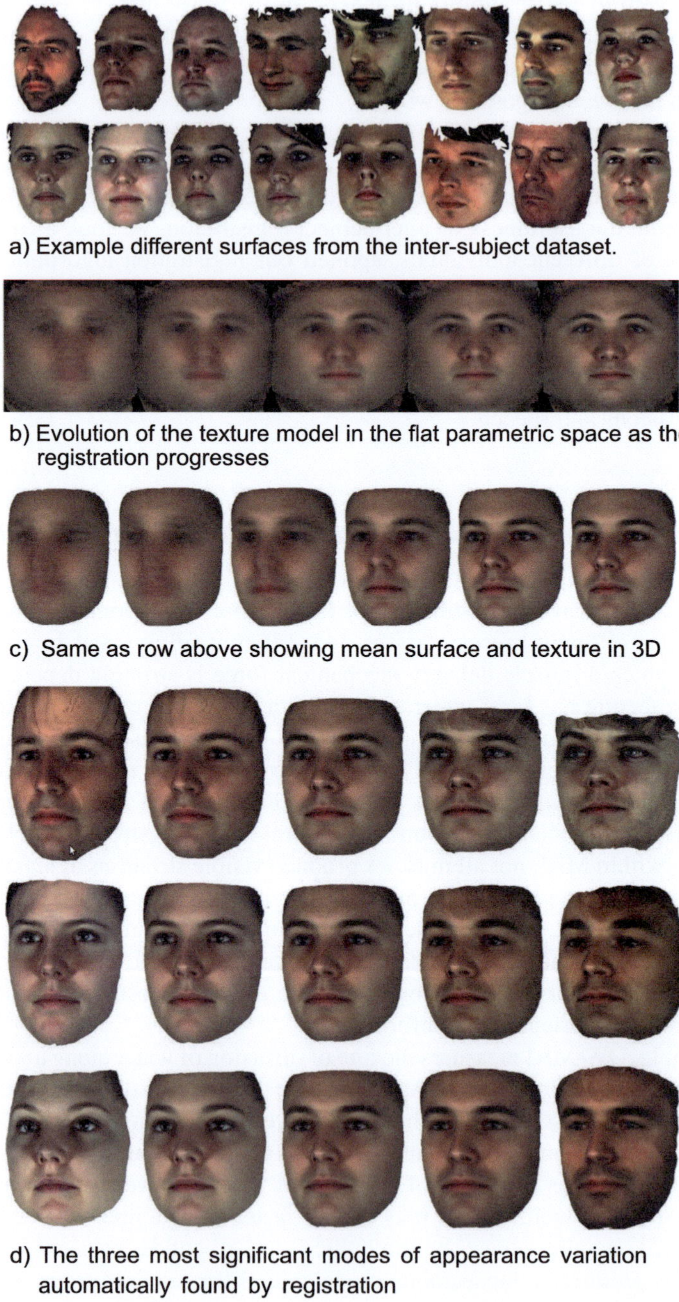

Fig. 5.14 Evolution of the reference model: (**a**) the original data; (**b**) the texture model in the flat parametric space; (**c**) mean surface and texture in 3D; (**d**) three most significant modes of appearance variation automatically found by registration and statistical modeling

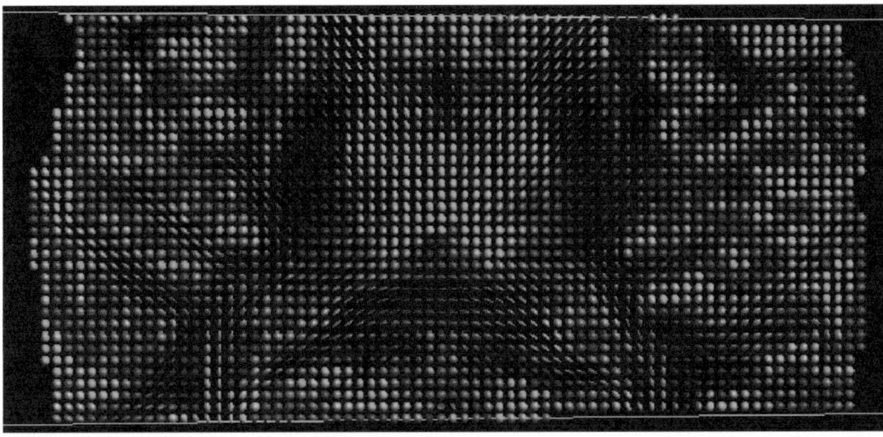

Fig. 5.15 Voxel-wise estimates of fiber orientation retrieved through DT-MRI (ellipsoidal representation). Image depicts a slice through the human brain. Direction is encoded through color with *blue* representing orientations into and out of the plane, *green* forwards/backwards and *red* left/right (otherwise known as directionally encoded color)

sumes that fibrous diffusion can be modeled as a three-dimensional Gaussian diffusion tensor (i.e. an ellipsoid with the axis of greatest diffusion pointed down the fiber trajectory); by fitting this model to observed DW-signals, Eigen-analysis can reveal fiber orientation (the first Eigenvector) and a host of other useful quantitative parameters such including Fractional Anisotropy (FA), a ratio of longitudinal to radial diffusion (provided by the Eigenvalues) that might be useful to in the analysis of tissue integrity (Basser and Pierpaoli, 1996).

A logical step from voxel-wise measurements of orientation is to attempt to retrieve some representation of connectivity; to determine where a particular fibrous structure begins, where it ends and the path it follows along the way. To achieve this goal we employ a class of techniques collectively known as tractography (Basser et al., 2000). An *extremely* basic algorithm would be as follows: Position seed points in a regular grid across the target image, from each seed point, anchor two streamlines (remembering that fibers are axially-symmetric). Each streamline takes the orientation of its host voxel (or its inverse) and follows that path until reaching a boundary with a new voxel; checking the angle between its own orientation and the dominant orientation within the new voxel, a streamline will either (1) terminate if the angle is above a predefined threshold or (2) proceed through the new voxel taking on that voxels orientation until it reaches another voxel boundary and repeats the process. Once all streamlines have terminated or reached an image boundary, those sharing a common start point can then be joined to create a single coherent path. In this way a streamline can follow an orientationally coherent string of voxel-wise orientations while filtering out un-natural reconstructions (it is highly unlikely that a muscle fiber will deviate more than 35–40° per 2–3 mm step). The streamline can then be rendered as a 3D line with vertices at visited voxel boundaries, facilitating a more intuitive visual inspection. In reality such a simplistic approach would never

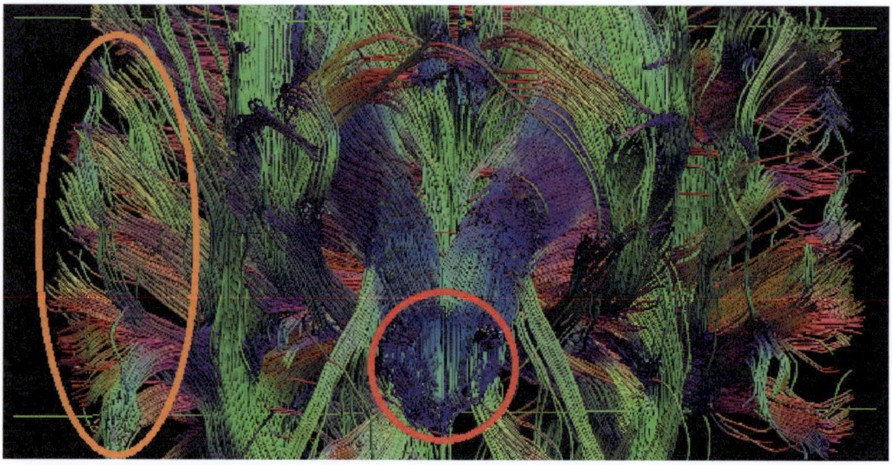

Fig. 5.16 Result of DT-MRI based tractography displaying all tracts originating from or traversing through the slice of human brain depicted in Fig. 5.15. Easily identifiable structures include sections of the brain stem (*red*) and *corpus callosum* (*orange*). Note that is far easier to identify connectivity through inspection of tractography than through voxel-wise data alone

be used, modern tractography will often employ techniques such as fiber orientation interpolation (placing vertices at fixed separations and computing point specific estimates of fiber orientation), probabilistic filtering (Parker et al., 2003) (to filter out erroneous streamlines) and support for more complicated DW-signal processing models (to be discussed shortly). An example of DT-MRI based tractography visualizing all tracts passing through the image slice is depicted in Fig. 5.16.

Unfortunately, DT-MRI is not without limitations. While DT-MRI derived estimates of fiber orientation can generally be considered reliable in voxels containing a single axially aligned fiber population, the tensor model is unable to resolve the 'crossing-fibers' problem that occurs when a voxel intersects two or more non-collinear fiber populations (Alexander et al., 2001). This is generally not a problem with larger muscles (relative to voxel dimensions)—explaining successful applications of DT-MRI to large muscle groups; legs (Heemskerk et al., 2010; Kan et al., 2009), heart (Kim et al., 2005; Zhukov and Barr, 2003) where one can derive important biomechanical properties such as the pennation angle (Damon et al., 2002; Heemskerk et al., 2005)—however as muscle size decreases relative to the size of a voxel, the frequency of intra-voxel orientational complexity increases (Fig. 5.17) and thus the tensor model fails more frequently.

Consequentially, when examining complex fiber architecture e.g. the tongue (Kim et al., 2005), successful DT-MRI often requires an image resolution that is not practical *in vivo* on clinical scanners (mostly due to SNR considerations at low field strengths 1.5–3 T).

The challenge for muscle reconstruction in particular originates from the shorter T_2 of muscle fiber (35–45 ms depending on activity; Rumeur et al., 1994) in comparison to that of white matter (80 ms) where study of complex fiber architecture is

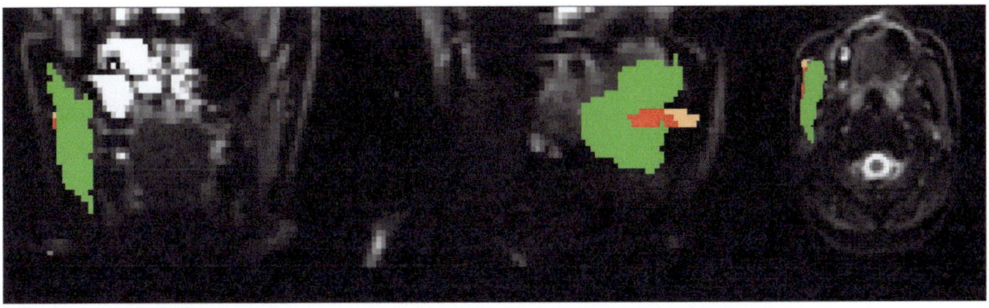

Fig. 5.17 A demonstration of crossing-fibers. Here we have segmented visible portions of the *masseter* (*green*) and risorius (*pink*), *red* denotes shared voxels. Note that the largest portion of the *risorius* lies within this shared region and thus the majority of the muscle would not be retrievable through DT-MRI. The *masseter* on the other hand is relatively easy to reconstruct, its relative size limits the effect of crossing fiber errors to smaller portions of its total volume

more prevalent. The resultant additional T_2 weighted signal losses, in combination with other factors more frequently encountered in *in vivo* studies of muscle (such as geometric distortions generated by magnetic inhomogeneities due to nearby air-tissue boundaries; Morgan et al., 2004), imposes greater restrictions on voxel dimensions to ensure that the diffusion-weighted signal intensities are above the Rician noise floor (Jones and Basser, 2004). While white matter studies may reliable image at high resolutions, SNR considerations with *in vivo* muscle have typically forced use of a coarser $3 \times 3 \times 3$ mm resolution (our own situation) or lower.

Where DT-MRI has been applied to muscle structure *in vivo*, e.g. Gilbert's study of the human tongue (Gilbert and Napadow, 2005), SNR considerations forced a spatial resolution of $3 \times 3 \times 6$–8 mm. This coarse resolution then prevented the extraction of meaningful fiber orientations and instead forced a reliance on fractional anisotropy to imply structure—i.e. voxels with low anisotropy imply the presence of crossing fiber, from which inferences can be made through comparison with classical anatomy. Compared to later work by the same author (Gilbert et al., 2006), which achieved successful lingual core tractography through diffusion spectrum imaging (DSI; Wedeen et al., 2005, one of many newer techniques designed to resolve crossing-fibers) of an *ex vivo* sample at voxel volumes ranging from 2 to 4 mm^3, it is clear that *in vivo* DT-MRI lacks the fidelity required to provide accurate subject specific biometric information. Unfortunately the high b-values required for DSI (a diffusion weighting affecting the weight of DW-signal attenuation with respect to measured diffusion weight) would result in unacceptably low *in vivo* SNR throughout the cranial-facial region on clinical hardware.

Constrained spherical harmonic deconvolution (CSHD; Tournier et al., 2004) provides one possible way forward. However, despite the increasing number of applications of CSD to white matter, use on other fibrous tissue is largely undocumented (either *in* or *ex vivo*). The principle assumption of all spherical deconvolution approaches (numerous examples exist) is that the fiber orientation distribution function (i.e., a set of vectors describing the principle orientations of fibrous tissue within the voxel) can be obtained through deconvolution of a 'common' single fiber

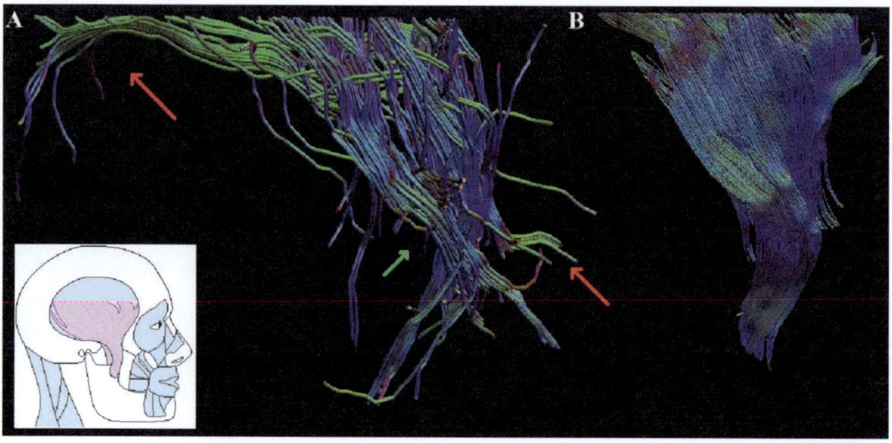

Fig. 5.18 The effects of calibration on CSHD derived estimates of fiber orientation, a look at the *temporalis* muscle. An example of inappropriate calibration (the selected response function was of higher anisotropy than muscle tissue), typical errors include spurious fiber tracts with no basis in anatomy (marked *red*) and premature tract termination, especially in regions with higher curvature (marked *green*) (*left*). Tractography applied through the same volume as A, but with appropriate CSHD response function selection. Note that the reconstruction appears fuller in general, premature tract termination is greatly reduced and additional detail is visible at the muscles insertions into the mandible. Tractography at the upper edge is prematurely terminated in both A and B due to limited image coverage (*right*)

response function (a representation of a DW-signal produced by a single-fiber population of the same tissue type) from the observed DW-signal—spherical deconvolution is no longer limited to one orientation per voxel. In practice, this common response function is not known *a priori* and thus an estimated/simulated fiber response must be used. Selection of an appropriate response is particularly important when applying CSDH as limitations inherent to its spherical harmonic data representation make it particularly unforgiving of errors at this point (Fig. 5.18 left) (Parker and Jones, 2011a). Fortunately however, our group has devised a simple, yet effective, automated response function selection technique (Parker and Jones, 2011b) allowing us to apply CSHD with reasonable success, achieving anatomically viable reconstructions of the *Temporalis* (Fig. 5.18 right), *Massetter* (Fig. 5.19a), *Buccinator* (Fig. 5.19b), *Risorius* and other smaller muscles where data quality permits (Fig. 5.20).

While advances have been made towards the signal-processing end our pipeline, image acquisition still remains problematic. Of the available imaging coils within our laboratory, the 8 channel brain imaging array provides the best coverage of our area of interest but, understandably, being optimized for brain imaging, tends to suffer from signal roll-off towards the below the subjects eyes. In combination with previously mentioned geometric distortions and T_2 related signal losses, data quality within the lower regions, particularly within the cheeks, about the lips and within the mandible can be particularly poor, resulting in incomplete or missing tractography. We are hopeful that with the addition of a new purpose built RF coil

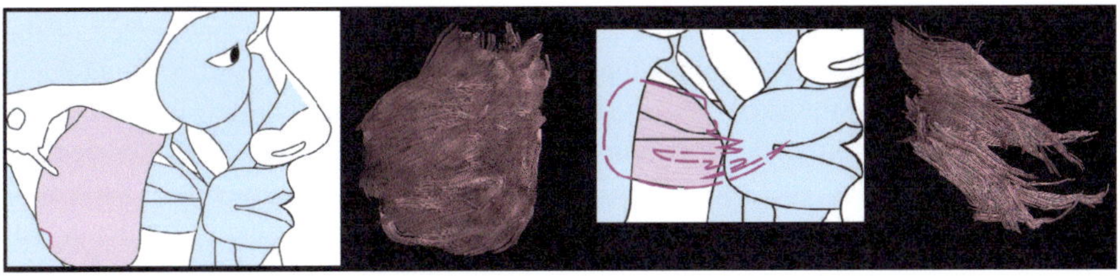

Fig. 5.19 Example of a near complete *masseter* muscle reconstruction achieved through CSHD tractography (*left*). Example of a partial *buccinator* reconstruction, while image distortion within the cheek prevents a complete reconstruction crossing fiber resolution has been successfully achieved at the *masseter-buccinator* intersection (*leftmost* segment of the image) and the three main muscle components are clearly distinguishable (*right*)

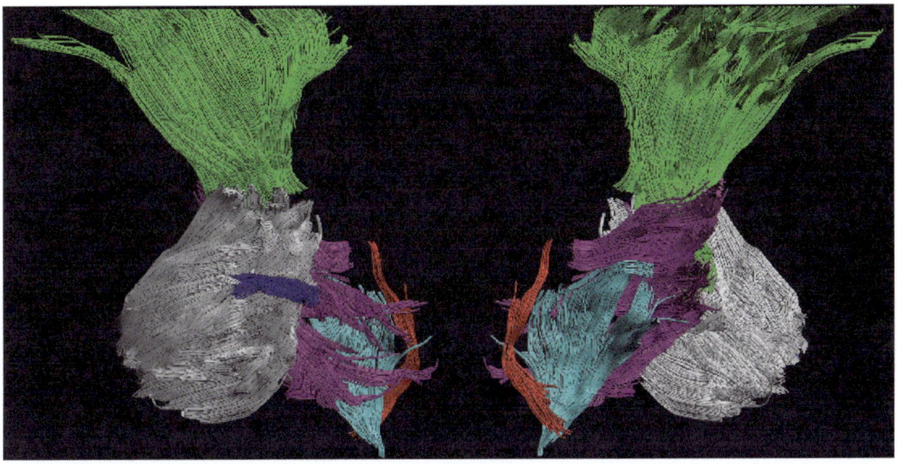

Fig. 5.20 Selection of muscles shown in context. *Green*: *Temporalis*, *grey*: *masseter*, *purple*: *buccinator*, *blue*: *risorius*, *cyan*: *genioglossus*, *red*: *depressor/levator anguli oris*. Unfortunately as we examine lower cranial-facial regions, DW-signal quality is such that reliable reconstruction is no longer achievable

and introduction of a susceptibility matched medium into the subject's oral cavity, data quality will improve.

5.7 Conclusion

There are many genetic and non-genetic factors that influence facial shape and it is likely that further genotype and phenotype associations as well as environmental influences will be discovered as soon as larger 3D facial databases combined with genetic information become established. Appreciating individual facial features is important when evaluating changes as a result of growth and surgical interventions.

A simple example of this is when a scalpel incision is made on the surface of the skin. The clinician often examines the lines on the skin surface and if the incision is made in line with the skin creases (Langer lines) scarring is often less visible as opposed to an incision made perpendicular to Langer lines. In the case of correcting facial disharmony the vast majority of surgery is performed intra-orally with minimal "invisible" scarring. However repositioning the bony surgical fragments will have an effect on the shape of the surface tissues and clinicians need to define the surface morphology and how the specific morphologies change with the magnitude of movement and spatial positioning. Surprisingly, with the wide variation in facial features, simple classifications such as, long/short, thin and wide still persist for individual facial features and shape is often ignored. Further work is needed to provide data for valid constituent modeling and to detail changes in the soft tissues during function. Nevertheless employing average parameters for soft tissues has provided an accurate model to predict facial surgery. Methods for automatic construction of craniofacial appearance models will in the future underpin much of craniofacial research, including realistic modeling of influences of non-invasive and invasive treatment modalities, management of facial injuries, predicting the effects of aging, simulation of surgical intervention, post-surgical evaluation of a patient's appearance leading to the optimization and refinement of surgical procedures. It is hoped that these significant advances will find their way into routine clinical practice in the near future.

References

Alexander AL, Hasan KM, Lazar M, Tsuruda JS, Parker DL (2001) Analysis of partial volume effects in diffusion-tensor MRI. Magn Reson Med 45(5):770–780

Basser PJ, Pierpaoli C (1996) Microstructural and physiological features of tissues elucidated by quantitativediffusion-tensor MRI. J Magn Reson 111:209–219

Basser PJ, Mattello J, Lebihan D (1994a) Estimation of the effective self-diffusion tensor from the NMR spin echo. J Magn Res 103:247–254

Basser PJ, Mattiello J, LeBihan D (1994b) MR diffusion tensor spectroscopy and imaging. Biophys J 66:259–267

Basser PJ, Pajevic S, Pierpaoli C, Duda J, Aldroubi A (2000) In vivo tractography using DT-MRI data. Magn Reson Med 44:625–632

Beldie L, Walker B, Lu YT, Richmond S, Middleton J (2010) Finite element modeling of maxillofacial surgery and facial expressions—a preliminary study. Int J Med Robot Comput Assist Surg 6(4):422–430

Bhatia SN, Leighton BC (1993) Manual of facial growth: a computer analysis of longitudinal cephalometric growth data. Oxford Medical Publications, Oxford

Bovendeerd PH, Huyghe JM, Arts T, Van Campen DH, Reneman RS (1994) Influence of endocardialepicardial of muscle fibers on left ventricular wall mechanics. J Biomech 27:941–951

Bryant JA, Drage NA, Richmond S (2008) Study of the scan uniformity from an i-CAT cone beam computed tomography dental imaging system. Dentomaxillofac Radiol 37(7):365–374

Cohen MM (2002) Malformations of the craniofacial region: evolutionary, embryonic, genetic, and clinical perspectives. Am J Med Genet C, Semin Med Genet 115:245–268

Cootes TF, Twining CJ, Petrovic VS et al (2010) Computing accurate correspondences across groups of images. IEEE Trans Pattern Anal Mach Intell 32(11):1994–2005

Cootes TF, Edwards GJ, Taylor CJ (1998) Active appearance models. In: Proceedings of the European conference on computer vision, pp 484–498

Damon BM, Ding Z, Anderson AW, Freyer AS, Gore JC (2002) Validation of diffusion tensor MRI-based muscle fiber tracking. Magn Reson Med 48:97–104

Djordjevic J, Richmond S, Toma A, Zhurov A (2010) Three-dimensional facial morphology and insulin sensitivity—a longitudinal study. In: 7th international orthodontic congress, Sydney, Australia, February 6–9

Drage N, Rout J (2010) Diagnostic imaging. In: Kau C, Richmond S (eds) Three-dimensional imaging for orthodontics and maxillofacial surgery. Wiley/Blackwell, New York. ISBN 978-0813806143

Dryden IL, Mardia KV (1998) Generalised Procrustes methods. In: Barnett V, et al (eds) Statistical shape analysis. Wiley, Chichester

Engstrom CM, Loeb GE, Reid JG, Forrest WJ, Avruch L (1991) Morphometry of the human thigh muscles. A comparison between anatomical sections and computer tomographical and magnetic resonance images. J Anat 176:139–156

Farkas L (1993) Anthropometry of the head and face. Raven Press, New York

Gilbert RJ, Napadow VJ (2005) Three-dimensional muscular architecture of the human tongue determined in vivo with diffusion tensor magnetic resonance imaging. Dysphagia 20:1–7

Gilbert RJ, Weeden VJ, Magnusson LH, Benner T, Wang R, Dai G, Napadow VJ, Roche KK (2006) Three-dimensional myoarchitecture of the bovine tongue demonstrated by diffusion spectrum magnetic resonance imaging with tractography. Anat Rec A 288:1173–1182

Heemskerk AM, Strijkers GJ, Vilanova A, Drost MR, Nicolary K (2005) Determination of mouse skeletal muscle architecture using three-dimensional diffusion tensor imaging. Magn Reson Med 53:1333–1340

Heemskerk AM, Sinha TK, Wilson KJ, Ding Z, Damon BM (2010) Repeatability of DTI-based skeletal muscle fiber tracking. NMR Biomed 23(3):294–303

Henderson J, Granell R, Heron J, Sherriff A, Simpson A, Woodcock A, Strachan DP, Shaheen SO, Sterne JA (2008) Associations of wheezing phenotypes in the first 6 years of life with atopy, lung function and airway responsiveness in mid-childhood. Thorax 63(11):974–980

Hill AV (1938) The heat shortening and the dynamic constants of muscle. Proc R Soc Lond B, Biol Sci 126:136–195

Hundley WG, Bluemke DA, Finn JP, et al (2010) ACCF/ACR/AHA/NASCI/SCMR 2010 expert consensus document on cardiovascular magnetic resonance: a report of the American College of Cardiology Foundation Task Force on Expert Consensus documents. Circulation 121(22):2462–2508

Jones DK, Basser PJ (2004) Squashing peanuts and smashing pumpkins: how noise distorts diffusion-weighted MR data. Magn Reson Med 52:979–993

Kan JH, Heemskerk AM, Ding Z, Gregory A, Mencio G, Spindler K, Damon BM (2009) DTI-based muscle fiber tracking of the quadriceps mechanism in lateral patellar dislocation. Magn Reson Med 29(3):663–670

Kang SH, Kim DK, Seo KM, Seo JH (2011) Usefulness of videofluoroscopic swallow study with mixed consistency food for patients with stroke or other brain injuries. J Korean Med Sci 26(3):425–430

Kau CH (2010) Three-dimensional surface acquisition systems for facial analysis. In: Kau C, Richmond S (eds) Three-dimensional imaging for orthodontics and maxillofacial surgery. Wiley/Blackwell, New York, pp 11–28. ISBN: 978-0813806143

Kau CH, Richmond S, Zhurov A, Ovsenik M, Tawfik W, Borbely P, English JD (2010) Use of 3-dimensional surface acquisition to study facial morphology in 5 populations. Am J Orthod Dentofac Orthop 137(4 Suppl):S56.e1-9

Kim S, Chi-Fishman G, Barnett AS, Pierpaoli C (2005) Dependence on diffusion time of apparent diffusion tensor of ex vivo calf tongue and heart. Magn Reson Med 54(6):1287–1296

Kim DS, Choi SC, Lee SS, Heo MS, Huh KH, Hwang SJ, Yi WJ (2010) Correlation between 3-dimensional facial morphology and mandibular movement during maximum mouth opening and closing. Oral Surg Oral Med Oral Pathol Oral Endo 110:648–656

Kohn LAP (1991) The role of genetics in craniofacial morphology and growth. Annu Rev Anthropol 20:261–278

LSTC (2007) LS-DYNA Keyword User's Manual, Version 971. Livermore Software Technology Corporation (LSTC), Livermore, CA, USA

Lu YT, Beldie L, Walker B, Richmond S, Middleton J (2011) Parametric study of a Hill-type hyperelastic skeletal muscle model. Proc Inst Mech Eng, Part H, J Eng Med 225(5):437–447

Lundström A (1984) Nature versus nurture in dentofacial variation. Eur J Orthod 6:77–91

Martin CJA, Alarcon JA, Palma JC (2000) Kinesiographic study of the mandible in young patients with unilateral posterior crossbite. Am J Orthod Dentofac Orthop 118:541–548

Mishima K, Yamada T, Sugii A, Matsumura T, Sugahara T (2009) Application of a novel method to analyze lip motion of cleft lip patients before and after lip repair. Dento-Maxillo-Facial Radiol 38:232–238

Morgan PS, Bowtell RW, McIntyre DJO, Worthington BS (2004) Correction of spatial distortion in EPI due to inhomogeneous static magnetic fields using the reversed gradient method. J Magn Reson Imaging 19(4):499–507

Nooreyazdan M, Trotman CA, Faraway JJ (2004) Modeling facial movement: II. A dynamic analysis of differences caused by orthognathic surgery. J Oral Maxillofac Surg 62:1380–1386

Oasys.PRIMER (2009) Oasys PRIMER9.3 & D3PLOT User Manual. Ove Arup & Partners Ltd: Solihull, UK

Okudaira M, Ono T, Kawamoto T, Moriyama K (2008) Three-dimensional analysis of lower lip movement during articulation in subjects with mandibular prognathism. Orthod Waves 67:93–103

Parker GJM, Haroon HA, Wheeler-Jingshott CAM (2003) A framework for a streamline-based probabilistic index of connectivity (PICo) using a structural interpretation of MRI diffusion measurements. J Magn Reson Imaging 18:242–254

Parker GD, Jones DK (2011a) Fibers at the magic angle generated by inappropriate calibration (MAGIC). In: Proc ISMRM 2011, p 1921

Parker GD, Jones DK (2011b) Towards automated modeling of maxillofacial musculature. In: Proc ISMRM 2011, p 1916

Paternoster L, Zhurov AI, Toma AM, Kemp JP, St Pourcain B, Timpson NJ, McMahon G, McArdle W, Ring SM, Smith GD, Richmond S, Evans DM (2012) Genome-wide association study of three-dimensional facial morphology identifies a variant in PAX3 associated with nasion position. Am J Hum Genet 90(3):478–485

Popat H, Henley E, Richmond S, Benedikt L, Marshall D, Rosin PL (2010) A comparison of the reproducibility of verbal and non-verbal facial gestures using three-dimensional motion analysis. Otolaryngol Head Neck Surg 142:867–872

Popat H, Richmond S, Marshall D, Rosin PL (2011) Facial movement in 3 dimensions: average templates of lip movement in adults. Otolaryngol Head Neck Surg 145:24–29

Riolo ML, Moyers RE, McNamara JA, Hunter WS (1979) An atlas of craniofacial growth, vol 2. Needham Press, Ann Arbor

Rumeur ELE, Carre F, Bernard AM, Bandard JY, Rochcongar P, Certained JDDE (1994) Multiparametric classification of muscle T1 and T2 relaxation times determined by magnetic resonance imaging. The effects of dynamic exercise in trained and untrained subjects. Br J Radiol 67:150–156

Richmond S, Beldie L, Lu Y, Middleton J, Walker B, Cronin A, Drage N, Zhurov A, Wilkinson C (2010) Predicting and managing surgical intervention in craniofacial disharmony—a biomechanical perspective. In: Three-dimensional imaging for orthodontics and maxillofacial surgery. Wiley/Blackwell, New York, pp 180–197. ISBN 978-0813806143

Saunders SR, Popovich F, Thompson GW (1980) A family study of craniofacial dimensions in the Burlington Growth Centre sample. Am J Orthod 78(4):394–403

Sidorov K, Richmond S, Marshall D (2009) An efficient stochastic approach to groupwise non-rigid image registration. In: Proc IEEE conf on comp vis and pat rec (CVPR '09), pp 2208–2213

Sidorov K, Richmond S, Marshall D (2011) Efficient groupwise non-rigid registration of textured surfaces. In: Proc IEEE conf on comp vis and pat rec (CVPR '11), pp 2401–2408

Sidorov K (2010) Groupwise non-rigid registration for automatic construction of appearance models of the human craniofacial complex for analysis, synthesis, and simulation. PhD Thesis, Cardiff University

Simpleware Ltd (2006) +ScanCAD, ScanIP, +ScanFE 3.1, Simpleware Ltd, Innovation Centre, University of Exeter, Rennes Drive, EX4 4RN, UK

Stjeskal EO, Tanner EJ (1965) Spin diffusion measurements: spin echoes in the presence of time-dependent field gradient. J Chem Phys 42:288–292

Toma AM, Zhurov AI, Playle R, Marshall D, Rosin PL, Richmond S (2011) The assessment of facial variation in 4747 British school children. Eur J Orthod (in press). PubMed PMID: 21934112

Tournier JD, Calamante F, Gadian DG, Connelly A (2004) Direct estimation of the fiber orientation density function from diffusion-weighted MRI data using spherical deconvolution. Neuroimage 23:1176–1185

Wedeen VJ, Hagmann P, Tsend WI, Reese TG, Weisskoff RM (2005) Mapping complex tissue architecture with diffusion spectrum magnetic resonance imaging. Magn Reson Med 54:1337–1386

Wood GD (1979) Recording the opening and closing cycle of the mandible. Br Dent J 146:305–309

Zhukov L, Barr AH (2003) Heart-muscle fiber reconstruction from diffusion tensor MRI. In: Proceedings of the 14th IEEE visualization conference. ISBN 0-7695-2030-8

Zhurov AI, Richmond S, Kau CH, Toma A (2010) Averaging facial images. In: Kau C, Richmond S (eds) Three-dimensional imaging for orthodontics and maxillofacial surgery. Wiley/Blackwell, New York, pp 126–146. ISBN 978-0813806143

Zitova B, Flusser J (2003) Image registration methods: a survey. Image Vis Comput 21(11):977–1000

Chapter 6
Computational Analysis of Flow and Stress Patterns in Patient Specific Thoracic Aortic Aneurysm Models

Alessandro Borghi, Nigel B. Wood, Raad H. Mohiaddin, and Xiao Yun Xu

Abstract Thoracic Aortic Aneurysms (TAAs) are associated with low frequency in a given population but high mortality rate. No reliable surgical criterion is available at present but internal wall stress has proved to be more reliable as a predictor of rupture than the maximum diameter in case of Abdominal Aortic Aneurysms (AAAs). However, few studies have been reported on the role of biomechanical factors in the development and rupture of TAAs. This chapter describes a computational mechanics model of TAA based on patient-specific anatomical and flow conditions, acquired from Magnetic Resonance Imaging (MRI). The model has been applied to five patients with TAAs at different locations of the aorta. The results showed no correlation between peak stress and aneurysm size such as the maximum diameter. The effects of intra-luminal thrombus (ILT) and its mechanical properties on wall stress patterns were investigated. It has been found that the shape, size and location of ILT have a significant effect on wall stress patterns. Peak stress calculated using a fully coupled fluid-structure interaction simulation was similar to that predicted by a static solid simulation, in agreement with previous studies of AAA. The work presented here serves as a first step towards developing a reliable predictive tool to allow improved prognosis and surgical decision making for TAA patients.

6.1 Introduction: Thoracic Aortic Aneurysms (TAAs)

6.1.1 Facts and Figures About TAAs

A Thoracic Aortic Aneurysm (TAA) is the swelling or ballooning of the thoracic aorta (the region of the aorta that extends from the aortic valve to the diaphragm). Although an aneurysm can occur in any artery of the body, it may become dangerous

A. Borghi · N.B. Wood · X.Y. Xu (✉)
Department of Chemical Engineering, Imperial College London, London, UK
e-mail: yun.xu@imperial.ac.uk

R.H. Mohiaddin
Royal Brompton and Harefield NHS Foundation Trust, London, UK

B. Calvo, E. Peña (eds.), *Patient-Specific Computational Modeling*,
Lecture Notes in Computational Vision and Biomechanics 5,
DOI 10.1007/978-94-007-4552-0_6,

Table 6.1 Summary of clinical features of Thoracic Aortic Aneurysms

	Diameter growth rate	Critical size	% Risk of rupture or dissection	% Surgical risk	Intervention diameter
Ascending TAA	0.07 cm/year	6 cm	31 %	2.5 %	5.5 cm
Descending TAA	0.19 cm/year	7 cm	43 %	8 %	6.5 cm

and symptomatic when it occurs in the thoracic aorta, abdominal aorta, iliac and cerebral arteries. The incidence of TAA in a population is 5.9 cases per 100,000 person-per year (Elefteriades, 2002). "Hinge points" in the aortic size, at which rupture or dissections occur, are 6 cm for the ascending aorta and 7 cm for the descending aorta respectively. By the time an aneurysm has reached the critical size, rupture or dissection has occurred in 31 % of the cases for ascending TAAs and 43 % of the cases for descending TAAs (Table 6.1). Aneurysm formation is normally chronic, though in some cases, mainly in case of infection, its formation can be acute (Fann, 2002).

Among the possible causes of aortic aneurysm are atherosclerosis, medial cystic degeneration and congenital disease. Family pedigrees confirm that 21 % of patients with TAA have first order family members with history of aortic aneurysm (Elefteriades, 2002; Pannu et al., 2006); the predominant mode of inheritance is autosomal dominant and familial TAAs tend to grow at a higher rate (Albornoz et al., 2006). Direct father to son transmission was found in a study in 38.5 % of the cases (Coady et al., 1999).

6.1.2 Clinical Management: The Lack of Reliable Surgical Criteria

At present, the only possible treatments for TAAs are open surgical repair (when a graft is used to replace part of the aorta) or endovascular graft repair (when a stent graft is inserted into the femoral artery through the groin and positioned at the aneurysm location, in order to support the dilated and weakened aorta).

All the criteria adopted so far to evaluate the risk of rupture for an aneurysm are based on aortic dimensions, growth rate or other geometrical indices. The diameter criterion has shown to be unreliable in case of both small and large aneurysms: aneurysms smaller than 5 cm rupture in 6.5 % of the cases (Elefteriades, 2002) and some abdominal aortic aneurysms (AAAs) have been shown to grow up to 8 cm without complications. Furthermore, it was found that aneurysm strength is not correlated with aneurysm dimension (Vorp et al., 2003). It has been shown for AAAs that the use of wall stress, calculated by means of the finite element method, correlates better than aneurysm size with rupture of the aneurysm (Fillinger, 2006). This is due to the nature of the rupture of the aortic wall in case of aneurysm; from a mechanical point of view, rupture occurs when the mechanical forces exerted on the aneurysm wall exceed the strength of the wall. Fillinger et al. (2003) reported that the peak wall stress in aneurysms had a higher sensitivity and specificity for predicting the rupture than maximum diameter (94 %, 81 % versus 81 %, 70 %). Venkatasubramaniam et al. (2004) analyzed 27 AAAs using finite element techniques, of which 15 had ruptured after the scan. The wall stress was found to be significantly higher in the ruptured aneurysms and the rupture site coincided with the area of maximum wall stress.

The analysis of the fluid dynamics has provided important information on the role of blood flow in aneurysm expansion, and studies have shown that blood flow patterns are generally abnormal in aortic aneurysms and aortic grafts and may create hydrodynamic irregularities (Bogren et al., 1995; Bogren and Buonocore, 1999). Furthermore, it was found that alteration in flow patterns was linked to the propagation of AAA owing to changes in shear stress on the aneurysm inner wall. Bluestein et al. (1996) investigated the role of disturbed flow on platelet deposition and thrombus formation in an aneurysm model using numerical as well as experimental methods, and showed that platelets with elevated shear histories and higher incidence of activation tended to adhere to the wall in areas of low wall shear stress. The effect of dynamic interactions between blood flow and wall motion in AAAs has been investigated and the first such work was performed by Di Martino et al. (2001), who analyzed the complex stress pattern and fluid dynamics in a patient-specific aneurysm model. In later studies the importance of coupled fluid structure interaction (FSI) was evaluated for calculating the stress pattern in patient-specific aneurysm models (Leung et al., 2004; Wolters et al., 2005; Papaharilaou et al., 2006). Wang and Li (2011) analyzed the physiological factors affecting the behavior of stented and non-stented thoracic aortic aneurysms, and they found that the performance of stent-grafts were affected by the presence and amount of ILT. The drag force exerted on stent grafts is not affected by aortic curvature, as demonstrated by Cheng et al. (2008).

The adoption of an engineering approach to predict the likelihood of aneurysm rupture requires knowledge about the strength of the aortic wall. At present, no reliable model of aneurysm strength is available. Vande Geest et al. (2006) proposed an equation for the AAA wall strength derived from a multiple linear regression of statistical models where wall strength was correlated with ILT thickness, age, normalized transverse diameter, family and sex. The ratio of local wall stress to strength provides the local Rupture Potential Index (RPI) of the aneurysm.

This chapter presents a study where the methodology developed for AAA is modified and applied to aneurysms of the thoracic aorta. The use of medical imaging together with an appropriate image segmentation technique allows the reconstruction of patient-specific models and the use of finite element method with fluid-solid interaction provides a tool to evaluate non-invasively the wall stress of the aneurysms.

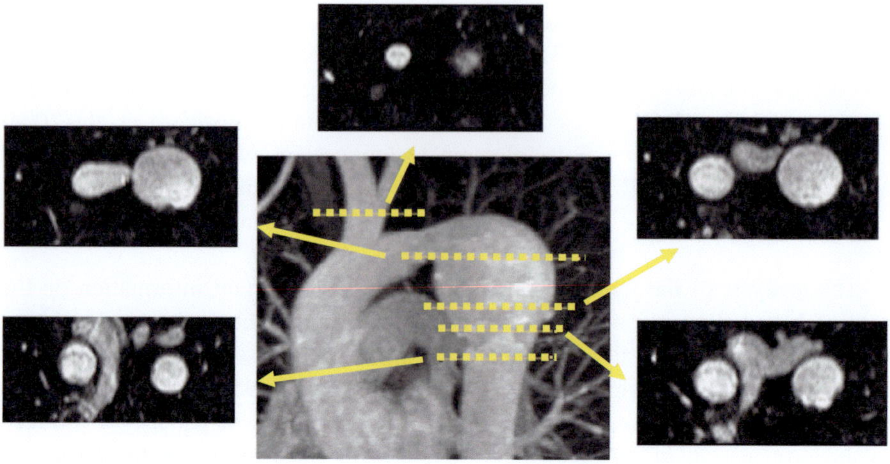

Fig. 6.1 Cross-sectional images of Patient 1 acquired using CE-MRA

6.2 Patient Specific TAA Model Creation

6.2.1 Population

The patient data for this study were provided by the Royal Brompton Hospital, London, where clinical sets of MRI images were acquired using a number of protocols. Three types of MRI image sets were used:

- CE-MRA (type A) (contrast-enhanced)
- HASTE (type B) (half Fourier single-shot turbo spin echo)
- PC Velo mapping (type C) (phase-contrast velocity imaging)

Figure 6.1 shows an example of type A images: the central image shows a frontal view of the arterial tree of the patient, centered on the TAA. The surrounding panels show cross-sectional images of the TAA acquired using the CE-MRA protocol. Figure 6.2 shows in a similar way cross-sectional images of the TAA of the same patient acquired using type B (HASTE) sequence.

Figure 6.3 shows samples of PC-Velo mapping images acquired from Patient 1 at three different times of the cardiac cycle.

6.2.2 Geometry Extraction

DICOM (Digital Imaging and Communication in Medicine) is the standard format for handling, storing, printing, and transmitting information in medical imaging. The images were pre-processed numerically before performing contour extraction by following the steps described below.

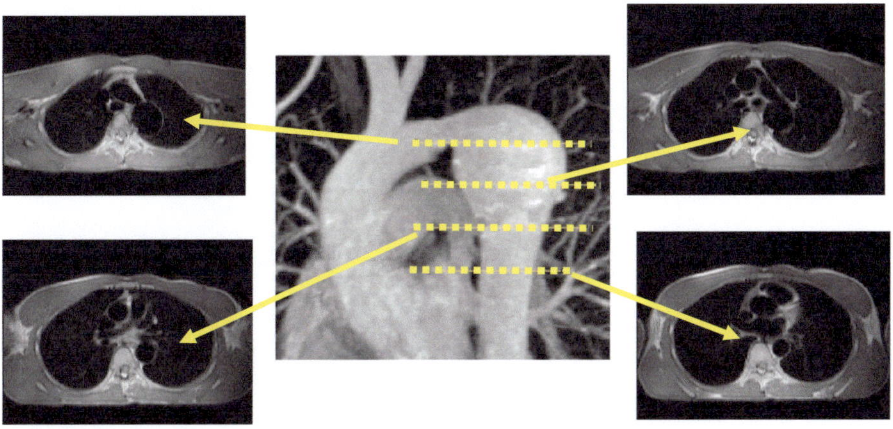

Fig. 6.2 Cross-sectional images of Patient 1 acquired using HASTE sequence

Fig. 6.3 Samples of PC-Velo mapping images (magnitude image on the *left*, phase image on the *right*) acquired from Patient 1 at different times of the cardiac cycle

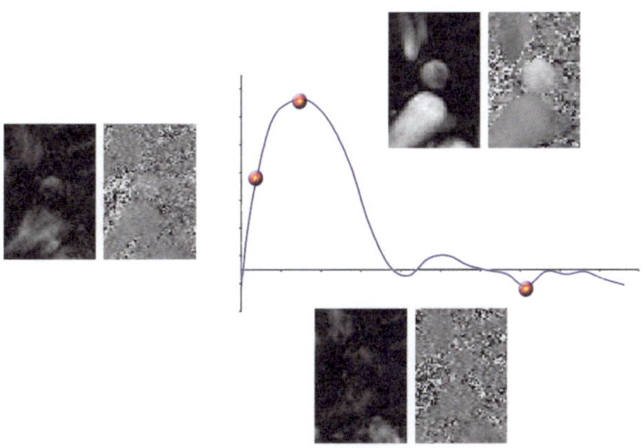

Image Filtering Noise in the images is due to the presence of magnetic and electric field of other appliances in the scanning room and to the internal noise of the scanner; numerical filtering is used to remove unwanted noise from the images. Median filtering is a non-linear smoothing enhancement technique that smooths images without edge blurring. The intensity of the pixel being processed is replaced by the median intensity of the neighborhood pixels:

$$\bar{f}(x, y) = \underset{(s,t)\in S_{xy}}{\text{median}}\left\{g(s, t)\right\} \tag{6.1}$$

where $g(s, t)$ is the neighborhood of the pixel in (x, y). Median filters provide excellent noise reduction capabilities, with considerably less blurring than linear filters of similar size (Gonzalez and Woods, 2002).

Segmentation For the extraction of anatomical features, various segmentation techniques have been developed in the past. In this study, different segmentation

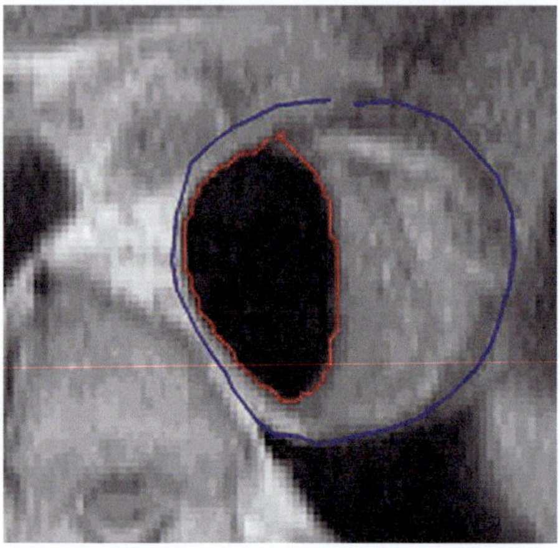

Fig. 6.4 Manual image segmentation of a HASTE image

methods were used for different types of images. CE-MRA shows very clearly the lumen boundaries, owing to the injection of a MR contrast agent. Showing the lumen boundary so clearly enables the use of an automatic segmentation method, such as the region growing method. The region growing technique segments images via pixel aggregation, based on predefined criteria. The results of segmentation are different regions with homogeneous parameters that are used to reflect pixel membership.

The HASTE images were cardiac gated and acquired during diastole; therefore, they were used to generate the reference configuration for patient geometries. HASTE images are suitable for delineation of the arterial wall and its composition (Jung et al., 2005; Hillenbrand et al., 2006). For these images, manual segmentation was performed for both the lumen and the outer wall boundaries owing to the lack of tissue contrast. Figure 6.4 gives an example of the segmentation of a HASTE image: the lumen contour is shown in red whereas the outer wall is in blue.

Wall Thickness Measurement 3 of the 5 TAA patients in this study presented intra-luminal thrombus (ILT) in their aneurysms; due to the low contrast between arterial wall and ILT in both types of images, it was not possible to distinguish the wall from thrombus for every slice. Therefore, a constant wall thickness was assumed along the entire length of the aneurysm. The wall thickness was determined from HASTE images using an average value of 12 measurements made at sections where wall thickness was clearly defined (usually in regions where the thrombus was not present). An average wall thickness of 3.38 ± 0.28 mm was found among these patients; this value is within the range found by Fukui et al. in their experimental work (Fukui et al., 2005).

Smoothing MATLAB routines were written to perform contour and surface smoothing, based on the use of least square cubic splines. Given a set of data (x, y)

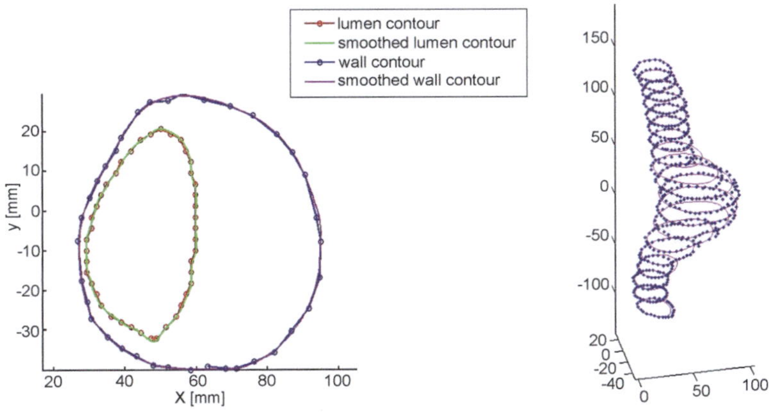

Fig. 6.5 Example of contour smoothing (*left*) and surface smoothing (*right*) (units in mm)

and a specified smoothing parameter p the smoothing spline s is the curve that minimizes

$$p\sum_i \left(y(i) - s\left(x(i)\right)\right)^2 + (1-p)\int D^2 st^2 dt \tag{6.2}$$

where p is a smoothing parameter which varies between 0 and 1 (1 returns the original curve, while 0 gives a straight line) (MATLAB Spline Toolbox User's Guide; The MathWorks I, 2001). A first step of contour smoothing was performed on each contour extracted from MRI, followed by contour re-sampling to increase the number of points. A final step of surface smoothing provides a suitable geometry for the creation of computational models. Figure 6.5 provides examples of the smoothing process.

6.2.3 Flow Information Extraction

The processing of flow images (cine PC-Velo mapping) allows important patient-specific flow conditions to be extracted. Each image set consists of paired magnitude and phase images corresponding to different time points in a cycle. From the magnitude image, it is possible to extract the contour of the flow region, in order to delineate the region of interest (ROI). Once the ROI is defined, the phase image is processed in order to extract the velocity values at each pixel in this region. The values of velocity are then determined by using the relation shown in this equation:

$$V = -V_{enc} + 2 \cdot \frac{V_{enc}}{(\lfloor R-1 \rfloor - I_{\min})} \cdot (I - I_{\min}) \tag{6.3}$$

where V_{enc} is the Velocity Encoding Value, embracing the expected velocity range, and R is the Rescale Intercept Value, available in the header of phase contrast images, whilst $I_{\min}$ is the minimum value of intensity of the images. The images were

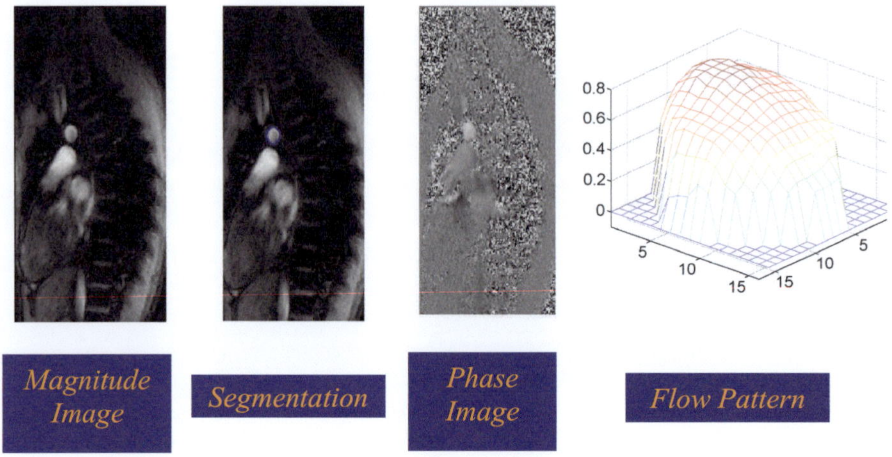

Fig. 6.6 Flow pattern extraction from PC-Velo mapping images

Fig. 6.7 Volumetric flow-rate for patients 1–4 as extracted from MRI images

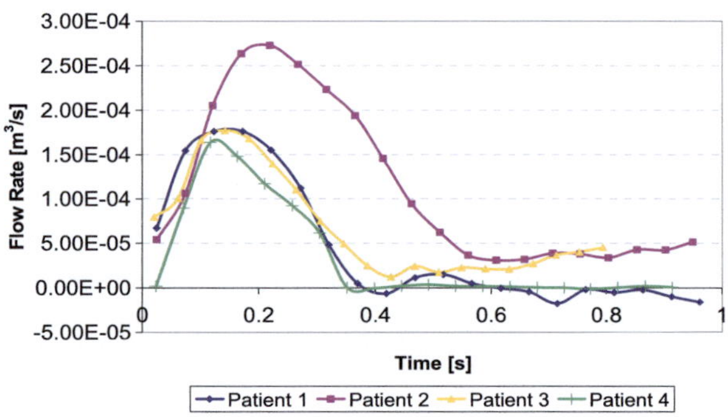

filtered using the median filter before segmentation. The overall process is shown in Fig. 6.6.

In order to derive the corresponding flow-rate from these images, the obtained velocity profiles were integrated using 2D Gaussian integration over the measured plane for each time point, yielding instantaneous volumetric flow-rates. Figure 6.7 shows the variation of volumetric flow-rate for patients 1 to 4, for whom flow measurement was made.

6.2.4 Creation of the Finite Element Model

6.2.4.1 Geometry Creation and Meshing

The points were imported into ADINA 8.4 using a point cloud. Lines were created by joining the points in order to define the outline shape of the aneurysm, thereafter internal surfaces and volumes were created subdividing each of the fluid and wall domains of a TAA model into four parts. For patients 1 to 4, both the blood domain and the arterial wall domain were created. Hexahedral volumes were used to form the wall domain while prismatic volumes were used for the lumen.

Structured mesh was adopted for the discretization of the wall model for each patient, and for the lumen models of patients 1–4. The wall models were subdivided into 8-node hexahedral elements, according to the methodology employed in other studies (Di Martino et al., 2001; Wolters et al., 2005; Leung et al., 2006; Li and Kleinstreuer, 2006; Borghi et al. 2006, 2008). Owing to convergence problems in the fluid-only model, different types of mesh were used for the four patients. 8-node hexahedral elements were used for patients 1 and 4, whilst 4-node tetrahedral elements were used for patients 2 and 3. In all cases, linear elements have been used. All the models have been tested for grid sensitivity; therefore the solution should be independent of the element choice.

6.2.4.2 Boundary Conditions and Loads

The boundary conditions and loads for the models were specified according to the type of simulation performed. Static structural analysis (S model) was performed for all the patients, since only the geometry and pressure are required for this type of analysis. For patients 1 to 4 flow information was available, therefore it was possible to perform flow simulation (F model) and, through coupling of the fluid and solid models via the ALE algorithm, to perform fluid-solid interaction simulation (FSI model).

The S model was designed for static structural analysis under a constant blood pressure without considering the interaction with the fluid flow. The model consists of the arterial wall domain for each patient, including both wall and thrombus where present. The boundary conditions were applied at the two ends, where rotations and translations were constrained in order to simulate the tethering to the rest of the aorta. At the wall-thrombus interface, the same number of elements was used; therefore the displacement was continuous across the two domains. At the two ends of the thrombus a tied interface condition was applied, in order to prevent sliding (this condition allows no sliding between the two surfaces in contact and can be used to connect surfaces having incompatible meshes). The algorithm used for the contact analysis is based on the segment method, which uses Lagrangian multiplier to enforce the contact condition and has been shown to be very robust (ADINA R&D, 2003).

The load applied on the internal surface of the model was equal to 40 mmHg (5.32 kPa, which represents the pulse pressure, i.e. the difference between the systolic and diastolic pressure in a normal subject). This value was chosen because the model was reconstructed from images acquired during diastole (where the pressure is 80 mmHg), therefore in order to reach the systolic configuration (where the pressure is 120 mmHg) only the difference in pressure needs to be applied.

6.2.4.3 Mechanical Properties

The mechanical characteristics of the aneurismal wall are different from those of the healthy aorta. It has been reported in several studies that aneurysm formation is associated with stiffening and weakening of the aortic wall, for both TAA and AAA (Bengtsson et al., 1996; Vorp et al., 2003), as a result of chronic inflammation, and that the aneurismal wall is heterogeneous, orthotropic and undergoes large deformation under the effect of the blood pressure (Raghavan, 1998). Evidence for the genetic basis of AAA was discussed by Ogata et al. (2005) and of TAA in Marfan syndrome by He et al. (2008); the comparison of TAA and AAA genomics was discussed by Absi et al. (2003).

Most studies report calculation of aneurysm material properties from ex-vivo wall tensile testing of abdominal aneurysms. The properties of TAA material were reported in only a limited number of studies, although the methodology used in these was the same. The main study on this subject was carried out by Raghavan and Vorp (2000) with an aim to develop a finite strain constitutive model for AAA strips from a group of 69 aneurysm specimens. They assumed that the wall was homogeneous, incompressible and isotropic, so that the strain energy function had the following form

$$W = W(I_B, II_B) \tag{6.4}$$

where W is the strain energy function and B is the left Cauchy-Green tensor. I_B and II_B are the first and second invariants.

The constitutive equation for such a material has the following form

$$T = -pI + 2\frac{dW}{dI_B}B + 2\frac{dW}{dII_B}B^{-1} \tag{6.5}$$

where T is the Cauchy stress tensor, p is the hydrostatic pressure and I is the identity tensor. They assumed that $W = W(I_B)$, and found from the experimental data that the derivative of W in respect of I_B varied linearly with $(I_B - 3)$:

$$\frac{dW}{dI_B} = \alpha + 2\beta(I_B - 3) \tag{6.6}$$

and

$$W = \alpha(I_B - 3) + \beta(I_B - 3)^2. \tag{6.7}$$

The results yielded the constitutive model for uniaxial extension:

$$T = \left[2\alpha + 4\beta\left(\lambda^2 + 2\lambda^{-1} - 3\right)\right]\left(\lambda^2 - \lambda^{-1}\right) \tag{6.8}$$

where α and β are constants derived from experimental data, T is the Cauchy stress and λ is the elongation of the strip.

The model was adjusted by Vorp et al. (2003) in order to fit it to the characteristics of a group of thoracic aorta strips tested with a loading machine. Longitudinal (LONG) and circumferential (CIRC) strips of ascending TAA tissues were extracted from a group of 26 patients. LONG-oriented tissue was found to be stiffer than CIRC-oriented tissue; wall strength was shown not to be related to diameter in either direction. They found that the TAA material was constitutively anisotropic, therefore the characterization of this material should be performed using biaxial tests. The model by Vorp et al. was used for the material properties of the TAA wall models of this study.

The constitutive model for the ILT was derived by Wang et al. (2001) using uniaxial tensile testing carried out on 50 specimens, including 14 longitudinally oriented and 14 circumferentially oriented from the luminal region, and 11 longitudinally oriented and 11 circumferentially oriented for the medial region. Using a similar methodology to that used by Raghavan and Vorp, a two parameter hyperelastic constitutive model was developed to describe the uniaxial behavior; in this case, the assumption was $W = W(II_B)$ and the resulting equation for uniaxial tension case is given by

$$T = 2\left[c_1 + 2c_2\left(2\lambda + \frac{1}{\lambda^2} - 3\right)\right]\left(\lambda - \frac{1}{\lambda^2}\right). \tag{6.9}$$

No significant difference in c_1 and c_2 was found between the longitudinal and circumferential directions. Therefore they concluded that ILT was an inhomogeneous and possibly isotropic material. The assumption of incompressibility was justified by Vorp et al. (1996), when a study on the compliance of AAAs showed a minimal difference between the ILT cross-sectional area at systole and diastole. Di Martino and Vorp (2003) demonstrated that the inhomogeneous characteristics of ILT could be neglected in computational models, since the use of different material properties for luminal and medial layers did not alter the stress distribution, and had minimal effect on the stress levels. They also showed that population mean parameters could be used to make reasonable estimates of the wall stresses in patient-specific aneurysm models, since the variation in peak stress in models having different ILT properties (varying in a physiological range) would only result in a peak stress variation of 5 %. The model by Wang et al. was used for the material properties of the TAA wall model in this study.

6.3 Results

6.3.1 Patient Population

Data for five patients with TAA were provided by the Royal Brompton Hospital where they had been scanned for routine examination. Patients 1 and 4 presented with the aneurysm located in the aortic arch, in an area distal from the subclavian artery. Concerning patient 4, the presence of the subclavian artery and the right carotid artery was neglected, as is usually done for the aortic arch (Mori and Yamaguchi, 2002; Morris et al., 2005; Gao et al., 2006).

Table 6.2 Summary of the patients used in this study and models created

Patient	Gender	Age (year)	TAA status	Models created		
				S	F	FSI
1	M	18	Operated	X	X	X
2	M	80	Unruptured	X	X	X
3	M	74	Unruptured	X	X	X
4	F	84	Unruptured	X	X	X
5	F	74	Unruptured	X		

Table 6.3 Summary of the main geometric features of the patients. Patients 1 and 4 have TAA located in the aortic arch and the height/length refers to centerline length; for patient 2, 3 and 5 height/length refers to the vertical axial length

Patient	Diameter (cm)	Wall thickness (mm)	Height/Length
1	5.1	3.61	91.5
2	7.0	3.44	156.8
3	6.2	3.05	145.6
4	6.6	3.74	94.0
5	7.0	3.07	108.8

As explained earlier, a similar methodology for the extraction of lumen and wall contours from medical images was used for patients 2, 3 and 5. In these cases lumen and wall contours were extracted manually and the wall thickness was calculated using an average value derived from the images. Lumen contours for patients 1 and 4 were delineated automatically using the segmentation algorithms described previously and the wall contours were obtained by inflating the lumen by a constant thickness. The absence of thrombus in these cases made this assumption possible. Table 6.2 shows a summary of the patients' information and medical conditions, as well as a summary of all the models created for each patient.

All the reconstructions were performed by including sufficient sections both proximal and distal to the aneurysm bulge. For the aneurysm of patient 4, it was necessary to extend the inlet and outlet in order to minimize the boundary effects. All the aneurysms located in the descending aorta showed the presence of intraluminal thrombus (ILT): this is a common feature in descending and abdominal aneurysms, and, as occurred in this study, the presence of eccentric thrombus is usually predominant in aneurysm groups (Hans et al., 2005). Table 6.3 shows a summary of the geometrical features of the patient models: the average diameter of the TAAs was 6.4 ± 0.7 cm and the average wall thickness was 3.38 ± 0.28 mm (mean $\pm$ SD). These values are consistent with those found by Tomohiro et al in their study (Fukui et al., 2005). The length of the aneurysms varied depending on the location of the aneurysm; in the cases of aortic arch aneurysm (patients 1 and 4) the arc length of

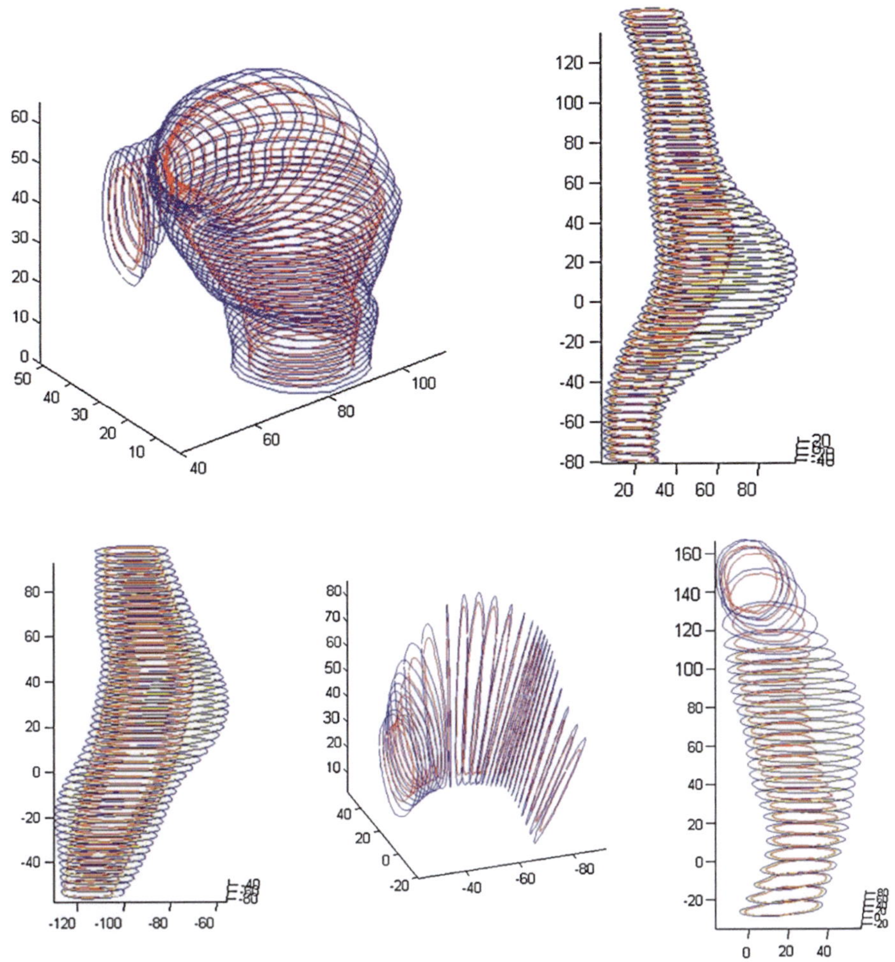

Fig. 6.8 TAA geometries of Patients 1, 2 (*top*), 3, 4, 5 (*bottom*). Units in mm

the aortic centerline in the aneurysm region was measured as an indication of the dimension of the aneurysm, for the other patients, the height refers to the vertical length of the aneurysm.

In Fig. 6.8, the boundary of the lumen is depicted in red, whilst the boundary of the outer wall is in blue. The aneurysms containing ILT have the boundary between the wall and the thrombus indicated in yellow. As can be observed, patients 2 and 5 had a large volume of thrombus located in one region of the aneurysm whilst the rest of the aorta was almost thrombus free. Patient 3 instead presented a continuous formation of thrombus over the length of the aneurysm, with thicker thrombus in the aneurysm bulge.

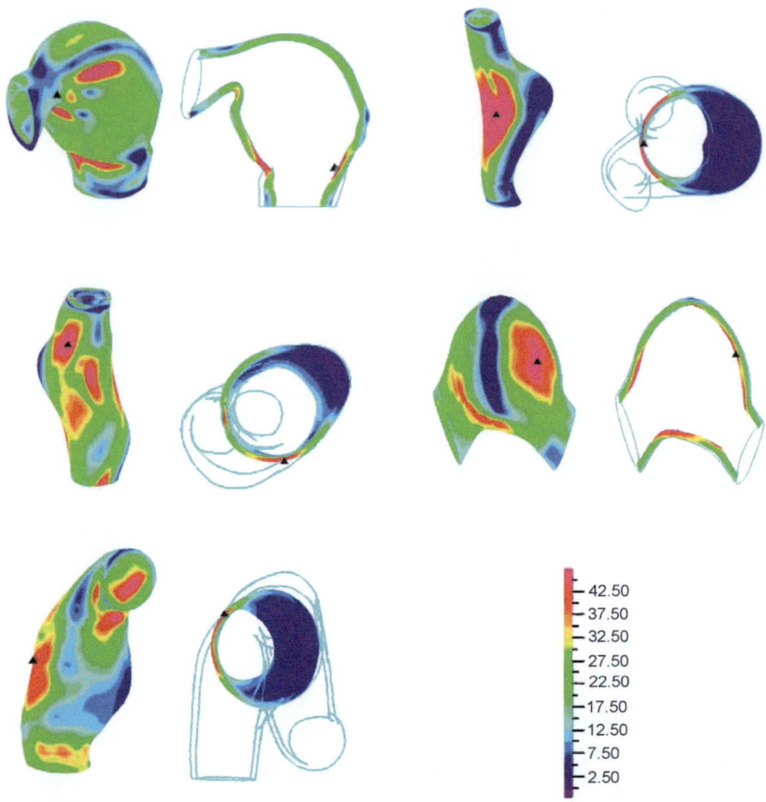

Fig. 6.9 Stress pattern for patients 1 to 5 (from top left to bottom right). For each patient the overall stress pattern (on the *left*) and the section of maximum stress (on the *right*) are reported (units in kPa)

6.3.2 Analysis of Stress Patterns in TAAs and Link to Geometrical Factors

All stress analyses were performed using ADINA 8.4, using material properties, boundary conditions and loads as described in the previous section. Figure 6.9 shows the stress patterns for the five patients, where stress is presented in terms of Von Mises stress, for consistency with other studies.

Table 6.4 summarizes the maximum aneurysm diameters and maximum stresses for all patients examined.

As shown in the table, patient 2 had the highest stress value, at 79.36 kPa, who also had the largest diameter. However, patient 5 had the same size but the lowest peak stress of the group. The smallest aneurysm (patient 1) had a peak stress value which was higher than patients 3, 4, and 5, whose aneurysms were larger. The stress levels of patients 1 and 4 were comparable to that of patient 2; however the dimensions were markedly different: a possible explanation is that the first 2 patients

Table 6.4 Summary of aneurysm diameters and maximum stresses for all patients examined

Patient	Diameter (cm)	Maximum stress (KPa)
P1	5.1	75.02
P2	7.0	79.36
P3	6.2	51.81
P4	6.6	74.42
P5	7.0	48.61

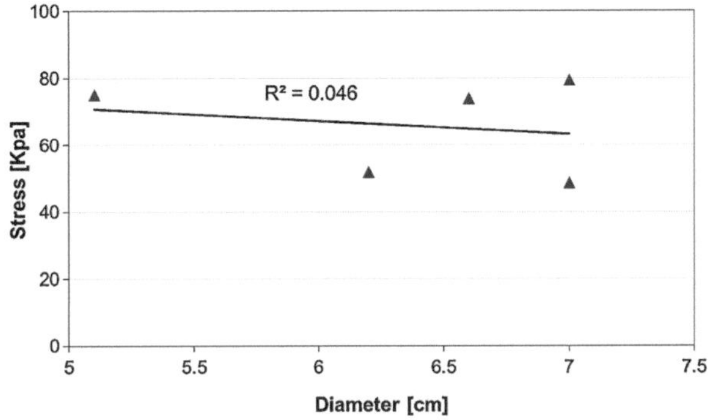

Fig. 6.10 Correlation between peak stress and maximum diameter for the patients analyzed in this study ($p = 0.729$)

had aneurysms in the arch and presented no formation of ILT, implying the importance of including ILT in accurate prediction of stress values in aneurysm models, as shown in previous studies (Mower et al., 1997; Wang et al., 2002; Thubrikar et al., 2003; Leung et al., 2006).

Detailed examination of the stress patterns in the TAA models shows similarities between patients 1 and 4, which had areas of high stress in the distal and proximal parts of the bulge (as shown by the vertical sections) and low levels in the bulge. However, the aneurysms having ILT showed low stress levels on the side of the bulge where the thrombus was present, and high stress on the other side where the thrombus was thin. This can be noticed particularly in patients 2, 3 and 5, that had similar geometrical features. In patient 5 the location of maximum stress matched that of the maximum diameter, opposite the highest thrombus thickness, and there was also a very close match in patient 2.

Figure 6.10 shows the correlation between maximum diameter and peak stress in the small aneurysm sample studied. As can be seen, the two parameters were very weakly correlated (Pearson correlation values, $r = 0.215$, $p = 0.729$).

6.3.3 Fluid-Solid Interaction Simulation of Wall Stress and Flow in TAA Models

Since velocity images were acquired for patients 1 to 4 (i.e. patient-specific flow waveforms can be derived), it was possible to perform fluid-solid coupled simula-

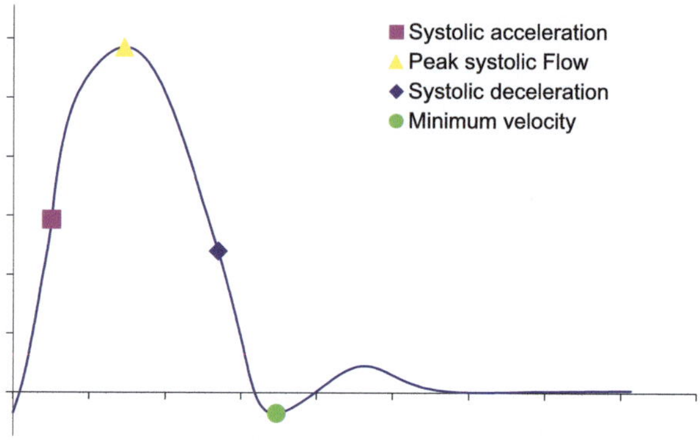

Fig. 6.11 Flow phases analyzed for the FSI results

tions in these cases. Fully coupled fluid-solid interaction simulation was performed using the ALE algorithm implemented in ADINA. The flow-rate information was extracted from the PC-MR image sets acquired at an upstream section of each aneurysm. In case of patient 3, the flow-rate curve was acquired in a section in the middle of the upper bulge, therefore the inlet was chosen at a different position in order to avoid boundary effects; however, no branches were present between these two locations and the measured flow-rate would still be valid. For patient 4, an extension of inlet and outlet was performed in order to minimize boundary effects. The flow phases analyzed for the FSI results are highlighted in Fig. 6.11.

The results are shown in Figs. 6.12, 6.13, 6.14 and 6.15. The vertical sections show the flow pattern along the aneurysm, while the transverse sections show the velocity distribution in the bulge. The flow in the vertical sections is shown in terms of velocity magnitude for patients 1 and 4, owing to the curvature of the model, while it is shown as vertical velocity for patients 2 and 3, since the aneurysms in these cases are located in the descending aorta. The flow in the transverse sections corresponds to the vertical component of the flow. The point of minimum velocity in patients 1 and 4 corresponds to the point of peak reverse flow, since for these patients the volumetric flow is reversed during part of the cardiac cycle.

In all the models flow recirculation is present during most of the cardiac cycle. Similarities are found between patients 1 and 4, where flow recirculation in the transverse section is visible from peak systole, while during systolic acceleration the flow is predominantly forward. The flow in patient 1 shows a consistent jet coming from the inlet towards the bulge and it follows the shape of the bulge. A central development of the flow inside the aneurysm of patient 4 is visible from Fig. 6.15. Partial recirculation remains inside the bulge of both patients also during the phase of reverse flow, though it is more visible in the model of patient 1, whose magnitude of reverse flow is higher. A FSI simulation of patient 1, incorporating a laminar-turbulent transition model, shows qualitatively similar effects, with some quantitative differences owing to the turbulence (see Sect. 6.4).

Similarities are also present between the flow patterns of patients 2 and 3, whose aneurysms are located in the descending aorta. The main stream of the flow bends towards the outlet in correspondence to the center of the aneurysm. In these patients,

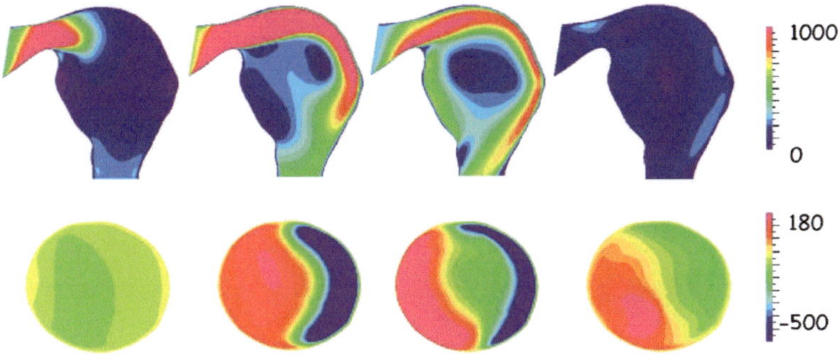

Fig. 6.12 Flow results for patient 1; velocity magnitude in an inferior-superior (IS) section of the model (*top row*); vertical velocity in a transverse section (*bottom row*), in this case the forward flow points downwards and has a negative value in the adopted coordinate system. Note different scales for top and bottom rows (units in mm/s)

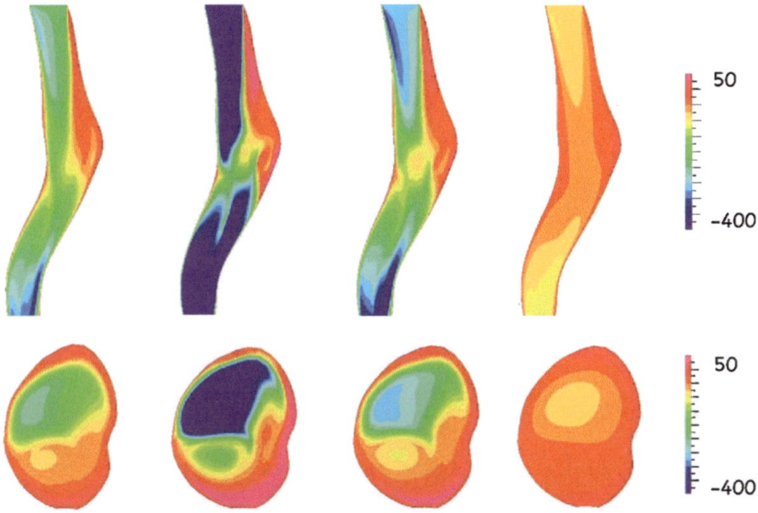

Fig. 6.13 Flow results for patient 2. See caption for Fig. 6.12 for details

small recirculation is already present during the acceleration part of the cardiac cycle. The presence of areas of reverse flow in the horizontal section is visible also during the deceleration, while only forward flow is present at the minimum velocity point. Qualitative similarity of results can be found between this study and that performed by Di Martino et al in 2001, where recirculation was found in the aneurysm bulge in the main characteristic instants of the cardiac cycle. Other studies analyzed the flow pattern in abdominal aneurysm models (Finol and Amon, 2001; Peattie et al., 2004; Leung et al. 2004, 2006; Scotti et al., 2005; Li and Kleinstreuer 2005, 2006; Khanafer et al., 2006) and patient specific models (Wolters et al., 2005; Papaharilaou et al., 2006). The presence of recirculation and vortices is confirmed by

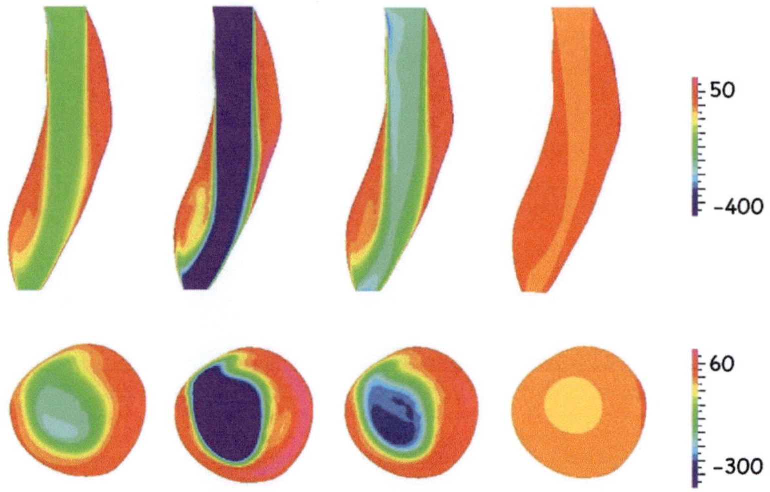

Fig. 6.14 Flow results for patient 3. See caption for Fig. 6.12 for details

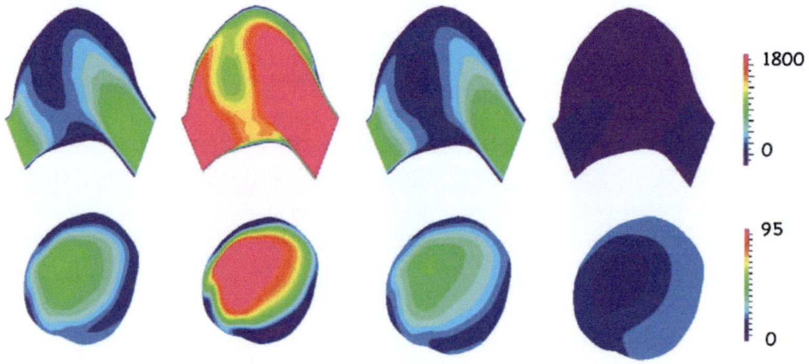

Fig. 6.15 Flow results for patient 4. See caption for Fig. 6.12 for details

these authors, although the recirculation is usually seen in models during the deceleration phase only. The main difference between these studies and the present is that, in case of patients 1 and 4, the aneurysm is located in the arch and the shape of the arch is predominant in determining the flow pattern. In case of patients 2 and 3, the presence of thrombus was included in the solid model; therefore the size of the lumen is smaller than that assumed in other studies (Wolters et al., 2005; Papaharilaou et al., 2006). Peattie et al. (2004) showed that larger aneurysms experienced higher level of flow disturbance and more evident flow separation during the cardiac cycle and that larger aneurysms in vivo might be subject to more frequent turbulence than smaller ones (possibly due to the greater area change that provokes a bigger spatial retardation and adverse pressure gradient). The bending of the aorta in these cases is likely to have a greater effect on the flow. Furthermore, as pointed out earlier, there

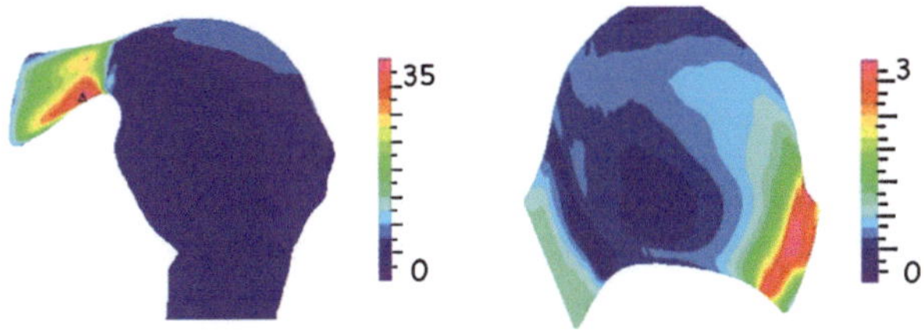

Fig. 6.16 WSS values for patient 1 (on the *left*) and patient 4 (on the *right*). Units in Pa

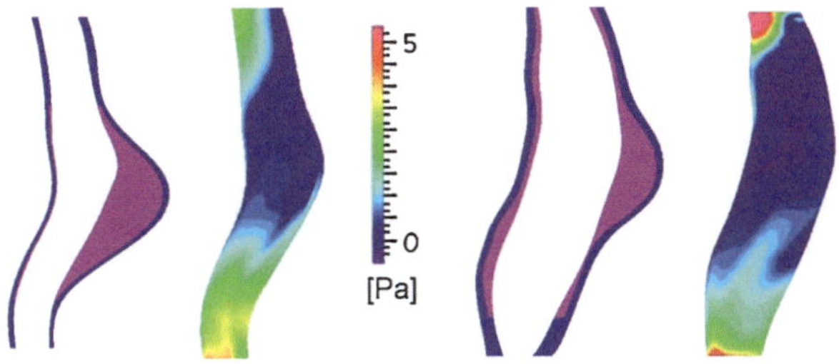

Fig. 6.17 WSS values for patient 2 and 3. Longitudinal sections of the wall domains for the two TA models are also shown to demonstrate the correspondence between low WSS regions and locations of thrombus (units in Pa). High values of WSS visible at inflow and outflow are related to boundary conditions

was no retrograde flow in the flow-rates measured from patients 2 and 3.

Wall shear stress patterns for the four patients at peak systole are shown in Figs. 6.16 and 6.17. Figure 6.16 shows the WSS patterns for patients 1, whose aneurysm are located in the proximal descending aorta and 4, whose aneurysm was in the aortic arch. For both patients higher WSS values are present at the inlet and the bulge shows relatively low values of WSS. Patient 1 presents much higher values of WSS at the inlet, owing to the presence of the stenosis. These simulations were performed under the assumption of laminar flow, whereas it is very likely that laminar-turbulent transition occurs in most aortic aneurysms, at least before thrombus formation. A summary of this phenomenon in patient 1, where the initiating flow instability is accentuated by the immediately proximal coarctation, is presented in the Sect. 6.4.

Different WSS patterns are found in patients 2 and 3, shown in Fig. 6.17. For both patients the area of low WSS coincides with the location of the thrombus (indicated by the longitudinal section of the wall model on the left). By comparing patients 2 and 3, it can be noted that for patient 3 low shear stress is present over the entire lumen/wall boundary, whilst for patient 2 the low WSS area is concentrated around the aneurysm bulge. Prior to thrombus formation, lower WSS would have been concentrated in the bulge, as a result of the separated and recirculating flow that would have been induced, probably promoting the thrombus formation. WSS in the normal aorta is relatively uniform with small spatial variation (not shown here). As can be seen from the contour plots, WSS values are in a similar range for both patients.

Overviews of the flow pattern at peak systole throughout the aneurysms of patients 2 and 3 are shown in Fig. 6.18 to examine the link between abnormal flow

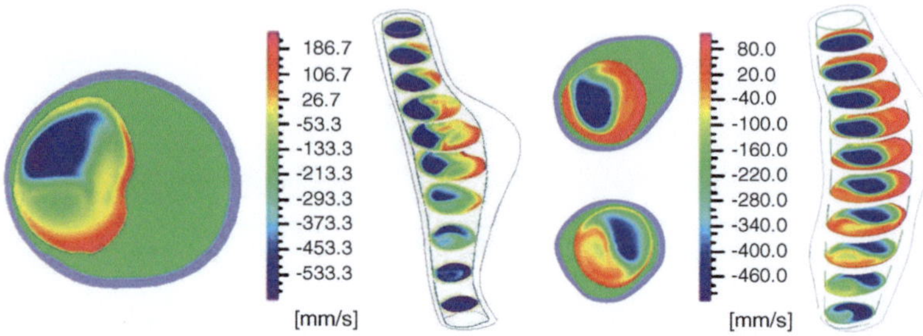

Fig. 6.18 Flow patterns inside the TAA models for patients 2 and 3. Note that forward flow points downwards and has a negative value in the adopted coordinate system. In each case, the flow pattern at the middle section of the aneurysm bulge is given on the *left* (forward flow is shown in *blue*), the thrombus layer is colored in *green* whilst the wall is in violet. Reversed flow (in *red*) occurs on the thrombus side (units in mm/s)

patterns and the presence of thrombus. As mentioned before, for both patients 2 and 3 flow recirculation is observed in the aneurysm bulge, located in the middle of the descending thoracic aorta of patient 2 and in two regions for patient 3 (as shown in the horizontal sections of Fig. 6.18). As shown by Bluestein et al. (1996) for AAA models, platelets trapped in recirculating zones tend to be deposited in areas of low shear stress, since this and the presence of vortices cause prolonged contact of the platelets with the surface in the layer of slow fluid motion (Bluestein et al., 2000). This can provide an insight into the mechanism that promotes the thrombus renewal and possibly enlargement inside the aneurysm.

The WSS patterns show that low shear stress is present in the bulge area, and patient 3 has a larger area of low WSS. This coincides with the location and distribution of thrombus in this patient, implying the role of low WSS in the formation and propagation of ILT. It has been reported that platelet activation is correlated with low WSS (Savage et al., 1996) and its deposition is enhanced by flow recirculation (Bluestein et al., 1996) and low WSS (Bluestein et al., 2000), that allow prolonged contact of the platelets with the lumen surface. It has also been found that interaction between the fibrinogen and platelet receptors occurs at low shear stress levels and the luminal layer of ILT is itself highly thrombogenic (Touat et al., 2006). These results imply that the areas of recirculation and low WSS may be susceptible to further thrombus renewal and propagation. A similar correspondence between low WSS and location of thrombus was found by Leung et al. (2006) in patient-specific AAA models.

6.3.4 Effect of Fully-Coupled Fluid-Solid Interaction on Stress and Flow Calculation

As explained previously, for patients 1 to 4 three models were created:

Table 6.5 Comparison of the peak stress calculated in the S and FSI models for patients 1–4 (units in kPa)

Max stress	FSI	S	Δ %
P1	71.64	73.89	−3.0
P2	82.25	79.36	3.4
P3	51.92	51.81	0.1
P4	75.14	74.42	1.0

- *the S model*, which contains the arterial wall for which a static structural analysis was performed under the assumption of a uniform internal pressure;
- *the F model*, which contains the fluid domain bounded by the aortic lumen for which the flow pattern was analyzed under the assumption of a rigid wall;
- *the FSI model*, where fully coupled blood flow and stress analysis was performed by coupling the wall domain of the S model with the fluid domain of the F model.

Comparison of the stress patterns for the S and FSI models shows that they are qualitatively very similar and the differences are negligible. Table 6.5 shows the differences in predicted maximum wall stress between the FSI and S models.

Quantitative comparison between results from the FSI simulations and static stress analyses shows that the difference in predicted peak wall stress is very small, ranging between −3.0 % for patient 1 to 3.4 % for patient 2. This agrees with other findings reported in the literature (Leung et al., 2006), where it is pointed out that the difference between stress levels in the fully coupled models and static models results from flow-induced pressure, which is negligible compared to the pulse pressure load. In 3 out of 4 models, the wall stress in the static analysis is underestimated in comparison with that obtained from the fully coupled solution. This finding also agrees with most studies of AAA in the literature. The difference in the behavior of the model for patient 1 can be explained by the geometry of the patient and the pressure drop along the aneurysm, which is higher than in other patients (see Table 6.6). This helps to understand why the area close to the inlet experiences a higher wall stress in case of the static structural model (where the exerted pressure is constant all over the aneurysm) in comparison with the FSI model, possibly owing to the flow-induced distortion of the wall.

The stress variation found here is higher than that found by Leung et al. but lower than that reported by Scotti et al. (2005) and Papaharilaou et al. (2006). In the first study, a higher relative internal pressure was used (120 mmHg, under the assumption that the unloaded model was removed from the circulation, compared with the 40 mmHg pulse pressure of the present study); hence the sensitivity of the computed stress to the fluid pressure drop along the vessel is lower than in the present study. In Scotti et al.'s work, a 1.5 mm wall was used to model a hypothetical abdominal aneurysm, as opposed to the wall thickness of approximately 3 mm measured from in vivo images of the patients in this study: a thinner wall is more sensitive to the internal pressure variation; therefore a larger difference between FSI and static analysis results can be expected. The same applies to Papaharilou et al.'s work which is based on a decoupled fluid and structure approach, so that the flow pattern and pres-

Table 6.6 Maximum pressure drop for patient 1 to patient 4 (units in mmHg)

Max pressure drop	FSI	F
Patient 1	13.3	17.3
Patient 2	1.98	2.05
Patient 3	3.33	3.89
Patient 4	1.07	1.21

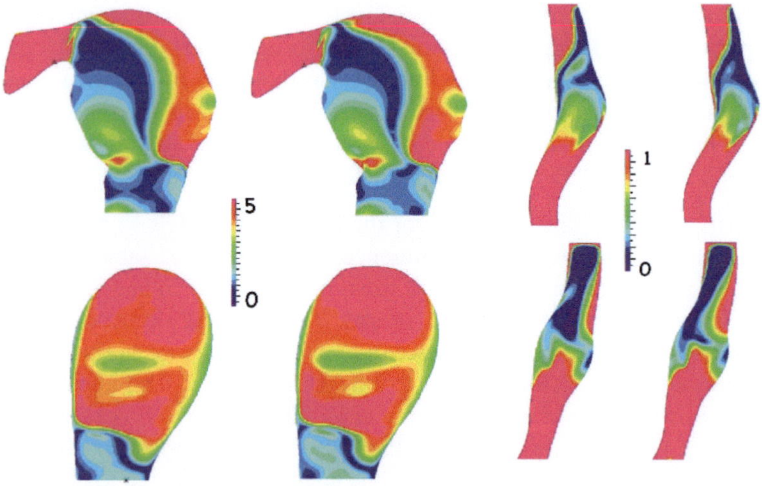

Fig. 6.19 Comparison between the WSS pattern in the F model (on the *left*) and FSI model (on the *right*) of Patient 1 and 2 (units in Pa)

sure drop calculated from the fluid model is not influenced by the wall motion since the wall was kept rigid.

The flow pressure drops between the inlet and the outlet of each model were calculated for both the F and FSI models. The main difference in pressure drop appears during the systolic part of the cardiac cycle, when the maximum expansion of the aneurysm occurs and the hydraulic resistance falls. The maximum pressure drop for each model is reported in Table 6.6. As can be seen, the pressure drop for patient 1 is very high, owing to the presence of the stenosis located in the area of the coarctation; in the FSI solution, the pressure drop was much lower, owing to the compliance of the wall that absorbs part of the kinetic energy of the blood flow during systole. The difference in pressure drop for the other patients is smaller in absolute term but the percentage difference was up to 14 % (in patient 3).

The differences in WSS were analyzed and no major differences were found between the F and FSI models for each patient. On average, the values of WSS for the F models were higher than those of the FSI model, owing to the distensibility of the wall. A comparison between the WSS patterns between the two models for the 4 patients is shown in Figs. 6.19 and 6.20.

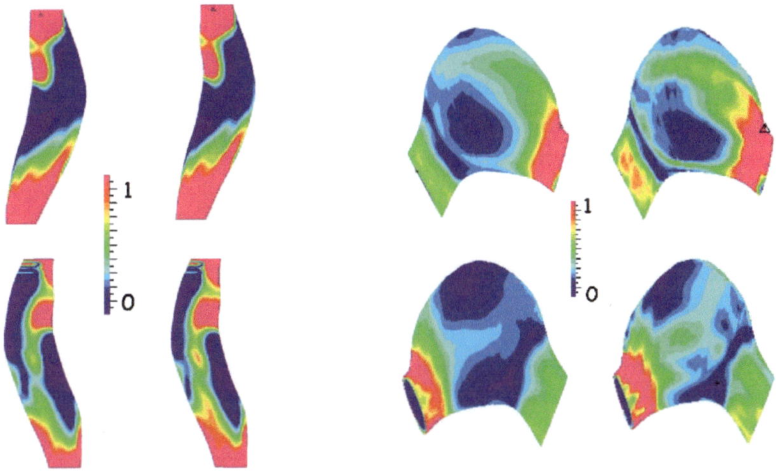

Fig. 6.20 Comparison between the WSS pattern in the F model (on the *left*) and FSI model (on the *right*) of Patient 3 and 4 (units in Pa)

The scale of the images has been chosen in order to highlight the areas of low wall shear stress. The main differences in WSS patterns cane be observed in the bulge for patients 1 and 4, with marked difference at the outlet of the bulge for patient 4 and visible difference in the descending part of the arch for patient 1. Smaller differences are present in patients 2 and 3, where the coincidence of minima of WSS and location of ILT is more evident in the FSI solutions.

6.4 Discussion and Conclusions

In this chapter, a methodology for the creation of patient specific TAA models has been developed and applied to a small group of patients. The ultimate goal of computational biomechanics research on aneurysm is to develop a clinically applicable tool that is able to predict the risk of aneurysm rupture with higher sensitively and specificity than the currently used criteria. The working hypothesis is that wall stresses predicted by means of finite element stress analysis based on patient-specific information are better risk indicators than those used till now, based on simple geometrical measurements. This hypothesis was tested in AAA patient groups (Fillinger et al., 2003; Venkatasubramaniam et al., 2004) and is likely to be also valid for aneurysms involving the thoracic aorta.

The procedure for the reconstruction of a TAA model from in vivo images has been developed, based on the methodology employed and validated for AAA models (Raghavan, 1998; Leung et al., 2006). Modification of the previous methods has been made in order to account for the different anatomical features of aneurysms involving the aortic arch and descending aorta, as well as the use of MR images to define geometry and boundary conditions. The FEM model has been created by importing patient-specific geometries into ADINA and defining suitable materials and boundary conditions. FSI models have been constructed for 4 patients, for which the flow pattern has been analyzed along with wall shear stress and possible link between recirculation and thrombus formation. The effect of coupled flow and stress analysis has been investigated in order to quantify the differences between FSI solution and decoupled solid analysis and fluid analysis. The solutions show similar values of wall stress, with a maximum difference of 3 %; the WSS patterns obtained by FSI simulations do not differ qualitatively from those obtained using the rigid-wall model, however local differences exist and in general the predicted WSS values are lower in the FSI model. The comparison of pressure patterns show similar results, with slightly higher pressure drop along the aneurysm calculated using the rigid-wall model.

It was mentioned earlier that the flow in most aortic aneurysms is likely to experience transition from laminar to turbulent flow. 'Turbulence' in this case means the classical breakdown of the laminar streamlines into chaotic patterns, representing a change in the subsequent character of the flow, as distinct from the 'disturbed' laminar flow patterns that are commonly described as turbulent. In turbulent fluid motion the various flow quantities display random variation in space and time coordinates, with a wide range of scales, such that statistically distinct average values may be discerned (Wilcox, 2006). The introduction of a new transitional turbulence model, incorporating correlations of the onset of transition (Menter et al., 2006), provided the opportunity of its application in cardiovascular flows and to evaluate or validate its efficacy. Following initial validation for an idealized 'carotid' stenosis (Tan et al., 2008), the method was applied to an FSI analysis of the TAA described earlier here as Patient 1 (Tan et al., 2009). In this case comparison between flow patterns in the outflow plane measured by PC-MRI and the patterns predicted by CFD-FSI indicated that the transitional turbulence model gave much better correspondence than either a simulation with an equivalent turbulence model without transition correlations or a pure laminar flow simulation.

In this chapter, the main methods adopted for biomechanical analysis of aortic aneurysms, specifically TAA, have been reviewed and typical results presented and discussed in detail. An interesting confirmation of the potential importance of the mechanical stress analysis was the study reported by Xu et al. (2010), where predicted patient-specific stress patterns were examined together with the corresponding images acquired by PET-CT scanning. Using 18F-FDG tracer (a form of fluorodeoxyglucose) as a marker, metabolic activities in a TAA, two thoraco-abdominal aneurysms, including one with aortic dissection, and two AAAs were obtained via PET (positron emission tomography). In the case of aneurysms or atherosclerotic lesions, 18F-FDG can be used to identify inflammation sites, where metabolic activity is high; in cases such as these it is indicated via strong macrophage activity. The PET scanner detects glycolysis of macrophages, highlighting very active regions. Here, it was found that the strongest signals were received from regions where the aneurysms were expanding. By comparing FE-derived wall internal stresses with the corresponding PET images, the regions of highest stresses were found to correspond to the sites of high FDG uptake, including rupture sites in two patients and the dissection site in another. This was an exciting and highly significant result, showing the potential of wall stress analysis combined with PET imaging to give more reliable prediction of the risk of aneurysm rupture.

The structural models of 5 patients have been built in order to analyze the factors that affect the wall stress in TAA patients. In a similar way to what was previously found for abdominal aneurysms, the stress pattern has been shown to be highly dependent on the geometry of the aneurysm. Perhaps the above two examples of recent investigations suggest the future direction of biomechanical analysis of aortic aneurysms.

Acknowledgement The work reported here was sponsored by the British Heart Foundation

References

Absi TS, Sundt TM 3rd, Tung WS et al (2003) Altered patterns of gene expression distinguishing ascending aortic aneurysms from abdominal aortic aneurysms: complementary DNA expression profiling in the molecular characterization of aortic disease. J Thorac Cardiovasc Surg 126:344–357. Discussion 357

ADINA R&D I (2003) ADINA theory and modeling guide volume I: ADINA solids and structures. ADINA R&D, Watertown

Albornoz G, Coady MA, Roberts M, Davies RR, Tranquilli M, Rizzo JA, Elefteriades JA (2006) Familial thoracic aortic aneurysms and dissections—incidence, modes of inheritance, and phenotypic patterns. Ann Thorac Surg 82(4):1400–1405

Bengtsson H, Sonesson B, Bergqvist D (1996) Incidence and prevalence of abdominal aortic aneurysms, estimated by necropsy studies and population screening by ultrasound. Ann NY Acad Sci 800:1–24

Bluestein D, Niu L, Schoephoerster RT et al (1996) Steady flow in an aneurysm model: correlation between fluid dynamics and blood platelet deposition. J Biomech Eng 118:280–286

Bluestein D, Rambod E, Gharib M (2000) Vortex shedding as a mechanism for free emboli formation in mechanical heart valves. J Biomech Eng 122:125–134

Bogren HG, Buonocore MH (1999) 4D magnetic resonance velocity mapping of blood flow patterns in the aorta in young vs. elderly normal subjects. J Magn Reson Imaging 10(5):861–869

Bogren HG, Mohiaddin RH, Yang GZ, Kilner PJ, Firmin DN (1995) Magnetic resonance velocity vector mapping of blood flow in thoracic aortic aneurysms and grafts. J Thorac Cardiovasc Surg 110(3):704–714

Borghi A, Wood NB, Mohiaddin RH (2006) 3D geometric reconstruction of thoracic aortic aneurysms. Biomed Eng Online 5(1):59

Borghi A, Wood NB, Mohiaddin RH (2008) Fluid-solid interaction simulation of flow and stress pattern in thoracoabdominal aneurysms: a patient-specific study. J Fluids Struct 24:270–280

Cheng SW, Lam ES, Fung GS, Ho P, Ting AC, Chow KW (2008) A computational fluid dynamic study of stent graft remodeling after endovascular repair of thoracic aortic dissections. J Vasc Surg 48(2):303–309; discussion, 309–310

Coady MA, Davies RR, Roberts M, Goldstein LJ, Rogalski MJ, Rizzo JA, Hammond GL, Kopf GS, Elefteriades JA (1999) Familial patterns of thoracic aortic aneurysms. Arch Surg 134(4):361–367

Di Martino ES, Vorp DA (2003) Effect of variation in intraluminal thrombus constitutive properties on abdominal aortic aneurysm wall stress. Ann Biomed Eng 31:804–809

Di Martino ES, Guadagni G, Fumero A, Ballerini G, Spirito R, Biglioli P, Redaelli A (2001) Fluid-structure interaction within realistic three-dimensional models of the aneurysmatic aorta as a guidance to assess the risk of rupture of the aneurysm. Med Eng Phys 23(9):647–655

Elefteriades JA (2002) Natural history of thoracic aortic aneurysms: indications for surgery, and surgical versus nonsurgical risks. Ann Thorac Surg 74:S1877–1880. Discussion S1892–1878

Fann JI (2002) Descending thoracic and thoracoabdominal aortic aneurysms. Coron Artery Dis 13:93–102
Fillinger M (2006) The long-term relationship of wall stress to the natural history of abdominal aortic aneurysms (finite element analysis and other methods). Ann NY Acad Sci 1085:22–28
Fillinger MF, Marra SP, Raghavan ML et al (2003) Prediction of rupture risk in abdominal aortic aneurysm during observation: wall stress versus diameter. J Vasc Surg 37:724–732
Finol EA, Amon CH (2001) Blood flow in abdominal aortic aneurysms: pulsatile flow hemodynamics. J Biomech Eng 123(5):474–484
Fukui T, Matsumoto T, Tanaka T, Ohashi T, Kumagai K, Akimoto H, Tabayashi K, Sato M (2005) In vivo mechanical properties of thoracic aortic aneurysmal wall estimated from in vitro biaxial tensile test. Biomed Mater Eng 15(4):295–305
Gao F, Watanabe M, Matsuzawa T (2006) Stress analysis in a layered aortic arch model under pulsatile blood flow. Biomed Eng Online 5:25
Gonzalez RC, Woods RE (2002) Digital image processing. Prentice-Hall, Upper Saddle River
Hans SS, Jareunpoon O, Balasubramaniam M et al (2005) Size and location of thrombus in intact and ruptured abdominal aortic aneurysms. J Vasc Surg 41:584–588
He R, Guo DC, Sun W et al (2008) Characterization of the inflammatory cells in ascending thoracic aortic aneurysms in patients with Marfan syndrome, familial thoracic aortic aneurysms, and sporadic aneurysms. J Thorac Cardiovasc Surg 136:922–929. 929 e921
Hillenbrand CM, Jesberger JA, Wong EY, Zhang S, Chang DT, Wacker FK, Lewin JS, Duerk JL (2006) Toward rapid high resolution in vivo intravascular MRI: evaluation of vessel wall conspicuity in a porcine model using multiple imaging protocols. J Magn Reson Imaging 23(2):135–144
Jung SE, Lee JM, Lee K, Rha SE, Choi BG, Kim EK, Hahn ST (2005) Gallbladder wall thickening: MR imaging and pathologic correlation with emphasis on layered pattern. Eur Radiol 15(4):694–701
Khanafer KM, Gadhoke P, Berguer R, Bull JL (2006) Modeling pulsatile flow in aortic aneurysms: effect of non-Newtonian properties of blood. Biorheology 43(5):661–679
Leung J, Wright A, Cheshire N, Thom SA, Hughes AD, Xu XY (2004) Flow patterns and wall shear stresses in Patient-specific models of the abdominal aortic aneurysm. In: International congress on medical and care compunetics, The Hague, June 2–4
Leung JH, Wright AR, Cheshire N, Crane J, Thom SA, Hughes AD, Xu Y (2006) Fluid structure interaction of patient specific abdominal aortic aneurysms: a comparison with solid stress models. Biomed Eng Online 5(1):33
Li Z, Kleinstreuer C (2005) Blood flow and structure interactions in a stented abdominal aortic aneurysm model. Med Eng Phys 27(5):369–382
Li Z, Kleinstreuer C (2006) Effects of blood flow and vessel geometry on wall stress and rupture risk of abdominal aortic aneurysms. J Med Eng Technol 30(5):283–297
Menter FR, Langtry R, Volker S (2006) Transition modelling for general purpose CFD codes. Flow Turbul Combust 77:277–303
Mori D, Yamaguchi T (2002) Computational fluid dynamics modeling and analysis of the effect of 3-D distortion of the human aortic arch. Comput Methods Biomech Biomed Eng 5(3):249–260
Morris L, Delassus P, Callanan A, Walsh M, Wallis F, Grace P, McGloughlin T (2005) 3-D numerical simulation of blood flow through models of the human aorta. J Biomech Eng 127(5):767–775
Mower W, Quinones W, Gambhir S (1997) Effect of intraluminal thrombus on abdominal aortic aneurysm wall stress. J Vasc Surg 26(4):602–608
Ogata T, Shibamura H, Tromp G et al (2005) Genetic analysis of polymorphisms in biologically relevant candidate genes in patients with abdominal aortic aneurysms. J Vasc Surg 41:1036–1042
Pannu H, Avidan N, Tran-Fadulu V, Milewicz DM (2006) Genetic basis of thoracic aortic aneurysms and dissections: potential relevance to abdominal aortic aneurysms. Ann NY Acad Sci 1085:242–255

Papaharilaou Y, Ekaterinaris JA, Manousaki E, Katsamouris AN (2006) A decoupled fluid structure approach for estimating wall stress in abdominal aortic aneurysms. J Biomech 40(2):367–377

Peattie RA, Riehle TJ, Bluth EI (2004) Pulsatile flow in fusiform models of abdominal aortic aneurysms: flow fields, velocity patterns and flow-induced wall stresses. J Biomech Eng 126(4):438–446

Raghavan ML (1998) Mechanical wall stress in abdominal aortic aneurysms: towards the development of a clinical tool to predict aneurysm rupture. PhD thesis, University of Pittsburgh, Pittsburgh

Raghavan ML, Vorp DA (2000) Toward a biomechanical tool to evaluate rupture potential of abdominal aortic aneurysm: identification of a finite strain constitutive model and evaluation of its applicability. J Biomech 33(4):475–482

Savage B, Saldivar E, Ruggeri ZM (1996) Initiation of platelet adhesion by arrest onto fibrinogen or translocation on von Willebrand factor. Cell 84:289–297

Scotti CM, Shkolnik AD, Muluk SC, Finol EA (2005) Fluid-structure interaction in abdominal aortic aneurysms: effects of asymmetry and wall thickness. Biomed Eng Online 4:64

Tan FP, Soloperto G, Bashford S et al (2008) Analysis of flow disturbance in a stenosed carotid artery bifurcation using two-equation transitional and turbulence models. J Biomech Eng 130:061008

Tan FP, Torii R, Borghi A et al (2009) Fluid-structure interaction analysis of wall stress and flow patterns in a thoracic aortic aneurysm. Int J Appl Mech 1:179–199

The MathWorks I (2001) Spline toolbox user's guide. The MathWorks, Natick

Thubrikar MJ, Robicsek F, Labrosse M, Chervenkoff V, Fowler BL (2003) Effect of thrombus on abdominal aortic aneurysm wall dilation and stress. J Cardiovasc Surg 44(1):67–77

Touat Z, Ollivier V, Dai J, Huisse MG, Bezeaud A, Sebbag U, Palombi T, Rossignol P, Meilhac O, Guillin MC, Michel JB (2006) Renewal of mural thrombus releases plasma markers and is involved in aortic abdominal aneurysm evolution. Am J Pathol 168(3):1022–1030

Vande Geest JP, Di Martino ES, Bohra A et al (2006) A biomechanics-based rupture potential index for abdominal aortic aneurysm risk assessment: demonstrative application. Ann NY Acad Sci 1085:11–21

Venkatasubramaniam AK, Fagan MJ, Mehta T, Mylankal KJ, Ray B, Kuhan G, Chetter IC, McCollum PT (2004) A comparative study of aortic wall stress using finite element analysis for ruptured and non-ruptured abdominal aortic aneurysms. Eur J Vasc Endovasc Surg 28(2):168–176

Vorp DA, Raghavan ML, Muluk SC, Makaroun MS, Steed DL, Shapiro R, Webster MW (1996) Wall strength and stiffness of aneurysmal and nonaneurysmal abdominal aorta. Ann NY Acad Sci 800:274–276

Vorp DA, Schiro BJ, Ehrlich MP, Juvonen TS, Ergin MA, Griffith BP (2003) Effect of aneurysm on the tensile strength and biomechanical behavior of the ascending thoracic aorta. Ann Thorac Surg 75(4):1210–1214

Wang X, Li X (2011) Fluid-structure interaction based study on the physiological factors affecting the behaviors of stented and non-stented thoracic aortic aneurysms. J Biomech 44:2177–2184

Wang DH, Makaroun M, Webster MW et al (2001) Mechanical properties and microstructure of intraluminal thrombus from abdominal aortic aneurysm. J Biomech Eng 123:536–539

Wang DH, Makaroun MS, Webster MW, Vorp DA (2002) Effect of intraluminal thrombus on wall stress in patient-specific models of abdominal aortic aneurysm. J Vasc Surg 36(3):598–604

Wilcox DC (2006) Turbulence modeling for CFD. DCW Industries, La Canada

Wolters BJ, Rutten MC, Schurink GW, Kose U, de Hart J, van de Vosse FN (2005) A patient-specific computational model of fluid-structure interaction in abdominal aortic aneurysms. Med Eng Phys 27(10):871–883

Xu XY, Borghi A, Nchimi A et al (2010) High levels of 18F-FDG uptake in aortic aneurysm wall are associated with high wall stress. Eur J Vasc Endovasc Surg 39:295–301

Chapter 7
Patient-Specific Biomechanical Framework for Aiding Clinical Decisions in Eye Surgery

E. Lanchares, M. Malvè, and B. Calvo

Abstract In this work we present the development of a patient-specific model of the eye for helping in different ophthalmologic surgical techniques. To build the model we use a simple general model on which we can add the patient specificities measured with proper equipment. The model of the eye is composed of several tissues that must be characterized to ensure that the model has a behavior similar to the real eye. Once the constitutive model is described and characterized for all the tissues included in the model, different surgical techniques can be accomplished. We present here the usefulness of this model to help in surgical planning of incisional surgery for the correction of astigmatism, the numerical analysis of the process of accommodation and the numerical simulation of the scleral buckling technique for retinal detachment.

7.1 Introduction

The human being is mainly visual. Evidences point to the existence of a connection between the evolutive development of the human brain and the manual and visual skills. The eye in the modern society is receptor of more than 90 % of the information arriving to the brain from the outside. Thus the influence of the more common refractive problems in the quality of life, productivity, driving safety, etc. is very important. The impact of refractive problems (myopia, astigmatism, etc.) is elevated

E. Lanchares · M. Malvè · B. Calvo (✉)
Aragón Institute of Engineering Research (I3A), University of Zaragoza, María de Luna s/n, Edif. Betancourt, 50018 Zaragoza, Spain
e-mail: bcalvo@unizar.es

E. Lanchares
e-mail: elanchar@unizar.es

M. Malvè
e-mail: mmalve@unizar.es

E. Lanchares · M. Malvè · B. Calvo
Centro de Investigación Biomédica en Red en Bioingeniería, Biomateriales y Nanomedicina (CIBER-BBN), C/Poeta Mariano Esquillor s/n, 50018 Zaragoza, Spain

B. Calvo, E. Peña (eds.), *Patient-Specific Computational Modeling*,
Lecture Notes in Computational Vision and Biomechanics 5,
DOI 10.1007/978-94-007-4552-0_7,

(about 40 % of the people) and presbyopia or cataract can affect almost 100 % of the elderly people, being cataract surgery one of the most performed. Corneal refractive surgery (PRK, LASIK, etc.) is increasingly performed and it may reach or even overpass the corneal cataract surgery record. Another refractive problem that affects most of the people from 45 years old on (at age 45 affects 70 % of the people, at age 60 almost 100 %) is presbyopia. Due to the large clinical and socioeconomic relevance of this sector, any improvement in products, techniques and procedures has an enormous and direct potential impact. Regarding common and frequent pathologies, the clinician's learning curve of proper treatments such as implants handling and new surgical techniques, improves greatly in a short period of time, establishing protocols which guarantee the successful result of the treatment. Other patients have severe ocular pathologies, infrequently presented. These cases require patient specific optical and anatomical solutions, whose success may be helped with computational tools to plan the surgery or even to design new implants, if necessary. On the other hand, the customized treatments are necessary to obtain an accurate optical quality. Currently this is possible due to the confluence of new technologies and products such as micro-optical devices, lasers, scanners, digital cameras, CAD and advanced behavior models of the tissues that allow the development of numerical models, involving both biomechanical and optical point of view, thus helping the surgeon in planning the successful treatment.

Finite element-based biomechanical models of the eye can be a powerful tool for a prediction of the effects of refractive surgeries and other treatments for eye pathologies (keratoconus, keratoplasties, glaucoma, etc.). The creation of *in silico* models, capable of reproducing the eye behavior by means of computational methods is of great interest nowadays. Numerical simulations using these models will allow a better knowledge of the physiological mechanisms of the eye, hence helping to develop new treatments or improving ones actually used.

Numerical models must be developed on base of its purpose. If the interest of the simulation is to determine the effect of a given treatment in a generic eye to extrapolate results to all the population, the geometry would be based on mean values of a group of patients. On the contrary, if a specific case has to be studied the eye of this patient must be reproduced as accurately as possible. The main difficulty is the modeling of the complex behavior of the tissues involved. One of the difficulties of studying a given treatment in degenerative pathologies is that the effect of the therapy strongly depends on each patient's damaged tissue characteristics.

Some recent treatments for specific pathologies are known to be effective under given conditions. Nevertheless, the influence of each parameter involved is not well known. Numerical simulation also allows sensitivity analysis of each parameter to learn its influence on the result of that treatment, hence making possible to estimate the more adequate value of each parameter for each patient.

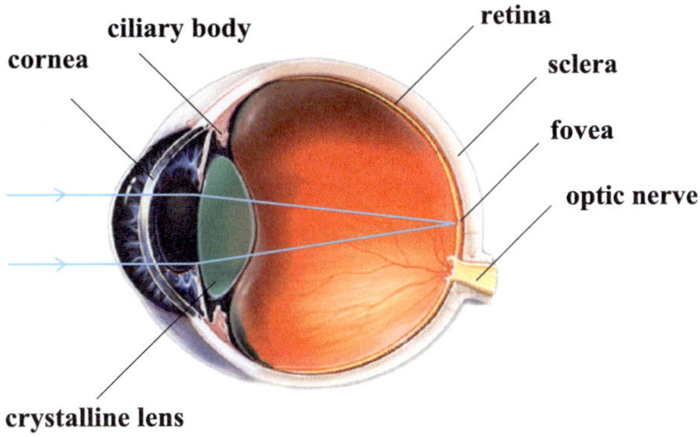

Fig. 7.1 The light goes through cornea, aqueous humor, crystalline lens and vitreous humor before reaching the retina

7.1.1 The Human Vision

The human vision is based on an optical phenomenon named *refraction*. The Snell's law describes refraction as the change in the direction of propagation of the light when it goes through the interface between two media whose indices of refraction are n_1 and n_2 respectively, being Θ_1 the angle of incidence and Θ_2 the angle of refraction:

$$n_1 \cdot \sin \Theta_1 = n_2 \cdot \sin \Theta_2. \tag{7.1}$$

The light in the human eye goes through four different media namely cornea, aqueous humor, crystalline lens and vitreous humor, modifying the direction of the light rays until it converges at the retina, where the image is formed (Fig. 7.1). The amount of rays entering the eye is restricted by the iris opening. The human eye has an optical power of 58 diopters (D). About 43 D correspond to the cornea, the component of the eye with the greatest optical power, and 15 D correspond to the crystalline lens. Thus, cornea and crystalline lens are the two main optical structures of the eye so the numerical model is mainly focused on these two structures.

The optical power in diopters can be calculated using the expression (Munnerlyn et al., 1988)

$$D \cong \frac{n-1}{R} \tag{7.2}$$

where n is the refractive index of the medium, whose value is 1.377 for the cornea, and R is the radius of curvature of the surface between media, in meters.

Depending on the pathology to study, the numerical model of the human eye will be differently defined. For example, for simulating refractive surgery the complexity of the cornea model should be correctly set. On the contrary, the rest of the model components does not need a high level of detail. For studying glaucoma, the most important aspect would be the stress or strain in the tissues of the optic nerve head, thus the cornea and the crystalline lens would be modeled in a simpler way.

Since refraction depends on the curvature of the interfaces crossed by the light rays, an accurate modeling of the geometry of the refractive components of the eye must be achieved to ensure a correct model of the eye. Some measurements must be taken from the patient to develop a patient-specific numerical model of the entire eye or of the different components as cornea, lens, etc.

7.1.2 Measurement and Diagnosis Equipment

Several devices allow measuring geometry of the refractive components of the eye with precision to estimate refractive errors and diagnose several pathologies, but the measurement of the material properties is not easy to be performed *in vivo* nowadays. For this reason there are many clinical devices to measure not only the cornea (anterior and posterior surface, thickness), but also the crystalline lens and the whole eyeball. The following equipments are usually present in the ophthalmologist's office and can be useful for the patient's specific numerical model development. The following briefly describes the most commonly devices.

- Tonometer. The tonometer is a device that determines de intraocular pressure (IOP), usually measured in millimeters of mercury (mmHg). The IOP is an essential parameter for the diagnosis of several pathologies. The numerical simulation of the human eye requires the application of the IOP inside the model, either a physiological healthy value (10–19 mmHg) or the patient's IOP measurement.
- Refractometer and Keratometer. Refractometers measure the optical power of the eye. Keratometers measure the corneal curvature in order to determine the corneal refractive power, and are usually integrated in the refractometer device. The corneal curvature is an essential geometrical parameter for the design of the model geometry to ensure the reproduction of the corneal optics in the model.
- Pachymeter. The pachymeter measures the corneal thickness (pachymetry). This function is actually integrated in other equipments (e.g. topographs).
- Topograph. This device estimates the irregularities of the anterior and posterior corneal surfaces, that are responsible for most visual aberrations of the eye. Other parameters measured by this system are the corneal power (keratometry), pachymetry, the anterior chamber depth, etc. All this information is presented in form of color maps (see Fig. 7.2). Topographs help for diagnosis of several pathologies, as well as for refractive surgery planning. Most of the parameters given by topographs are necessary for building the numerical model.
- Scheimpflug camera. Equipments with a rotating Scheimpflug camera take images of the anterior segment of the eye. This device is specially interesting to obtain information on geometry of the crystalline lens. Some topographs include a rotating Scheimpflug camera (see Fig. 7.3).
- OCT (Optical Coherence Tomography). This non-invasive technique gives transversal images of the living eye useful for the study of both corneal and retinal pathology.
- Ocular Response Analyzer (*Reichert Ophthalmic Instruments, Inc., Depew, NY, USA*) is a recently appeared system which measures IOP and some parameters related to corneal biomechanics. The procedure consists of the ejection of an air

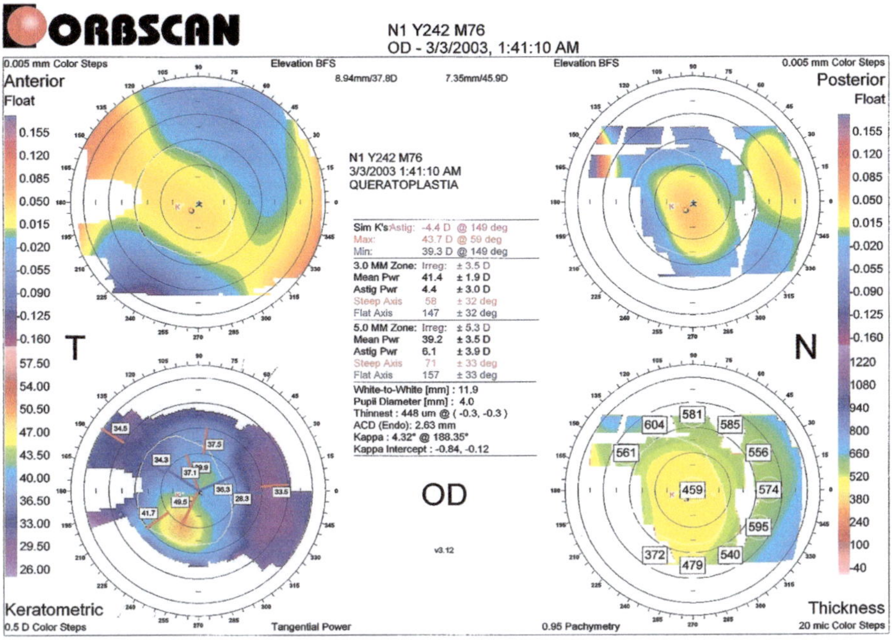

Fig. 7.2 Color maps (Orbscan II, *Bausch&Lomb, Rochester, NY, USA*) corresponding to anterior elevation (*top left*), posterior elevation (*top right*), keratometry (*bottom left*) and pachymetry (*bottom right*)

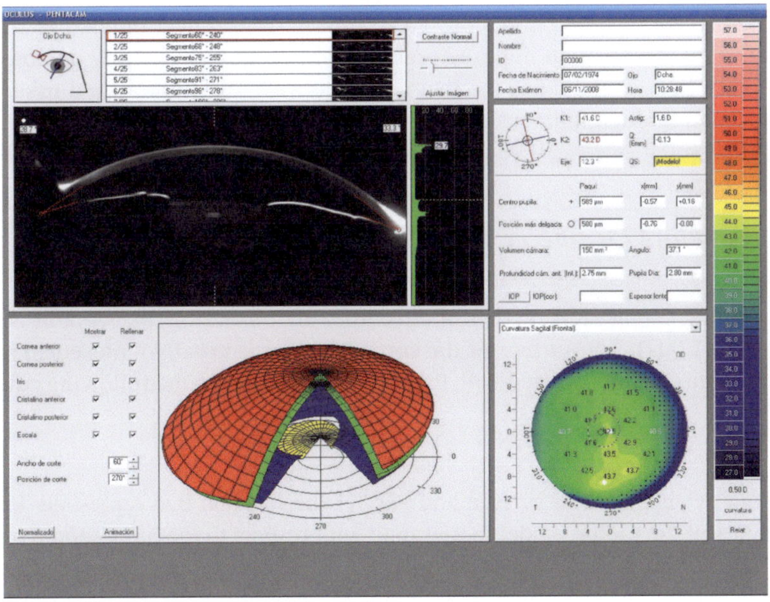

Fig. 7.3 Picture taken with a Scheimpflug camera and optical model of the eye (Pentacam, *Oculus Inc., Germany*)

pulse against the central cornea. The corneal movement is registered by means of an ultrasound system and used to compute several graphics and parameters. Among all the outputs, corneal hysteresis (CH) and corneal resistance factor (CRF) are the most significant of our interest since they are related to the viscohyperelasticity of the corneal tissue. Moreover, these parameters are taken *in vivo* in a non-invasive form directly from the patient's eye. These data could then be used to estimate the material parameters of the corneal constitutive model.

7.2 Finite Element Model of Human Eye

In order to develop a human ocular globe model there are basically two main strategies available. The most general, a generic model that can be used as baseline to extract results that can be applied to a large population of patients or predict *ad hoc* results using patient specific models that can be directly used for helping refractive surgery.

We present both strategies since the generic model which presents radial symmetry can be easily adapted to a patient specific human eye moving the grid nodes. In summary, firstly we will present different generic models of a healthy eye based on different geometries, starting from the easiest case i.e. a sphere and ending with a non-revolution ellipsoid.

The main parts considered to build this human eye model are the cornea, the crystalline lens, the sclera and the optic nerve. The aqueous and vitreous humor are currently not included in the presented model. Their effect on the eye tissue is introduced by means of an imposed pressure which can be clinically obtained (see Sect. 7.1.2). In further studies the interaction between eye humors and tissues will be considered through fluid-structure (FSI) coupled models.

7.2.1 Baseline Geometry Model of Cornea

The following geometrical models of the cornea are taken from the work of Navarro et al. (2005, 2007). The surface of the cornea $S(x, y)$ is usually represented assuming the sagitta z ideally aligned with the optical axis, through the following equation:

$$z \equiv S(x, y) = b(x, y) + r(x, y) \tag{7.3}$$

where $b(x, y)$ is the basal surface and $r(x, y)$ the residual that represents local irregularities of the global model topography with respect to the basal model $b(x, y)$. In this way, through $b(x, y)$ one guarantees a satisfactory global topography of the cornea while the residual is normally adjusted according with the Zernike polynomial function. Since $r(x, y)$ is patient specific, it will be added to the basal model once the Zernike polynomial function is estimated.

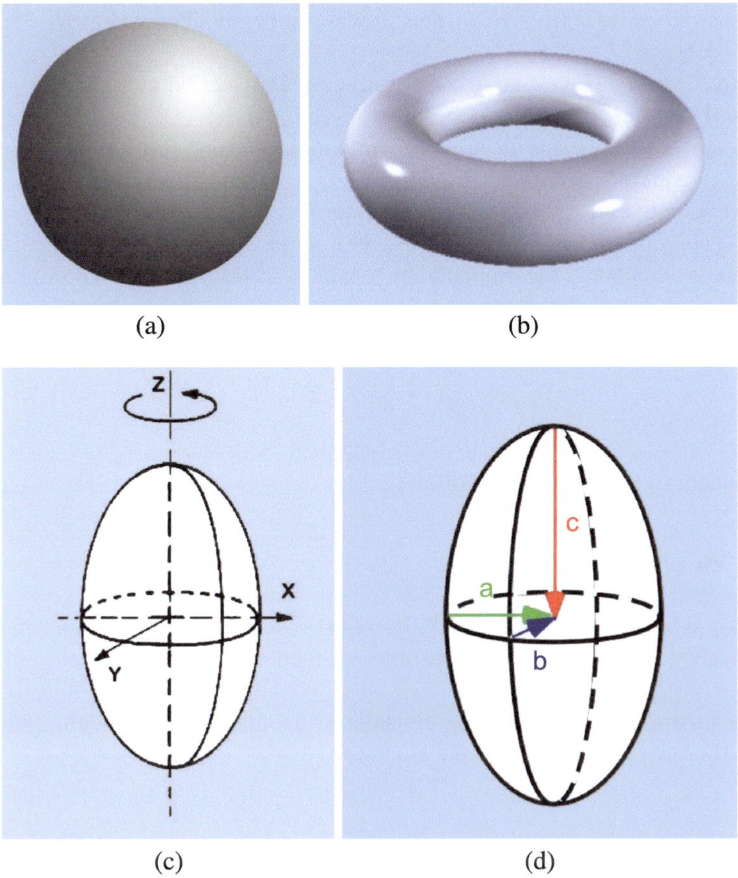

Fig. 7.4 Conical surfaces used for modeling the cornea geometry: (**a**) sphere, (**b**) toroid surface, (**c**) revolution ellipsoid, (**d**) non-revolution ellipsoid

We use a biconical model for $b(x, y)$:

$$z = \frac{c_x x^2 + c_y y^2}{1 + \sqrt{1 - (1 + Q_x)c_x^2 x^2 - (1 + Q_y)c_y^2 y^2}}. \tag{7.4}$$

In this equation, the sagittal coordinate z is represented as a function of four parameters: the horizontal and vertical curvature (c_x and c_y, respectively) that can be obtained using the following expressions: $c_x = \frac{1}{R_x}$ and $c_y = \frac{1}{R_y}$ with R_x and R_y the curvature radius, and, the conic constant factors Q_x and Q_y. Modifying the polynomial function (7.4) different models can be obtained:

- *Spherical model* (Fig. 7.4(a)). In this case, $R_x = R_y = R$, $Q_x = Q_y = 0$. The baseline sphere that consists in the easiest model is normally called BFS (Best Fit Sphere).

- *Corneal ellipsoid* (Fig. 7.4(c)). This model can be obtained when: $R_x = R_y = R$ y $Q_x = Q_y = Q$.
- *Toroidal surface* (Fig. 7.4(b)). Due to the circular section along x and y: $Q_x = Q_y = 0$.
- *Biconical model*. This is the most general model since no restrictions are imposed to the considered parameters. Equation (7.4) represents this surface supposed that the astigmatic axis (that with more curvature) is oriented at 0° or at 90°.
- *Non-revolution ellipsoid* (Fig. 7.4(d)). This surface, which can be visualized as a melon, is completely determinated by means of its three orthogonal semiaxis a, b and c according to the expression:

$$\frac{x^2}{a^2} + \frac{y^2}{b^2} + \frac{z^2}{c^2} = 1. \tag{7.5}$$

This case is a particular one of the biconical model assuming two constants as dependent of the semiaxis as follows:

$$R_x = \frac{a^2}{c}, \qquad R_y = \frac{b^2}{c}, \qquad Q_x = \frac{a^2}{c^2} - 1, \qquad Q_y = \frac{b^2}{c^2} - 1. \tag{7.6}$$

Finally it has to be noted that even having two dependent parameters which limit its generality, the ellipsoid is a two-order surface while the biconical is of fourth order.

In this work we present two of the anterior geometries for the definition of the cornea: the spherical and the elliptical model.

7.2.1.1 Spherical Geometry

The human eye does not present a spherical geometry even in case of emmetropia. This means that a small amount of astigmatism always exists so the horizontal corneal axis possesses more curvature than the vertical one (Navarro et al., 2009). Nevertheless the spherical geometry is a good approximation of the elliptical since the differences between the aforementioned axis are in the order of [μm]. For this reason, in the literature the axisymmetric model is widely used to model the human cornea (Pandolfi et al., 2009; Pinsky and Datye, 1991), especially in case of emmetropia (Calossi, 2007).

Although the axisymmetric model is very simple, it can be easily used for simulating the incisional surgery to correct astigmatism or to induce in the geometry the required level of astigmatism which must be corrected through the surgery (Lanchares et al., 2008). It would be in fact possible to create a different model changing in each model the surgical parameter which one wants to analyze. In the same way, it would be possible to simulate the myopia surgery. Cornea, sclera and limbus were modeled using the geometry of revolution. After that, the optical lens, the surrounding muscles and the optic nerve were adapted to this geometry. In Fig. 7.5 the complete model and its main components are shown.

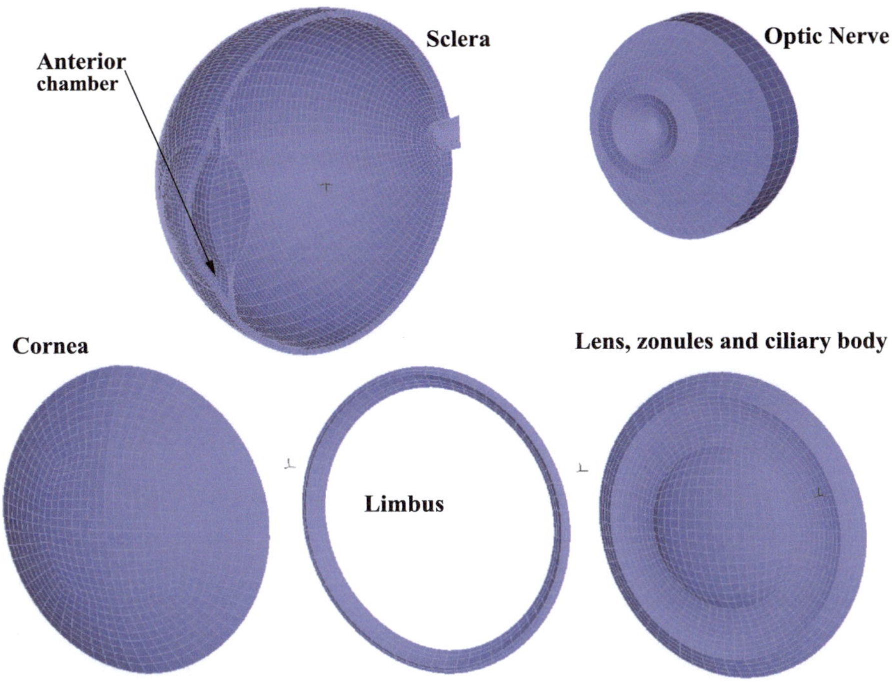

Fig. 7.5 3D view of the modeled human eye parts: cornea, limbus, sclera, lens, zonules, ciliary body and optic nerve

The global ocular radius was determined according with (Cabrera et al., 2006) and is $R = 7.5$ mm. To the ocular surface was assigned the diameter of 12 mm (Pinsky and Datye, 1991), axial thickness of 550 μm while the peripheral corneal thickness was 650 μm (Pinsky and Datye, 1991). In this way, the posterior surface possesses an apical radius of 6.04 mm with a conicity $Q = -1.35$ (see Fig. 7.6). The limbus, sketched in Fig. 7.5 consists in a ring which surrounds the cornea. The intern limbus diameter is 12 mm while the external is 12.5 mm. Its thickness shows an increase of 0.65 mm along the corneal direction and 1 mm along the scleral direction. The scleral geometry can also be considered as of revolution. The external radius is 13 mm with a thickness of 1 mm (see Figs. 7.5 and 7.6).

The geometry and the computational grid were performed with the commercial software Ansys Icem CFD (*Ansys, Inc., Software, Canonsburg, PA, USA*). In order to be able to perform numerical simulations of the surgery especially in case of ocular incisions of different lengths and variable distances with respect to the ocular axis (axis z in Fig. 7.6) the mesh is composed only of hexahedral elements. The total node and element number is 34,430 and 27,456 respectively. The computational grid of the cornea was built using the known topological structure *O-Grid* (see Fig. 7.5) so that the aforementioned surgical situations can be simulated.

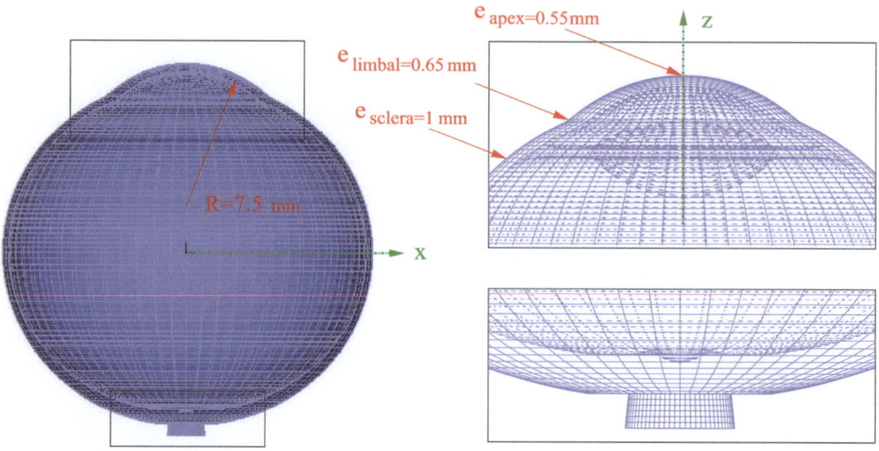

Fig. 7.6 2D view of the computational grid with zoom on the cornea and optical nerve. The cornea is modeled assuming sphericity

7.2.1.2 Ellipsoidal Geometry

This model is capable of representing the astigmatism through the different curvatures between the merian axis and its perpendicular. The merian axis is that with more refractive power.

As said before, healthy corneas always present a light astigmatism. Generally, the axis with greater curvature radius is the horizontal one (x axis), being the horizontal semiaxis (nasal-temporal axis) greater than the vertical one (superior-inferior axis). In Fig. 7.7 the process to obtain the corneal surface starting from the non-revolution ellipsoid is depicted. The final surface is a geometrical shape with an elliptical basis with semiaxis a', b' in which the biggest axis is equal to the corneal biggest diameter ($2a' = \phi_{cornea}$). The direction identified with the biggest ellipse semiaxis is then taken as ($a' = \frac{\phi_{cornea}}{2}$) horizontal axis ($x$-axis). The light astigmatism of healthy corneas is due to this difference. Finally, the (z-axis) is taken to be the optical axis.

According with the study of Navarro et al. (2005) for a healthy cornea, in this work we assign to the principal semiaxes a, b and c the values of 10.43 mm, 10.27 mm and 14.26 mm, respectively. For the corneal diameter $\phi_{cornea} = 2a'$ the value of 12 mm was assumed (Bryant and McDonnell, 1996).

The corneal diameter $2b'$ in the direction y is smaller than that in horizontal direction. This was determinated by means of the relationship between the corresponding ellipsoid semiaxis a, b: $\frac{a'}{b'} = \frac{a}{b}$. For the posterior corneal surface as well as the spherical model, the apical thickness of 550 μm was considered while at the end of the limbus the thickness was 660 μm.

As it will be clarified in the next sections, this model can be used in the simulations of corneal incisional surgery for astigmatism correction. The computational grid of the elliptical geometry was built basically using the same process described in the previous section. It is composed by the same element and node number and

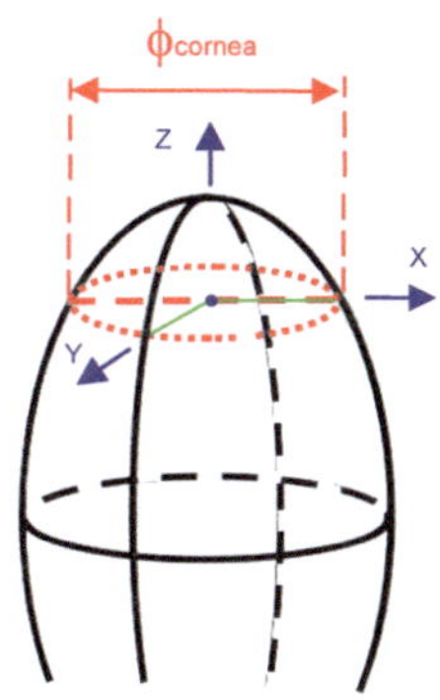

Fig. 7.7 The basal surface of the cornea was obtained cutting with a coronal plane the ellipsoid. The obtained geometrical shape possesses an elliptical base which main axis is the corneal diameter (ϕ_{cornea}). The direction of the principal semiaxis of this surface ($\frac{\phi}{2}$) is taken as horizontal x axis. In this way a little astigmatism is produced. The z axis defines the optical axis

it is topological identical in every aspects to the spherical grid. This model allows in fact to get back from the spherical surface to the elliptical inducing in a spherical cornea the degree of astigmatism of interest.

7.2.2 Patient Specific Model of Cornea

The most important application of the shown methodology is the possibility to predict for a patient the corrected and most adequate treatment, analyzing for example the consequences of different treatments for this single patient. For this reason, the cornea should be reproduced the more detailed as possible for a specific patient and simulate directly in this geometry the different treatments. In this section we propose a methodology for developing a patient specific cornea model.

The patient specific corneal model starts from the ocular topography which can be obtained from the patient corneal surface by means of an ocular topographer. This device performs a scan of the anterior surface of the cornea. Measuring the different elevation of the points composing the anterior and posterior surface it is able to depict a color map of the different elevation of these points (see Fig. 7.2). In addition, the corneal topographer is able to give an estimation of the corneal thickness, the curvature radius and the position of the lens. In Fig. 7.2 are shown the corneal informations obtained using the device Orbscan II (*Bausch&Lomb, Rochester, NY, USA*) which was used in the present work. The upper panel shows the elevation map of the anterior (on the left) and posterior surface (on the right). The basal surface used for the scan is the best fitting (BSF) which radius is reported beside each scan of the figure. The bottom panel shows the keratometric map (optical power of the corneal surface) and the pachymetric map (estimation of the corneal thickness).

Starting from the patient specific corneal elevation map, using the commercial software Matlab (*The MathWorks, Inc.*), the surface was generated through a bidi-

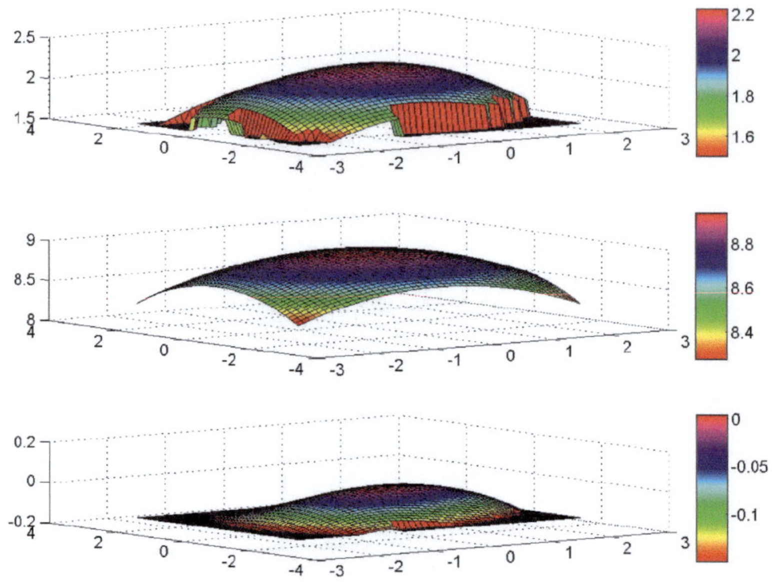

Fig. 7.8 Posterior surface of a patient specific cornea. The surface data were extracted from the scan performed by the topographer Orbscan II of *Bausch&Lomb* (see Fig. 7.2). The *subfigure in the middle* represents the BFS which radius is 7.35 mm. This was used to depict the surface starting from the posterior elevation map. The *lower subfigure* represents the elevation, the difference between the points composing the anterior surface and the BFS. In a second stage, to this data were adapted the biomechanical model

mensional grid. For this case, a matrix of 101 × 101 points included between −5 and 5 mm centered in the apex along the directions X and Y at interval of $\Delta x = \Delta y = 0.1$ mm. Each point is assigned its measured elevation. Depending on its position with respect to the BFS this elevation can assume positive or negative values.

The upper subpicture of Fig. 7.8 shows the reproduced surface. The color scale represents the elevation of the points composing the surface with respect to the BFS. The BFS is shown in the middle subfigure. The radius adopted to build this surface (7.35 mm) is that reported in Fig. 7.2. The lower subpicture of Fig. 7.8 shows the difference of the elevation between the first two surfaces, the corneal surface and the BFS. It has to be noted that the color pattern of the lower subpicture perfectly matches that of Fig. 7.2 (upper panel on the right) showing a slightly enlarged area with a small eccentricity.

Finally, the anterior and posterior elevations obtained through the scan and reproduces by means of geometrical surface are use to adapt the selected numerical model, the spherical one or the elliptical. The numerical model of the cornea is adapted adding or subtracting the elevation, depending on the position of every point of the measured surface with respect to the BFS by means of a projection. This process is sketched in Fig. 7.9.

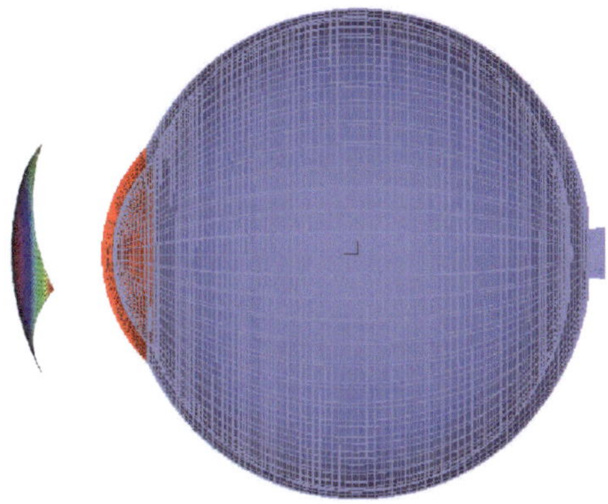

Fig. 7.9 Coupling between the patient specific cornea surface and the general numerical model of the human eye

7.2.3 Crystalline Lens

In order to develop a human crystalline lens model we adopted the method proposed by Hermans et al. (2008). This method represents the anterior and posterior curvature around the optical axis based on optical models in order to adapt the equatorial radius to the right estimated measures following the patient age and the reached accommodation. The crystalline lens is modeled starting from the Orbscan II images. From this device it is possible to detect the approximate position of the lens inside the eye. Using this information, we modeled the lens through a parametric model with aim to be able to perform the aforementioned age accommodation. Differently from Hermans et al. (2008), the external surface of the lens was built merging three parts as results of the combination of different experimental measures in the central (Dubbelman and der Heijde, 2001) and equatorial (Schachar et al., 1993) area. The in-between area was estimated by interpolation in order to guarantee surface continuity. The central part of the anterior and posterior surfaces of the lens (characterized by red lines in Fig. 7.10) are conicoid surfaces with revolution symmetry (see (7.7)) where C is the curvature and Q is the conic constant:

$$z_1 = z_0 + \frac{Cx^2}{1+\sqrt{1-(Q+1)C^2x^2}}. \tag{7.7}$$

According to Schachar et al. (1993), the equatorial edge (green curve in Fig. 7.10) is modeled as an arc of circumference with radius r_e (equation (7.8)). This connects the anterior and posterior surfaces and it is positioned at the equator at the previously established lens radius R_{lens}

$$z_3 = \sqrt{r_e^2 - (x - R_{lens} + r_e)^2}. \tag{7.8}$$

The ratio between r_e and R_{lens} is constant ($\frac{r_e}{R_{lens}} = 0.1208$), as well as the values of the anterior and posterior angles which determine the length of the equatorial arc ($\theta_{ant} = 63°$, $\theta_{pos} = 37°$) (Schachar et al., 1993).

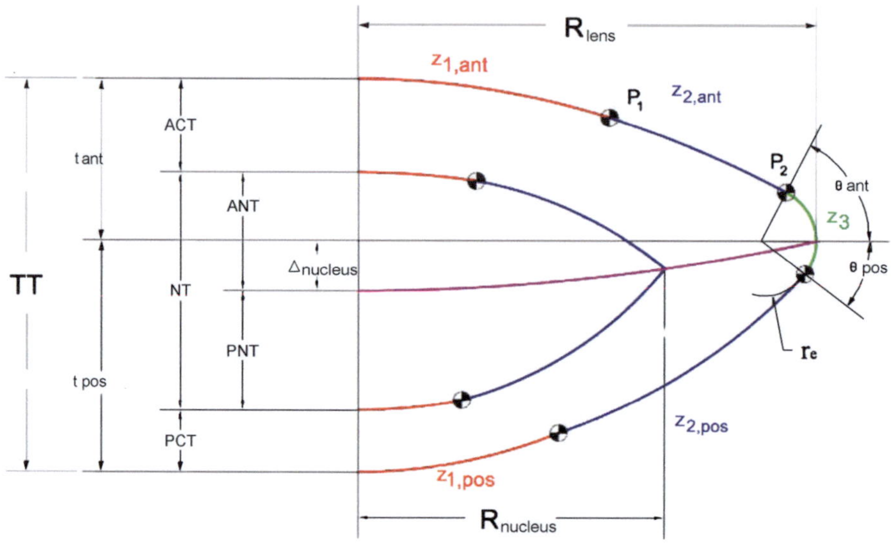

Fig. 7.10 Parametric geometry of the lens used to define the FE model. Lens thickness (*TT*), anterior half lens thickness (t_{ant}), posterior half lens thickness (t_{pos}), anterior cortex thickness (*ACT*), posterior cortex thickness (*PCT*) and nucleus thickness (*NT*) as the sum of anterior nucleus thickness (*ANT*) and posterior nucleus thickness (*PNT*)

The central part of the lens (red curves) and the equatorial edge (green curves) must be connected through an intermediate surface (colored in blue in Fig. 7.10) to complete the outer geometry of the lens. The blue curves, z_2, are conic, and were designed to guarantee continuity with the red and green curves. The connecting points are named P_1, between the red and blue curves, and P_2, between the blue and green curves. Following Hermans et al. (2008), P_1 is set at $x = 2.5$ mm for the anterior part and $x = 2$ mm for the posterior surface. As previously explained, P_2 is fixed by θ_{ant} and θ_{pos}, using the cited values (Schachar et al., 1993). The computed values for $C_{2,ant}$ and $Q_{2,ant}$ were 0.1021 mm^{-1} and 1.1302, respectively. The expressions for $z_{2,pos}$, $Q_{2,pos}$ and $C_{2,pos}$ can be obtained similarly to $z_{1,ant}$, $Q_{1,ant}$ and $C_{1,ant}$. The computed values for $C_{2,pos}$ and $Q_{2,pos}$ were 0.0036 mm^{-1} and 53.5284, respectively.

The interface between the anterior and posterior halves of the lens is not modeled as an equatorial plane but as a conicoid surface of revolution (Jones et al., 2005). We used the conicoid proposed by Navarro et al. (2007). From this curve we obtained a quadratic surface of revolution.

The interfaces between nucleus and cortex, both anterior and posterior, are assumed to be concentric with the outer surfaces of the cortex. No equatorial circumference is used for the equator of the nucleus.

Rosen et al. (2006) found a nearly constant ratio of 0.7 between anterior and posterior thicknesses, measured as the distances from the anterior and posterior poles to the equator. This factor, along with the expression for the lens thickness *TT* in

Table 7.1 Geometrical parameters used for the design of the numerical model of the 30 year-old crystalline lens: anterior cortex thickness (*ACT*), nucleus thickness (*NT*), posterior cortex thickness (*PCT*), total thickness (*TT*). *A* is the age (years) and *D* (diopters) represents the range of accommodation (Brown, 1973; Dubbelman et al., 2003; Rosen et al., 2006)

	Regression function	$7.5D$	$0D$
ACT [mm]	$0.51(\pm 0.04) + 0.0116(\pm 0.007)A + 0.0040D$	0.89	0.87
NT [mm]	$2.11(\pm 0.04) + 0.0030(\pm 0.001)A + 0.0400D$	2.49	2.19
PCT [mm]	$0.33(\pm 0.04) + 0.0082(\pm 0.007)A + 0.0006D$	0.58	0.57
TT [mm]	$2.95 + 0.0228A + 0.045D$	3.96	3.63
$R_{nucleus}$ [mm]	$3.05 + (0.5542 - 0.0091A)(1 - \frac{D}{15-0.25D})$	3.05	3.33
R_{lens} [mm]	$0.0069(\pm 0.001)A + 4.35(\pm 0.07)$	4.56	4.84

Table 7.1 was used here to compute the thickness of nucleus and cortex for different ages and accommodations.

To design the geometry of the nucleus we used *in vivo* experimental data obtained by Dubbelman et al. (2003). The growth rate of the cortex with aging is greater than that of the nucleus, which is consistent with the fact that new fibers are continuously formed in the outermost layer of the cortex.

The equatorial radius of the nucleus was estimated by the expression proposed by Brown (1973) for $R_{nucleus}$. Since the anterior and posterior cortex-nucleus interface and the outer surface of the lens are coaxial in the optical zone, the geometry of the nucleus is completed with two anterior and posterior curves which extend the central parts to the point of the medium surface situated at $R_{nucleus}$ from the optical axis (see Fig. 7.10).

The capsular thickness varies with the radial position and grows with age (Fisher and Pettet, 1972). We followed the equations proposed by Burd et al. (2002), based on Fisher-Pettet data (Fisher and Pettet, 1972) to estimate the capsular thickness as a function of the radial position. The anterior capsular thickness is greater than the posterior. It has to be noted that take advantage of the parametric modeling performed on the crystalline lens, the capsular thickness in the presented model can be adapted to the age.

Once the lens geometry is assessed and the patient age is selected or available by means of Orbscan II, the computational mesh can be accomplished. The geometry surface of the lens (in IGES format) is exported by a commercial CAD (SolidWorks©) and imported in FEMAP (Siemens PLM Software, Plano, TX, USA) were a fully hexahedral mesh was built. In Fig. 7.5 the complete eye model also shows the lens grid, which is fixed to the inner surface of the sclera. In Fig. 7.11 this mesh is plotted evidencing the main modeled components: the ciliary body, the zonules and the muscular tissue responsible for the lens movement. The ciliary body is modeled as a coronal volume joint with the zonules.

The resulting FE model is composed of 24,000 solid hexaedrical elements, 12,000 of which belong to the cortex and the other 12,000 to the nucleus. The capsule is modeled independently using 2,000 shell elements of variable thickness. The

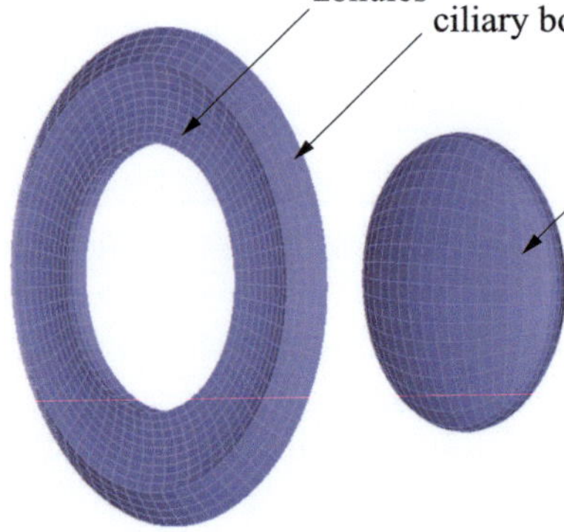

Fig. 7.11 3D view of the crystalline lens numerical grid. The model also includes the zonules of Zinn and the ciliary body

value of the thickness is assigned to each capsule element according to its radial position, as previously explained.

7.2.4 Optic Nerve Head

The geometry of the optic nerve head (ONH) was approximated using the geometry models of Sigal et al. (2010). The nerve head was modeled as circular, and asymmetry in its position with respect to the eye geometry axis is assumed. In this way, both right and left eye can be modeled with a simple geometrical modifying i.e. moving the optic nerve axis slightly to the left and to the right respectively.

The ON was divided in three main parts: the optic nerve head, an intermediate part, the lamina cribosa, and an inferior part, the optic nerve body. The scleral cup is defined to connect the optical nerve, the lamina cribosa and the optic nerve. In Fig. 7.12 the computational grid of this main components is shown. The geometry was meshed by means of 6,080 elements: 1,088 wedge and 4,992 hexaedrical elements, respectively.

7.3 Constitutive Behavior of Eye Tissues

Biological soft tissues in generally and eye tissues in particular are subjected to large deformations with negligible volume changes due to high water content and show an anisotropic mechanical response due to their internal structure. The extra-cellular matrix is composed of a network of collagen fibrils and elastin fibers embedded in a viscous and isotropic ground substance. Their mechanical stiffness and ultimate tensile strength have been shown to depend on the length of collagen fibrils; longer fibrils permit a greater number of inter-fibrillar connections, resulting in a more efficient force transmission. Experimental evidence shows that eye's tissues such as cornea, sclera and lens subjected to axial tensile stresses (Downs et al., 2003;

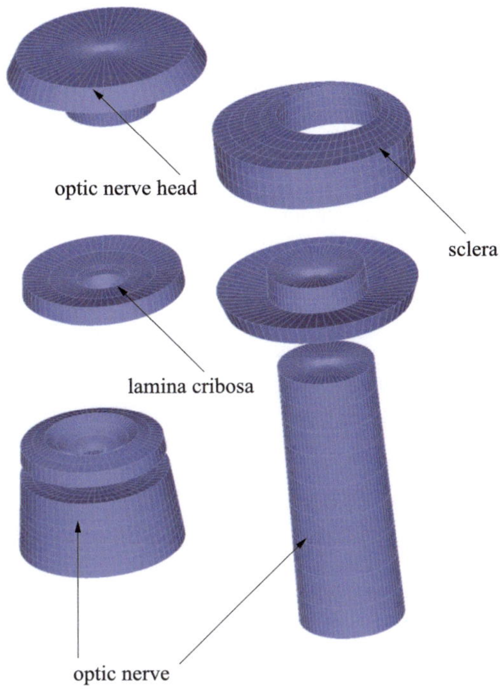

Fig. 7.12 3D view of the optic nerve head computational grid. It is composed of the optic nerve head, sclera, lamina cribosa and the optic nerve

Dubbelman et al., 2003; Fung, 1993; Pinsky and Datye, 1991) have a typical non-linear response, with an initial low stiffness toe region, a linear part with approximately constant stiffness, and a third region corresponding to progressive failure of the composing fibers.

Usually, the description of the constitutive behavior of this type of material relies on the identification of an appropriate strain energy density function from which stress-strain relations and local elasticity tensors are derived.

To define the strain energy density function that characterizes the mechanical behavior of the tissue experimental tests are needed. Even though different strain energy density functions have proved to be successful for particular applications and for describing many of the material properties, their use is limited, in most cases, to the range of physiological loads. This section have been limited to describe the mechanical response of eye tissue into the toe and linear regions, that is, the behavior of soft tissue under normal physiological loads and their mechanical response at long-term, viscoelasticity is despised.

7.3.1 Anisotropic Hyperelastic Behavior of Fibered Tissue

This section provides a brief review of basic concepts in finite deformation continuum mechanics and constitutive behavior of fibered materials, as cornea, limbus or the capsule of lens.

Consider a continuum body with reference configuration Ω_0 at the initial reference time $t = 0$. Then, an assumed motion χ maps this configuration to the current configuration Ω at each time t. Hence, a point $\mathbf{X} \in \Omega_0$ transforms to a point $\mathbf{x} \in \Omega$, where $\mathbf{X}$ and $\mathbf{x}$ define the respective positions of a particle in the reference and current configurations relative to a fixed set of axes. The direction of a collagen fiber at a point $\mathbf{X} \in \Omega_0$ is defined by a unit vector field $\mathbf{m}_0(\mathbf{X})$, $|\mathbf{m}_0| = 1$. It is usually assumed that, under deformation, the fiber moves with the material points of the continuum body. Therefore, the stretch λ of the fiber defined as the ratio between its lengths at the deformed and reference configurations can be expressed as

$$\lambda \mathbf{m}(\mathbf{x}, t) = \mathbf{F}(\mathbf{X}, t)\mathbf{m}_0(\mathbf{X}) \tag{7.9}$$

where $\mathbf{m}$ is the unit vector of the fiber in the deformed configuration

$$\lambda^2 = \mathbf{m}_0 \cdot \mathbf{F}^T \mathbf{F} \cdot \mathbf{m}_0 = \mathbf{m}_0 \cdot \mathbf{C}\mathbf{m}_0. \tag{7.10}$$

In (7.9) and (7.10), $\mathbf{F} = \frac{d\mathbf{x}}{d\mathbf{X}}$ and $\mathbf{C} = \mathbf{F}^T\mathbf{F}$ are the standard deformation gradient and the corresponding right Cauchy-Green strain measure. A multiplicative decomposition of $\mathbf{F}$ into *volume-changing (dilational)* and *volume-preserving (distortional)* parts is usually established as in Flory (1961) and Simo and Taylor (1991) with $\mathbf{J} = \det \mathbf{F}$

$$\mathbf{F} = J^{\frac{1}{3}}\bar{\mathbf{F}}, \qquad \mathbf{C} = J^{\frac{2}{3}}\bar{\mathbf{C}}. \tag{7.11}$$

The introduced kinematics for one family of fibers can be applied to other fiber families in an analogous manner. We shall denote a second preferred fiber direction by the unit vector field $\mathbf{n}_0(\mathbf{X})$.

To characterize isothermal processes, we postulate the existence of a unique decoupled representation of the strain-energy density function Ψ (Simo and Taylor, 1985). Because of the directional dependence on the deformation, we require that the function Ψ explicitly depends on both the right Cauchy-Green tensor $\mathbf{C}$ and the fibers direction $\mathbf{m}_0$ and $\mathbf{n}_0$ in the reference configuration. Since the sign of $\mathbf{m}_0$ and $\mathbf{n}_0$ is not significant, Ψ must be an even function of $\mathbf{m}_0$ and $\mathbf{n}_0$ and so it may be expressed by $\Psi = \Psi(\mathbf{C}, \mathbf{M}, \mathbf{N})$ where $\mathbf{M} = \mathbf{m}_0 \otimes \mathbf{m}_0$ and $\mathbf{N} = \mathbf{n}_0 \otimes \mathbf{n}_0$ are structural tensors (Spencer, 1954). Based on the kinematic description (7.11), the free energy can be written in decoupled form as

$$\Psi(\mathbf{C}, \mathbf{M}, \mathbf{N}) = \Psi_{vol}(J) + \bar{\Psi}(\bar{\mathbf{C}}, \mathbf{M}, \mathbf{N}) \tag{7.12}$$

where $\Psi_{vol}(J)$ and $\bar{\Psi}(\bar{\mathbf{C}}, \mathbf{M}, \mathbf{N})$ are given scalar-valued functions of J, $\bar{\mathbf{C}}$, $\mathbf{m}_0$ and $\mathbf{n}_0$ respectively that describe the volumetric and isochoric responses of the material (Holzapfel, 2000). In terms of the strain invariants (Spencer, 1954) Ψ can be written as

$$\begin{aligned}\Psi = {} & \Psi_{vol}(J)\bar{\Psi}\big(\bar{I}_1(\bar{\mathbf{C}}), \bar{I}_2(\bar{\mathbf{C}}), \\ & + \bar{I}_4(\bar{\mathbf{C}}, \mathbf{m}_0), \bar{I}_5(\bar{\mathbf{C}}, \mathbf{m}_0), \bar{I}_6(\bar{\mathbf{C}}, \mathbf{n}_0), \bar{I}_7(\bar{\mathbf{C}}, \mathbf{n}_0), \bar{I}_8(\bar{\mathbf{C}}, \mathbf{m}_0, \mathbf{n}_0), \bar{I}_9(\mathbf{m}_0, \mathbf{n}_0)\big)\end{aligned} \tag{7.13}$$

with $\bar{I}_1$ and $\bar{I}_2$ the first two modified strain invariants of the symmetric modified Cauchy-Green tensor $\bar{\mathbf{C}}$ (note that $I_3 = J^2$ and $\bar{I}_3 \approx 1$). Finally, the invariants $\bar{I}_4, \ldots, \bar{I}_9$ characterize the constitutive response of the fibers (Spencer, 1954):

$$\begin{aligned} &\bar{I}_4 = \mathbf{C} : \mathbf{M}, \qquad \bar{I}_5 = \mathbf{C}^2 : \mathbf{M}, \qquad \bar{I}_6 = \mathbf{C} : \mathbf{N}, \qquad \bar{I}_7 = \mathbf{C}^2 : \mathbf{N}, \\ &\bar{I}_8 = (\mathbf{m}_0 \cdot \mathbf{n}_0)\mathbf{m}_0 \cdot \bar{\mathbf{C}}\mathbf{n}_0, \qquad \bar{I}_9 = (\mathbf{m}_0 \cdot \mathbf{n}_0)^2. \end{aligned} \tag{7.14}$$

While the invariant $\bar{I}_4$ and $\bar{I}_6$ have a clear physical sense, the square of the stretch λ in the fiber directions, the influence of $\bar{I}_5$, $\bar{I}_7$ and $\bar{I}_8$ is difficult to evaluate due to the high correlation among the invariants. For this reason and the lack of sufficient experimental data it is usual not to include these invariants in the definition of Ψ (Spencer, 1954). Finally, $\bar{I}_9$ does not depend of the deformation and therefore is not relevant to the constitutive behavior.

We now define the constitutive equation for quasicompressible hyperelastic materials in the standard form

$$\mathbf{S} = 2\frac{\partial \Psi(\mathbf{C}, \mathbf{M}, \mathbf{N})}{\partial \mathbf{C}} = \mathbf{S}_{vol} + \bar{\mathbf{S}} \tag{7.15}$$

where the second Piola-Kirchhoff stress $\mathbf{S}$ consists of a purely volumetric contribution ($\mathbf{S}_{vol}$) and a purely isochoric one ($\bar{\mathbf{S}}$). The associated decoupled elasticity tensor may be written as

$$\mathbb{C} = \mathbb{C}_{vol} + \bar{\mathbb{C}} = 2\frac{\partial \mathbf{S}_{vol}}{\partial \mathbf{C}} + 2\frac{\partial \bar{\mathbf{S}}}{\partial \mathbf{C}}. \tag{7.16}$$

The Cauchy stress tensor $\boldsymbol{\sigma}$ and the elasticity tensor in the spatial description $\mathbb{c}$ is $1/J$ times the push-forward of $\mathbf{S}$ or $\mathbb{C}$ respectively (Holzapfel, 2000)

$$\boldsymbol{\sigma} = J^{-1}\chi_*(\mathbf{S}), \qquad \mathbb{c} = J^{-1}\chi_*(\mathbb{C}). \tag{7.17}$$

For a more detailed derivation of the material and spatial elasticity tensors for completely incompressible or quasi-incompressible fibered hyperelastic materials and their explicit expressions, see i.e. Spencer (1954) or Holzapfel (2000).

7.3.2 Experimental Characterization of the Tissues

Tensile tests are performed to estimate the material model $\Psi = \Psi(\mathbf{C}, \mathbf{M}, \mathbf{N})$ and the material parameters for each eye tissue. Since *in vivo* material parameters of the tissues in a non-invasive way cannot be measured, we resort to tests *ex vivo*, despite the tissue is not under physiological conditions thus the mechanical behavior may be affected. The only way to estimate *in vivo* the corneal material properties would be using the ORA equipment. Then parameters such as CH and CRF can be measured (see Sect. 7.1.2) and an optimization algorithm can be used to determine the parameters of the constitutive model that reproduce the tissue behavior.

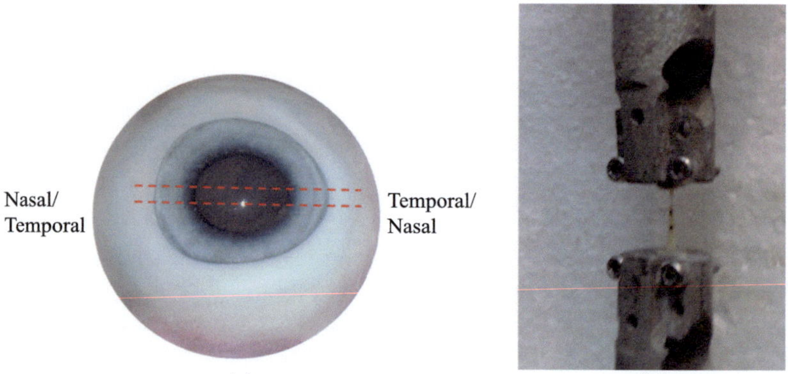

Fig. 7.13 (**a**) Image of a porcine eye. A central strip of the cornea is cut to obtain the sample. (**b**) Total rupture of the sample after the tensile test

The process to carry out the sample obtention and the developing of the test is described next.

Human corneas not viable for transplant due to a damaged endothelium are retrieved from the local tissue bank. All of them must present an intact epithelium. For a good maintenance, during the whole process all the samples must be preserved at 4 °C in a moist chamber. To prepare the specimen, a central strip (2 mm wide, 20 mm long) is extracted from the tissue explanted (including central cornea and sclera) in a nasal-temporal fashion using a double-bladed scalpel (see Fig. 7.13(a)). In order to preserve the hydration of the corneal tissue and to prevent the swelling caused by the moist environment, a preparation of hydroxypropyl methylcellulose (METHOCEL® 2 %, *OmniVision, Puchheim, Germany*) is applied on both the anterior and posterior surfaces of the corneal strip. The thickness of the samples is measured and the cross-sectional area is then estimated. Before placing the sample in the testing machine, each specimen is attached using cyanoacrylate cement to sandpaper tabs to avoid slippage between the tissue and the clamps.

To perform the stress-strain measurement, the specimens must be tested directly after preparation. Uniaxial tensile tests are performed under displacement control on an INSTRON 5548 Microtester (*Illinois Tool Works Inc., Glenview, IL, USA*) with a 10 N full scale load cell. In order to avoid specimen drying, an ultrasonic humidifier is used. This provided a subcooling steam, allowing a constant temperature of 25 °C. A testing velocity estimated as $0.2L \times \frac{60}{100}$ mm·min^{-1}, where L is the initial sample length and 0.2 is the deformation rate, is maintained throughout the test and for all specimens. The corneal strip is then clamped vertically between the jaws of the test machine. Specimens are subjected to three loading/unloading cycles up to a load of 0.3 N before testing them to fracture. The elongation of the strip can be expressed in both stretch (λ) and percentage elongation: $(\lambda - 1) \times 100$ %. Stretch data is obtained as $\lambda = (L_0 + \Delta L) \times L_0^{-1}$ where L_0 is the initial length between clamps, ΔL is the clamp displacement, and Cauchy stress is obtained as $\sigma = \frac{N\lambda}{A_0}$, where N

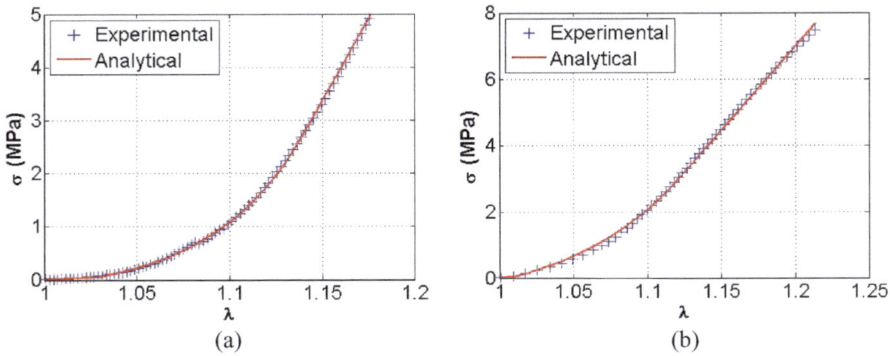

Fig. 7.14 Stress-stretch curves of human tissue (*blue markers*) and fitting using the constitutive model presented in Sect. 7.3.2.1 (*red line*). (**a**) Cornea; (**b**) Sclera.

is the applied load and A_0 the initial cross-sectional area of the specimen. Load and displacement data were recorded until complete specimen rupture (see Fig. 7.13(b)).

Using the expression (7.19) the parameters of material can be estimated to fit the stress-stretch curve. Figure 7.14 shows the stress-stretch curves obtained with corneal and scleral human tissue, which have been fitted with the constitutive model. The model achieves accurate fitting of both curves.

7.3.2.1 Constitutive Law for the Different Eye Tissues

- Cornea. Human cornea is highly porous and filled with biological fluid. It is divided into five layers parallel to its surface. From outside to inside they are as follows: the epithelium, Bowman's membrane, stroma or substantia propia, Descemet's membrane,and the endothelium. The stroma forms about 90 % of the thickness and is divided into 300–500 sheets of collagenous material, the stromal lamellae, parallely distributed to the corneal surface. Lamellae appear to run uninterruptedly from limbus to limbus. It is composed of long collagen fibrils embedded in a ground substance, mainly formed of proteoglycans and water. Collagen fibrils lie parallel and run along the whole length of the lamella. In the central region of the cornea, fibrils run predominantly in the inferior-superior and nasal-temporal directions (Meek and Newton, 1999). This microstructure and the different distributions of collagen fibrils imply an anisotropic behavior for the cornea (Alastrue et al., 2006; Elsheikh et al., 2008; Komai and Ushiki, 1991; Pinsky and Datye, 1991).

  The anisotropic hiperelastic response of the cornea tissue will be assumed to arise from the resistance of the collagen fibrils and the matrix, that is, from a unique strain energy function defined as in (7.12). Following other authors (Gardiner and Weiss, 2003), we have considered

$$\Psi_{vol} = \frac{1}{D}\big(\mathrm{Ln}(J)\big)^2 \tag{7.18}$$

which quasi-enforces the null volumetric change depending on the value of the penalty coefficient $1/D$. We have applied Holzapfel's constitutive model (Holzapfel and Gasser, 2000) to model corneal behavior

$$\begin{aligned}\Psi_{iso} &= \Psi_{iso}^{matrix} + \Psi_{iso}^{fibrils} \\ &= \frac{C_1}{2}(\overline{I}_1 - 3) + \frac{C_2}{2}(\overline{I}_2 - 3) \\ &+ \frac{k_1}{2k_2}\{\exp[k_2(\overline{I}_4 - 1)^2] - 1\} + \frac{k_1}{2k_2}\{\exp[k_2(\overline{I}_6 - 1)^2] - 1\}.\end{aligned} \tag{7.19}$$

- Limbus. The collagen fibrils in the limbus are mainly disposed in a circumferential fashion (Meek and Newton, 1999). So a preferential direction of deformation is considered for the limbal tissue modeling.
- Sclera. The collagen fibrils of the sclera form bundles, present various diameters ranging from 25–230 nm and lay not parallel among them (Komai and Ushiki, 1991). For these reason the scleral tissue can be considered as an isotropic material therefore Ψ_{iso} corresponds to a Mooney material.
- Crystalline lens. The crystalline lens is composed of nucleus, cortex and capsule. The newest tissue is formed in the outer cortex, where the fibers are clearly arranged, running parallel between them, so this part of the lens would be considered anisotropic. Nevertheless, there is no empirical way to characterize the material properties of the fibers of the cortex *in vivo*, so we must assume isotropy. On the other hand, the oldest fibers stay in the nucleus, where they degrade progressively and are no longer aligned. So the nucleus can be considered as an isotropic material. The capsular tissue shows a increasingly stiffer behavior in the circumferential direction than the meridional direction towards the equator (Pedrigi et al., 2007), so a family of fibers is considered in this preferred direction of deformation.
- Optic nerve. In spite of the clearly arranged direction of the nerval cells, we assumed isotropy behavior for this tissue.

The experimental curves for the eye tissues are taken from the literature (Fisher, 1971; Krag et al., 1997; Sigal et al., 2004) and are fitted with the generally strain energy function (equation (7.19)). All these parameters are shown in Table 7.2.

7.4 How Can Numerical Modeling Help in Clinical Treatments?

In this section some applications of the biomechanical model of the eye are presented. To begin with, corneal incisions for the correction of astigmatism are simulated to observe how the biomechanical model could help in the planing of refractive surgery for a patient instead of using the guidelines given by *nomograms*, a set of tables of corrected values or graphics compiling surgical outcomes, which are

Table 7.2 Material parameters for the anisotropic fibered model (7.19) for the eye tissue

Tissue	C_1 (MPa)	D (MPa^{-1})	C_2 (MPa)	k_1 (MPa)	k_2	k_3 (MPa)	k_4
Cornea	0.1	0.00001	0.0	0.234	29.917	0.234	29.917
Limbus	0.1	0.00001	0.0	0.234	29.917	0.000	0.000
Sclera	35	0.00001	−32	0.000	0.000	0.000	0.000
Cortex	0.00058295	34.54	0.000	0.000	0.000	0.000	0.000
Nucleus	0.000093667	214.96	0.0	0.000	0.000	0.000	0.000
Capsule	0.2160	0.2835	0.0	0.0339	9.7406	0.000	0.000
Nerve	0.0050335	4	0.0	0.000	0.000	0.000	0.000

used to plan the surgery. Then, the mechanism of accommodation is simulated to investigate the causes of presbyopia and the patient-specific design of intraocular lenses. Finally, the technique of scleral buckling for retinal detachment is analyzed by means of numerical simulation with the purpose of customizing this procedure for a patient.

All of these simulations are carried out using the biomechanical model of the ocular globe described previously.

Once the patient-specific model is created, the boundary conditions of the problem must be established. The boundary conditions for the eye model are depicted in Fig. 7.15. Those nodes located at the muscles insertions are allowed to move in the direction of that muscle.

Before any simulation, the physiological conditions of the human eye must be reproduced in the model. The stress-free configuration is not known *a priori*. However, the configuration deformated by the IOP, which can be measured directly from the patient's eye (see Sect. 7.1.2) is known. An iterative process was used to incorporate into the model the initial strain distribution (Lanchares et al., 2008) (see Fig. 7.16). This iterative method guarantees that the geometry of the final configuration under IOP will match the initial (stress free) configuration.

7.4.1 Incisional Surgery for the Correction of Astigmatism

Astigmatism is an optical defect in which refractive power is not uniform in all meridians. Refractive surgery techniques modify the corneal curvature in order to repair the refractive error of the eye. If the corneal astigmatism is the only refractive defect, it may be corrected by making the cornea as spherical as possible. In order to achieve emmetropia, corneal incisions and cataract surgery are often performed at the same time. According to the optical power to be corrected, different sorts of cuts can be performed: radial, arcuates (43 D) or limbal relaxing incisions (13 D). When curved incisions are made, the incised meridian flattens; therefore, they have to be performed in the most curved meridian. It also causes the perpendicular meridian

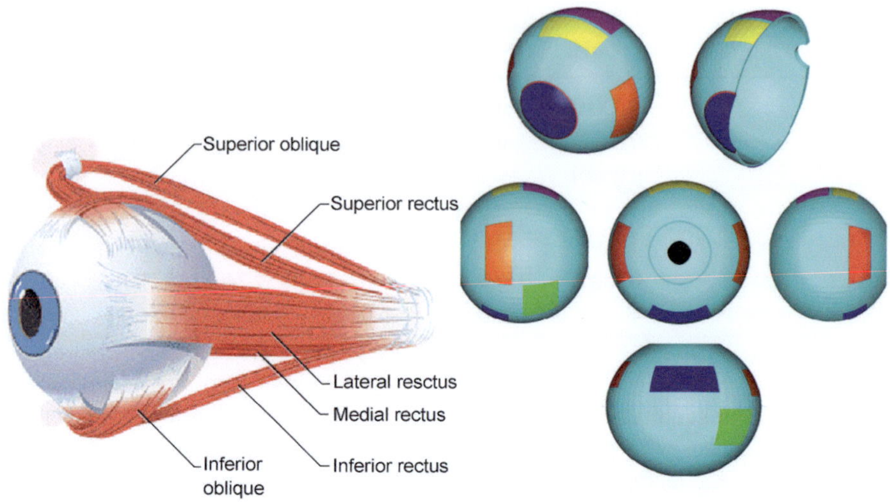

Fig. 7.15 *Left*: muscles of the eye. *Right*: their insertions can be used to define the boundary conditions of the FE model: medial rectus (*red*), lateral rectus (*orange*), superior rectus (*yellow*), inferior rectus (*blue*), superior oblique (*magenta*), inferior oblique (*green*)

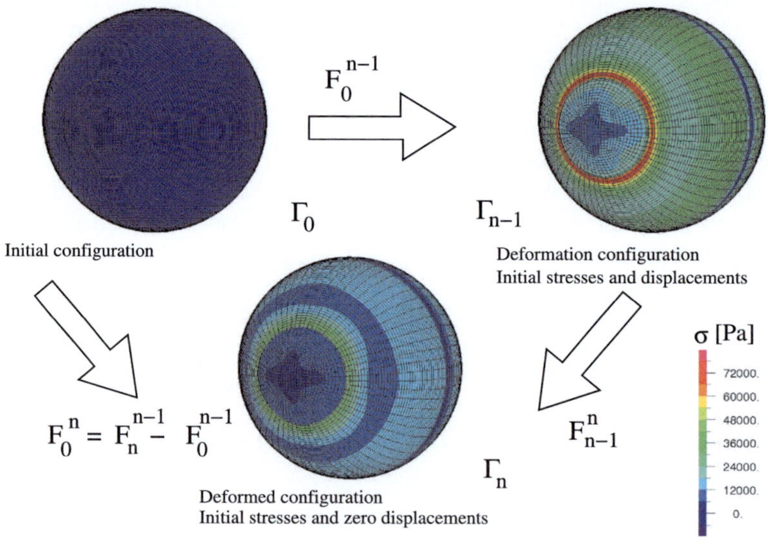

Fig. 7.16 Iterative process to introduce the initial strain distribution into the model, which allows the definition of the reference geometry under the IOP

to be steepened. This effect is usually named by surgeons as *coupling*. The surgeon plans the surgery according to the relation between the amount that the incised meridian flattens and how much the perpendicular one steepens, predicting the optimal result. The parameters to be decided before surgery (number of incisions, angle,

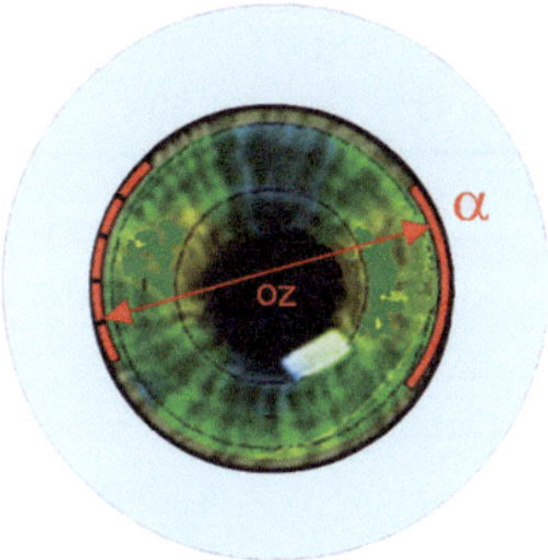

Optical zone (oz)	N incisions	$\alpha = 45°$	$\alpha = 60°$	$\alpha = 90°$
7 mm	1	1.0 D	1.50 D	2.0 D
7 mm	2	2.0 D	3.00 D	4.0 D
6 mm	1	1.5 D	2.25 D	3.0 D
6 mm	2	3.0 D	4.50 D	6.0 D

Fig. 7.17 Incisional parameters in Lindstrom's nomogram (Chu et al., 2005)

depth, shape, symmetry, optical zone) are compiled, according to the optical power to be corrected, in statistically obtained *nomograms* (see Fig. 7.17). Nevertheless, an accurate nomogram to be used as an universal reference to achieve a spherical equivalent and astigmatism correction as expected is very complex to be obtained (Cristóbal et al., 2006). Moreover, the same surgical technique (same angle, optical zone, etc.) usually leads to different results for different patients because the nomograms do not include all the factors related to the effect of the incisions such as the human factor (surgeon) and the patient-specific biomechanical properties of the cornea.

The object of this work is to study the effect, by numerical simulation, of some of the parameters considered in nomograms for relaxing incisions, both non-penetrating arcuates and limbal incisions, by varying only one of the parameters and the rest remaining constant. Thereby, a new approach apart from the clinical experience is supplied for a better knowledge of the incisional surgery. As said before, the use of nomograms leads to unpredictability and scarce reproducibility of the results. Numerical simulation of the incisional surgery allows us to obviate these aspects and focus just on the parameters of the incisional surgery.

7.4.1.1 Curved Incisions in Clear Cornea: Arcuates

For the simulation of this surgery, a mesh was developed following a radial pattern to achieve the open angles of the arcuates to be simulated: 90°, 60° and 45°. All the incisions were performed at 3 mm from the corneal center (*apex*).

After surgery simulation, the optical power, measured in diopters, was estimated. The incised astigmatic principal meridian and the secondary one, defined by the final position of the nodes belonging to the corneal anterior surface and inside the optical zone, a circular area centered in the apex of 3 mm radius, was fitted by means of least squares. Two radii of curvature were obtained, one for each meridian. Then the diopters were calculated using the expression (7.2).

The estimated optical power in diopters for the simulated incisions is shown in Table 7.3. The results match those of the Lindstrom's nomogram (Chu et al., 2005)

Table 7.3 Astigmatic change surgically induced in the six cases of simulation and expected values according to the Lindstrom's nomogram (Chu et al., 2005). Optical zone of 6 mm for all the incisions

N incisions	1	1	2	1	2	1
Length	45°	60°	45°	90°	60°	90°
D Simulation	1.47	2.13	3	2.72	4.5	5.95
D Nomogram	1.5	2.25	3	3	4.5	6
% Error	2.0	5.3	0.0	9.3	0.0	0.8

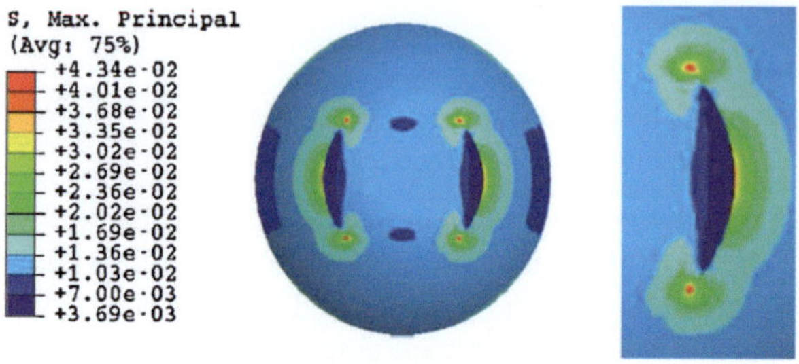

Fig. 7.18 Maximum principal stress distribution (MPa). Paired incisions 90 % depth, 90°. Front view of the cornea and zoom of the area of the incision

therefore, the model is considered suitable for the simulation of incisional refractive surgery at least as a first approach.

With respect to the maximum principal stress, as expected, the longer the cut the greater values of stress appear. For paired incisions of 90 % of the corneal thickness depth, simulation of 45°, 60° and 90° length incisions gave maximum values of 3.26×10^{-2}, 3.88×10^{-2} and 4.34×10^{-2} MPa, respectively. In Fig. 7.18, the maximum principal stress distribution is shown for paired incisions of 90° length. The greater values of stress turn up in the outer lip of the cut and at the extremes of the incision.

7.4.1.2 Limbal Relaxing Incisions

Limbal relaxing incisions were reproduced in the biomechanical model of the eye, in order to estimate the effect of each isolated incisional parameter (length of the incision, depth and optical zone). The other factors are forced to remain constant. Since all the cases of simulation are performed on an eye with precisely the same biomechanical characteristics, there is no influence of human factors (surgeon or patient) on the outcomes.

It is important to clarify that the length of the incisions is not measured in millimeters. Since the size of the cornea is different for each patient, the length of the incision has to be given in degrees of arc (Wang et al., 2003). The corneal diameter, thus the position of the limbal limit, imposes the position of the limbal incisions. The biomechanical simulation allows predicting the amount of diopters that would be surgically induced for a specific patient because both the corneal diameter and the degrees of arc of the incision can be inputs for the simulation.

The process of surgical simulation is similar to that described previously for arcuate simulation. The initial strain distribution and a 15 mmHg IOP are introduced in the model before any simulation.

The outcomes of numerical simulation show that the greater the length of the incisions, measured either as an arc (degrees) or as the length of the chord (millimeters), the greater the astigmatic change induced. Astigmatic changes of 1.2, 1.4, and 1.9 D were obtained for incisions of 45, 60, and 90 degrees, at an optical zone of 10 mm and depth of 90 % of the corneal thickness.

The depth of the cut has a big influence on the induced astigmatism change. The greater the depth, the greater the resulting effect. Paired incisions were simulated at a 7.5-mm optical zone and 90 degrees of length, astigmatic changes of 0.7, 2.6, and 4.4 D for 40 %, 75 %, and 90 % depth, respectively, were obtained. A regression curve, an exponential function, is used to fit them.

The optical zone is the parameter that shows higher influence. The closer the incision to the apex, the bigger the effect regarding astigmatic change. Comparing the previous results for paired incisions of 90-degree length and 90 % depth, for two different optical zones, 10 and 7.5 mm, the results were 1.9 and 4.4 D, respectively.

Numerical simulation provides a wide range of possibilities in addition to the data compiled in nomograms. The effect of each isolated parameter related to the incisions can be customized for a specific case. For example, if an astigmatic level of 1.5 D must be corrected (Fig. 7.19) and the surgeon decides to perform 90-degree length paired incisions at an optical zone of 7.5 mm, numerical simulation prescribes a depth of incision of 60 % to induce the target astigmatism. As it was previously mentioned, the correlation of all the outcomes of simulation is not linear, so an exponential function, which fits the three simulated cases, was considered. Obviously, each specific case can also be numerically reproduced and the induced astigmatic change is then obtained. Moreover, the numerical model allows coupling with an optical model which allows estimation of low- and high-order aberrations of the numerical model after the surgery (Navarro et al., 2009).

7.4.2 The Process of Accommodation

Accommodation is the ability of the human eye to change its optical power to focus far and near objects. The mechanism of this process is not yet well known. The loss of the accommodation capability with age is named as *presbyopia* and 100 percent population suffers from it at the age of 60 (Glasser and Campbell, 1998; Weale, 1992).

Numerical models of the crystalline lens and other structures involved in the process of accommodation (ciliary body, zonule of Zinn) allow us to improve knowledge of the mechanism of accommodation and its decline with age.

For the development of a patient specific model of the human crystalline lens only geometries are available, both in fully accommodated and unaccommodated states (near and far vision, respectively). From these data we use mathematical expressions to design the geometry of the model, as it was explained before (Sect. 7.2).

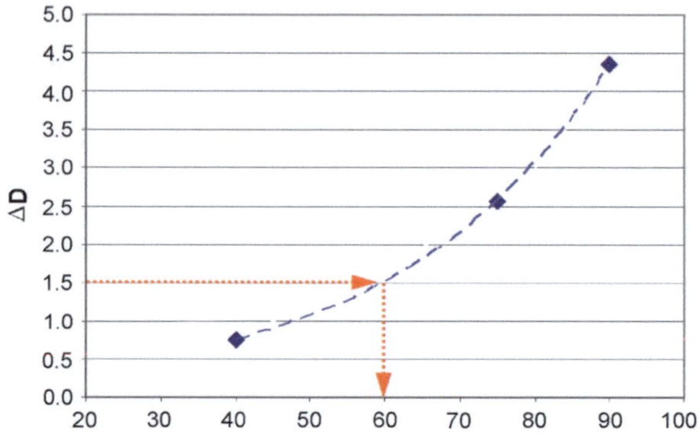

Fig. 7.19 Paired incisions: length 90°, optical zone 7.5 mm. A regression curve, an exponential function, fits the values obtained by numerical simulation for 40 %, 75 %, and 90 % of the corneal thickness depth to correct 0.7, 2.6, and 4.4 D, respectively. According to these outcomes of the numerical simulation, an astigmatic change of 1.5 D would be induced by paired incisions, 60 % of the corneal thickness depth

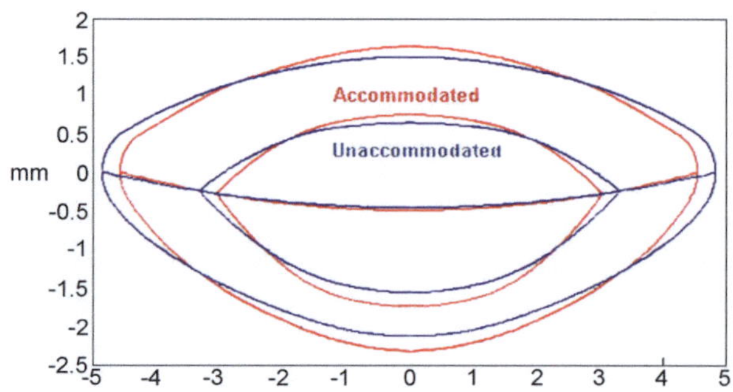

Fig. 7.20 The geometry of the human lens in the fully accommodated state (*red*) is more incurved than in the unaccommodated state (*blue*)

Numerical simulation with this model allows estimation of the zonular forces, which are responsible for the antero-posterior movement of the crystalline lens during the process of accommodation, assuming the material properties of the tissues at the age of study are known, and also the determination of the material properties of the tissues at any age in case the zonular forces are known. With this outcomes, the patient specific model is ready for the analysis of customized techniques.

Figure 7.20 shows the periphery of the lens before and after the simulation of the mechanism of accommodation, corresponding to the fully accommodated and unaccommodated states, of a 30 year-old finite element model. The fully accommodated state happens for near vision and corresponds to the steepest curve which has a greater optical power. Figure 7.21 shows the outcomes of the numerical simulation of the accommodation process. The nucleus can be clearly distinguished from the cortex since this two tissues show different behavior both in the stress distribution and in the displacement map.

By means of an inverse algorithm the zonular forces acting at the equatorial band of the lens can be computed, being known the initial and final geometries and the

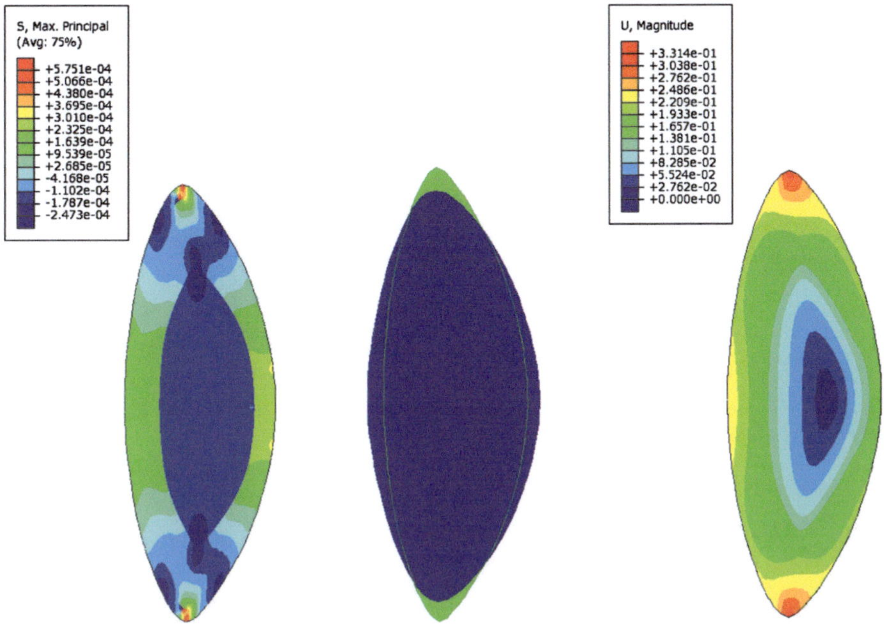

Fig. 7.21 Cross-sectional view of the numerical model of the crystalline lens at the age of 30 after the simulation of the accommodation process. *Left*: maximum principal stress distribution [MPa]. *Center*: deformed (*green*) and undeformed (*blue*) geometries (unaccommodated and fully accommodated, respectively). *Right*: displacement distribution [mm]

material properties at this age. The zonular forces obtained by numerical simulation were 0.078 N, which is close to the values estimated by other authors (Krag and Andreassen, 1996; Manns et al., 2007).

Following a similar process, the material properties of the tissues of the crystalline lens (nucleus, cortex and capsule) at any age can be estimated. The zonular forces are supposed to decrease with age, but it would be needed the measurement or estimation of this fall, or it could be assumed that they remained constant with age (Hermans et al., 2008).

In the last few years, with the development of technique for cataract surgery, intraocular lenses have been continuously improved. Numerical simulation can help in design of intraocular lenses, both in geometry and optics. The geometry of the lens could be optimized not only for the fixation of the optic zone to the capsule, but also for the implantation process. On the other hand, the optics of the intraocular lens could be determined for a given case if a patient specific numerical model is developed. Then, the estimation of parameters such as the antero-posterior displacement of the lens and the zonular forces will help in determining the best optic design of an accommodative lens for that patient.

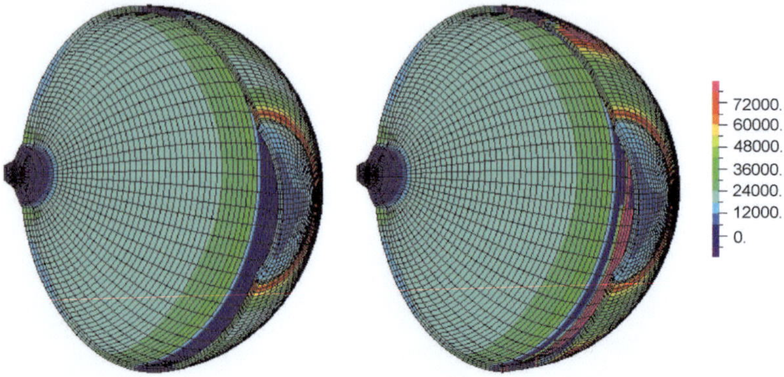

Fig. 7.22 Simulation of the scleral buckle surgery: Stress distribution (in [Pa]) before (*left*) and after (*right*) surgery

7.4.3 Scleral Buckling

A scleral buckle is a surgical procedure that can be used to repair a retinal detachment. The scleral buckling consists of a silicone strip sewn onto the sclera at the site of a retinal tear to push the sclera toward the detached retina. The buckle holds the retina against the sclera.

We used the biomechanical model of the eyeball to simulate the scleral buckle surgery in order to observe the displacement and stress distributions turned up in the different parts of the model.

Figures 7.22 and 7.23 show the outcomes of the simulation of the surgery of scleral buckle. In both figures a stress concentration can be observed at the limbus, which is the stiffest tissue of the model. Regions with high displacements show a minimum value of stress (Fig. 7.23). The greater displacements happen in the scleral ring where the circling band is placed, at the periphery of the optic nerve head, and also in the cornea. This procedure also modifies the axial length, which is the distance from the front central point on the cornea to the center of the retina at the back of the eye. This parameter, together with the optical power of the refractive structures of the eye, determines the level of myopia. In Fig. 7.23 an elongation of this distance caused by the buckling surgery can be observed. The increase in the eye's axial length has a myopic refractive effect.

The proposed simulation can be used before surgery for improving the clinical outcome. Through numerical simulation the radial force needed to make the retina attached to the sclera can be estimated before surgery and at the same time the necessary displacement can be computed. In addition, some important variables which are not assessable *in vivo* before or after surgery can be evaluated by means of the presented finite element model. Local stress distributions, compression of the optic nerve or abnormal elongation of the axial length are example of post operatory problems which could be numerically analyzed before surgery.

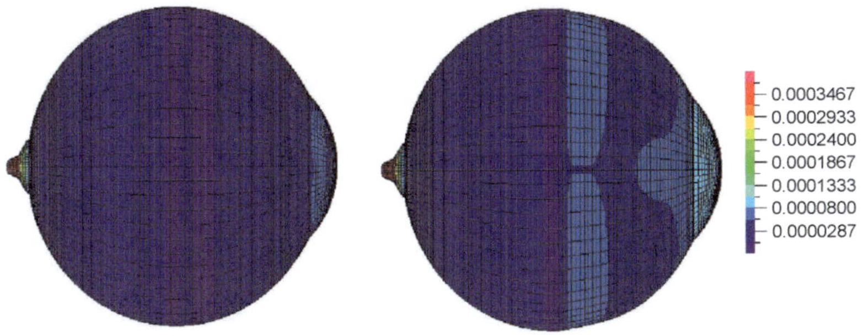

Fig. 7.23 Simulation of the scleral buckle surgery: Displacement distribution (in [mm]) before (*left*) and after (*right*) surgery

7.5 Conclusions

The biomechanics of the human eye is complex and crucial for understanding related pathologies as for instance astigmatism, myopia and glaucomatous optic neuropathy. Recently many studies have addressed eye pathologies (Kapnisis et al., 2009; Norman et al., 2010; Sigal et al., 2010). However, biomechanical studies in the literature try to address clinical problems studying each single eye component separately. In this way, the global view of the human eye biomechanical behavior is completely lost. The principal appeal of modeling the human eye biomechanics presented in this chapter is that it provides a powerful framework that can be used in the clinical practice for explaining several aspects of eye diseases. We focused our attention in the human cornea without neglecting the connected parts such as sclera, crystalline lens and optic nerve. Every component is properly associated to the corresponding biomechanical material behavior obtained through experimental tests. In particular, we demonstrated that the behavior of the proposed material tissue models, which include anisotropy, is capable to reflect the response of the physiological tissues. The framework was finally tested for several pathologies and it is feasible to be adapted to patient specific applications. We showed how it is possible to predict with the proposed model the effects of different surgical techniques. Firstly, the constitutive model of the tissues of each eye main part was described and characterized separately. For this goal, we started from a generic model, based on a defined geometrical shape. Then, an entire human eye was built and numerically simulated in order to test its capability to reproduce pathologies, surgeries (astigmatism correction) and patient specific situations (through medical images). Such numerical model offers the possibility to help clinical outcomes extracting from computational results physical variables not assessable in vivo. Finite element computation can be performed rapidly before surgery giving to the surgeons possible choices in the surgical strategies.

Acknowledgements The authors gratefully acknowledge the Instituto de Salud Carlos III (ISCIII) and the CIBER-BBN (Centro de Investigación Biomédica En Red en Bioingeniería, Biomateriales y Nanomedicina) initiative, and also the research support of the Spanish Ministry of Education and Science through the research project DPI2008-02335.

References

Alastrue V, Calvo B, Peña E, Doblare M (2006) Biomechanical modelling of refractive corneal surgery. J Biomech Eng 128:150–160
Brown N (1973) Change in shape and internal form of the lens of the eye on accommodation. Exp Eye Res 15:441–459
Bryant MR, McDonnell PJ (1996) Constitutive laws for biomechanical modeling of refractive surgery. J Biomech Eng 118:473–481
Burd H, Judge S, Cross J (2002) Numerical modelling of the accommodating lens. Vis Res 42:2235–2251
Cabrera D, Niazy A, Kurtz RM, Djotyan GP, Juhasz T (2006) A finite element model for ultrafast laser-lamellar keratoplasty. Ann Biomed Eng 34:69–83
Calossi A (2007) Cornea asphericity and spherical aberration. J Refract Corneal Surg 23:505–514
Chu Y, Hardten D, Lindquist T, Lindstrom R (2005) Astigmatic keratotomy. Duane's ophthalmology. Lippincott Williams and Wilkins, Philadelphia
Cristóbal JA, del Buey MA, Mateo A (2006) Astigmatismo y catarata. In: Centurión V, Nýcoli C, Villar-Kuri J (eds) El libro de cristalino de las Américas. Ed. Santos, Brazil, pp 10–13
Downs JC, Suh JK, Thomas KA, Bellezza AJ, Burgoyne CF, Hart RT (2003) Viscoelastic characterization of peripapillary sclera: material properties by quadrant in rabbit and monkey eyes. J Biomech Eng 125(1):124–134
Dubbelman M, Van der Heijde GV (2001) The shape of the aging human lens: curvature, equivalent refractive index and the lens paradox. Vis Res 41:1867–1877
Dubbelman M, van der Heijde GV, Weeber H, Vrensen G (2003) Changes in the internal structure of the human crystalline lens with age and accommodation. Vis Res 43:2363–2375
Elsheikh A, Brown M, Alhasso D, Rama P, Campanelli M, Garway-Heath D (2008) Experimental assessment of corneal anisotropy. J Refract Surg 24(2):178–187
Fisher RF (1971) The elastic constants of the human lens. J Physiol 212(1):147–180
Fisher R, Pettet B (1972) The postnatal growth of the capsule of the human crystalline lens. J Anat 112(2):207–214
Flory PJ (1961) Thermodynamic relations for high elastic materials. Trans Faraday Soc 57:829–838
Fung YC (1993) Biomechanics. Mechanical properties of living tissues. Springer, New York
Gardiner JC, Weiss JA (2003) Subject-specific finite element analysis of the human medial collateral ligament during valgus knee loading. J Orthop Res 21:1098–1106
Glasser A, Campbell MCV (1998) Presbyopia and the optical changes in the human crystalline lens with age. Vis Res 38:209–229
Hermans EA, Dubbelman M, van der Heijde GL, Heethaar RM (2008) Change in the accomodative force on the lens of the human eye with age. Vis Res 46:119–126
Holzapfel GA (2000) Nonlinear solid mechanics. Wiley, New York
Holzapfel GA, Gasser TC (2000) A new constitutive framework for arterial wall mechanics and a comparative study of material models. J Elast 61:1–48
Jones C, Atchison D, Meder R, Pope J (2005) Refractive index distribution and optical properties of the isolated human lens measured using magnetic resonance imaging (MRI). Vis Res 45:2352–2366
Kapnisis K, Doormaal MV, Ethier CR (2009) Modeling aqueous humor collection from the human eye. J Biomech 42(15):2454–2457
Komai Y, Ushiki T (1991) The three-dimensional organization of collagen fibrils in the human cornea and sclera. Investig Ophthalmol Vis Sci 32(8):2244–2258
Krag S, Olsen T, Andreassen TT (1997) Biomechanical characteristics of the human anterior lens capsule in relation to age. Investig Ophthalmol Vis Sci 38:357–363
Krag S, Andreassen T (1996) Biomechanical measurements of the porcine lens capsule. Exp Eye Res 62:253–260
Lanchares E, Calvo B, Cristóbal JA, Doblaré M (2008) Finite element simulation of arcuates for astigmatism correction. J Biomech 41(4):797–805

Manns F, Parel JM, Denham D, Billotte C, Ziebarth N, Borja D, Fernandez V, Aly M, Arrieta E, Ho A, Holden B (2007) Optomechanical response of human and monkey lenses in a lens stretcher. Investig Ophthalmol Vis Sci 48:3260–3268
Meek KM, Newton RH (1999) Organization of collagen fibrils in the corneal stroma in relation to mechanical properties and surgical practice. J Refract Surg 15(6):695–699
Munnerlyn CR, Koons SJ, Marshall J (1988) Photorefractive keratectomy: a technique for laser refractive surgery. J Cataract Refract Surg 14:46–52
Navarro R, Gonzalez L, Hernandez JL (2005) Representación canónica de la superficie corneal: topografía promedio. Ver Oir 24:594–606
Navarro R, Palos F, Gonzalez L (2007) Adaptive model of the gradient index of the human lens. I. Formulation and model of aging ex vivo lenses. J. Opt. Soc. Am. A, Opt. Image Sci. Vis. 24(8):2175–2185
Navarro R, Palos F, Lanchares E, Calvo B, Cristóbal JA (2009) Lower- and higher-order aberrations predicted by an optomechanical model of arcuate keratotomy for astigmatism. J Cataract Refract Surg 35(1):158–165
Norman RE, Flanagan JG, Rausch SMK, Sigal IA, Tertinegg I, Eilaghi A, Portnoy S, Sled JG, Ethier CR (2010) Dimensions of the human sclera: thickness measurement and regional changes with axial length. Exp Eye Res 90(2):277–284
Pandolfi A, Fotia G, Manganiello F (2009) Finite element simulations of laser refractive corneal surgery. Eng Comput 25:15–24
Pedrigi RM, David G, Dziezyc J, Humphrey JD (2007) Regional mechanical properties and stress analysis of the human anterior lens capsule. Vis Res 47:1781–1789
Pinsky P, Datye V (1991) A microstructurally-based finite element model of the incised human cornea. J Biomed Eng 10:907–922
Rosen A, Denham DB, Fernandez V, Borja D, Ho A, Mannis F, Parel J, Augusteyn R (2006) In vitro dimensions and curvatures of human lenses. Vis Res 46:1002–1009
Schachar R, Huang T, Huang X (1993) Mathematic proof of Schachar's hypothesis of accommodation. Ann Ophthalmol Clin 33(2):103–112
Sigal IA, Flanagan JG, Tertinegg I, Ethier CR (2004) Finite element modeling of optic nerve head biomechanics. Investig Ophthalmol Vis Sci 45(12):4378–4387
Sigal IA, Fanagan JG, Tertinegg I, Eithier CR (2010) 3D morphometry of the human optic nerve head. Exp Eye Res 90:70–80
Simo JC, Taylor RL (1985) Consistent tangent operators for rate-independent elastoplasticity. Comput Methods Appl Mech Eng 48:101–118
Simo JC, Taylor RL (1991) Quasi-incompressible finite elasticity in principal stretches. Continuum basis and numerical algorithms. Comput Methods Appl Mech Eng 85:273–310
Wang L, Misra M, Koch DD (2003) Peripheral corneal relaxing incisions combined with cataract surgery. J Cataract Refract Surg 29:712–722
Weale RA (1992) The senescence of human vision. Oxford University Press, Oxford
Spencer AJM (1954) Theory of invarinats. In: Continuum physics. Academic Press, New York, pp 239–253

MIX
Papier aus verantwortungsvollen Quellen
Paper from responsible sources
FSC® C105338

If you have any concerns about our products,
you can contact us on
ProductSafety@springernature.com

In case Publisher is established outside the EU,
the EU authorized representative is:
Springer Nature Customer Service Center GmbH
Europaplatz 3, 69115 Heidelberg, Germany

Printed by Libri Plureos GmbH
in Hamburg, Germany